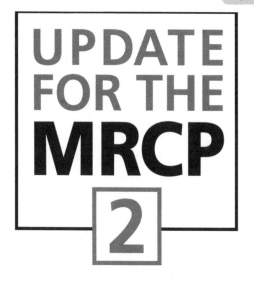

UPDATE FOR THE MRCP 2

Thomasin Andrews BSc MRCP
Specialist Registrar in Neurology, Guy's, King's College and St Thomas' Hospitals,
London, UK

Peter Arlett BSc MRCP
Senior Medical Assessor, Medicines Control Agency, Department of Health,
London, UK

Bernard Brett BSc MRCP
Clinical Research Fellow in Gastroenterology,
Royal Free and University College Medical School,
London, UK

Rebecca Jones BA MRCP
DDF/BSG Clinical Research Fellow and Specialist Registrar,
Liver Research Laboratories and Queen Elizabeth Hospital,
University of Birmingham, Birmingham, UK

Foreword by Professor Roy E. Pounder MA MD DSc(Med) FRCP

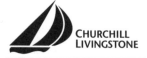

CHURCHILL
LIVINGSTONE

EDINBURGH LONDON NEW YORK PHILADELPHIA ST LOUIS SYDNEY TORONTO 2000

CHURCHILL LIVINGSTONE

An imprint of Harcourt Publishers Limited

© Harcourt Publishers Limited 2000

 is a registered trade mark of Harcourt Publishers Limited

The right of Thomasin C. Andrews, Peter R. Arlett, Bernard T. Brett and Rebecca L. Jones to be identified as authors of this work has been asserted by them in accordance with the Copyright, Designs and Patents Act 1988.

First published 2000

ISBN 0 443 06257 9

British Library Cataloguing in Publication Data
A catalogue record for this book is available from the British Library.

Library of Congress Cataloging in Publication Data
A catalog record for this book is available from the Library of Congress.

Medical knowledge is constantly changing. As new information becomes available, changes in treatment, procedures, equipment and the use of drugs become necessary. The authors, contributors and the publishers have, as far as it is possible, taken care to ensure that the information given in this text is accurate and up to date. However, readers are strongly advised to confirm that the information, especially with regard to drug usage, complies with current legislation and standards of practice.

The opinions offered in this book are those of the authors and contributors and do not necessarily reflect the opinions of the organisations for whom they work.

The
publisher's
policy is to use
paper manufactured
from sustainable forests

Typeset by IMH(Catrtif), Loanhead, Scotland
Printed in the UK

Foreword

This is the second volume of the innovative *Update for the MRCP*, which has been written by junior doctors for junior doctors. It is now two years since the publication of the first volume, and the original quartet of authors has now been joined by nine other Specialist and Senior Registrars.

The authors have constructed groups of multiple choice questions relating to the top fifteen sub-specialties of general medicine. Important articles published over the last five years are the basis of the questions, and this is revealed to the reader in the second part of the book. The bulk of the book is made up of short essays that explain the correct and incorrect answers to the multiple choice questions. Finally, if the reader has any remaining strength, the authors have constructed a range of supplementary viva questions but provide no more answers!

This book is very challenging, extremely interesting, and a really excellent way to have a broad review of many recent advances in the field of general medicine. Whilst the book is designed for the MRCP, it would be valuable reading for every general physician.

Roy Pounder
London 2000

Preface

Following the success of Update for the MRCP, we have produced Update for the MRCP: 2 which contains new material on topics not addressed in the first volume. The books are intended to be complementary and as such provide a comprehensive guide to recent advances in the understanding and management of many medical conditions.

This book is aimed at candidates preparing for both MRCP parts 1 and 2 examinations. The fast pace of change in medicine and basic science means that textbooks quickly become out of date. Both parts 1 and 2 of the examination increasingly emphasise a knowledge of basic science and of recent scientific and medical literature. In recent years the results of large multi-centre trials have influenced changes in clinical practice and led to a drive towards evidence-based medicine. This book reviews and references the seminal papers. We have invited doctors from various specialties to contribute to the book to ensure that major advances of clinical relevance are included.

MRCP: 2 follows the popular layout of the first volume with multiple choice questions followed by extended answers. These answers review the recent advances in each subject. There are viva questions to help candidates preparing for the Part II clinical. The major papers are included in a list of references, which should guide your further reading.

We wish you the very best of luck.

T. Andrews
P. Arlett
B. Brett
R. Jones   2000

Contributors

Thomasin Andrews BSc MRCP
Specialist Registrar in Neurology, Guy's, King's College and St Thomas' Hospitals, London, UK

Peter Arlett BSc MRCP
Senior Medical Assessor, Medicines Control Agency, Department of Health, London, UK

Bernard Brett BSc MRCP
Clinical Research Fellow in Gastroenterology, Royal Free and University College Medical School, London, UK

Kate Cwynarski BSc MRCP
Specialist Registrar in Haematology, Hammersmith Hospital, London, UK

Robin Fox BSc MRCP
Lecturer in Medical Education / Specialist Registrar in Rheumatology, Royal Free and University College Medical School, London, UK

Neil Goldsack BSc MRCP
Specialist Registrar in Respiratory Medicine, Royal Free Hospital, London, UK

Rebecca Jones BA MRCP
DDF/BSG Clinical Research Fellow and Specialist Registrar, Liver Research Laboratories and Queen Elizabeth Hospital, University of Birmingham, Birmingham, UK

Jattinder Khaira BA MRCP
Clinical Research Fellow in Endocrinology, Department of Medicine, Queen Elizabeth Hospital, University of Birmingham, Birmingham, UK

Clive Lewis MA MRCP
Research Fellow and Honorary Specialist Registrar in Cardiology, Addenbrooke's Centre for Clinical Investigation, University of Cambridge, Cambridge, UK

Elinor Sawyer BSc MRCP FRCR
Clinical Research Fellow in Oncology, Imperial Cancer Research Fund, and Guy's and St Thomas' Hospitals, London, UK

Claire Sharpe BSc MRCP
Clinical Research Fellow and Honorary Specialist Registrar, Department of Renal Medicine, Guy's, King's College and St Thomas' Hospitals School of Medicine, London, UK

Christopher J M Whitty MA MSc MRCP DTM&H
Senior Registrar in Infectious and Tropical Medicine, Hospital for Tropical Diseases, London; Honorary Lecturer, London School of Hygiene and Tropical Medicine, London, UK

Sarah Woodrow BSc MRCP
MRC Clinical Training Fellow and Honorary Specialist Registrar in Dermatology, Dept of Dermatology, Addenbrooke's Hospital, University of Cambridge, Cambridge, UK

Contents

Part 1: Questions

BASIC SCIENCE, IMMUNOLOGY AND GENETICS

1. **In comparing mechanisms of cell death (apoptosis, necrosis and cytotoxicity)**
    A. Cytotoxicity refers to the ability of a chemical or cell to specifically activate apoptosis
    B. Apoptosis is energy independent, whereas necrosis is energy dependent
    C. Mitochondrial changes are seen early in apoptosis
    D. In apoptosis there is an influx of water and electrolytes across the plasma membrane, leading to cell membrane rupture
    E. During necrosis nuclear morphology is preserved until late in the process

2. **In T-cell activation**
    A. Activated cytotoxic T cells recognize the MHC class 1 molecule
    B. Interleukin 2 downregulates T-cell proliferation
    C. Antigens are recognized by the CD3/T-cell receptor complex
    D. Th1 cells produce interferon-γ on activation
    E. Th2 cells produce interleukin 10 on activation

3. **T helper 2 (Th2) cells**
    A. Are implicated in T-cell mediated cellular immunity
    B. Secrete interferon-γ
    C. Differentiation is produced by the action of interleukin 4
    D. Are the predominant T helper subtype found in rheumatoid arthritis synovium
    E. Are the predominant activated T helper subtype found in asthma

4. **Chemokines**
    A. Are cytokines
    B. Chemokine secretion is increased in inflammation
    C. Interleukin 8 acts predominantly on monocytes
    D. Chemokines facilitate leucocyte migration through endothelial cells
    E. Chemokines have a role in the regulation of angiogenesis

5.   Chemokines and HIV-1 receptors

A. Macrophage-tropic strains of HIV-1 gain entry to host cells by binding of GP120 to the CD4 molecule
B. Macrophage-tropic strains of HIV-1 gain entry to host cells by binding to the CCR5 chemokine receptor
C. T lymphocyte-tropic strains of HIV-1 gain entry to host cells by binding to the CXCR4 chemokine receptor
D. Mutations of the CCR5 chemokine receptor may reduce susceptibility to HIV-1 infection
E. Stromal derived factor-1 (SDF-1) is the main ligand for CCR5

6.   IgE in asthma

A. Binds to specific $F_\varepsilon SR1$ receptors on mast cells
B. Binds to $F_\varepsilon SR2$ receptors on lymphocytes
C. Monoclonal antibodies to the Fab portion of IgE have been used to treat asthma successfully
D. Is involved in both early and late asthmatic responses
E. Asthma symptoms correlate with serum IgE levels

7.   Allergen immunotherapy

A. Is performed by exposing an allergic patient to a gradually increasing dose of allergen
B. Is most effective in patients with severe asthma
C. Following successful treatment, the release of histamine is reduced on repeat allergen testing
D. Following successful treatment, the serum IgE response is reduced on repeat allergen testing
E. Is more effective in children

8.   Vaccination for hepatitis B virus (HBV)

A. Recombinant hepatitis B surface antigen vaccination produces neutralizing antibodies in 90% of recipients
B. Smokers are at risk of lower response to vaccination than non-smokers
C. Egg allergy is a contraindication to recombinant HBV vaccine
D. Immunogenicity is reduced if HBV vaccine is given simultaneously with HBV immunoglobulin
E. The preferred site for administration is gluteal injection

9.   Flow cytometry

A. Can be used to count CD4 cells in patients with HIV infection
B. Can be used to measure the DNA content of a cell nucleus
C. Can provide information on cell morphology
D. Can provide information on cell viability
E. Can provide information on spatial relationships of cells to each other

10. The Human Genome Project

A. There are three million base pairs
B. 97% of human DNA is involved in encoding proteins
C. Genetic markers should have low heterozygosity
D. One centimorgan is equivalent to a 1% chance that two markers will be separated in meiosis by recombination
E. The sequencing of genes and proteins has resulted in new treatments for many genetic diseases

11. Which of the following statements about neurogenetics are true?

A. Genetic imprinting is a technique used for creating physical maps of chromosomes
B. Angelman syndrome and Huntington's disease result from different defects within the same gene
C. Prader–Willi syndrome is characterized by macro-orchidism and cerebellar ataxia
D. Expanded trinucleotide repeats were first identified as pathogenic in Kennedy's disease
E. All pathogenic trinucleotide repeat sequences consist of CAG repeats

12. The mitochondrial genome

A. There are 37 genes in human mitochondrial DNA
B. Complex II of the respiratory chain is encoded entirely by mitochondrial DNA
C. The maternal inheritance of mitochondrial DNA explains the male preponderance of Leber's hereditary optic neuropathy
D. Leber's hereditary optic neuropathy presents with painful bilateral visual loss and optic atrophy
E. The clinical presentation of Leber's hereditary optic neuropathy is influenced by alcohol and tobacco consumption

13. The following statements are true about the prothrombin-gene G20210A mutation:

A. It occurs in an untranslated region of the gene
B. Lower prothrombin levels are noted in individuals with the mutation
C. The mutation is present in 1–2% of the population
D. It is the most common genetic determinant of deep vein thrombosis
E. It has been identified as an important risk factor for cerebral vein thrombosis

14.   In the assessment of nutritional requirements

A. Basal metabolic rate constitutes between 20 and 50% of total energy expenditure
B. Energy expenditure is reduced in severe disease
C. The thermic effect of food constitutes approximately 10% of total energy expenditure
D. Physical activity normally constitutes only 15–20% of total energy expenditure
E. A 70 kg man with mild disease would require approximately 70 g of nitrogen per day to maintain nitrogen balance

PHARMACOLOGY AND DRUG DEVELOPMENT

15.   In drug development

A. On average, of 10 newly synthesized chemicals, only one will become a licensed medicine
B. No biotechnology product has yet been licensed
C. All toxicology studies must be completed before a potential drug is used in humans
D. In Phase I clinical studies, single doses of the drug are tested in patients
E. Phase III clinical studies rarely involve more than 1000 patients

16.   The Yellow Card Scheme for reporting suspected adverse drug reactions (ADRs)

A. For new drugs designated by a black triangle symbol, all suspected ADRs should be reported
B. For older (non-black triangle) drugs only serious reactions should be reported
C. Invites reports from hospital pharmacists
D. Invites reports from patients
E. Has not identified safety issues that were not apparent from clinical trials

17.   The following study designs are appropriate:

A. Cohort study of a rare disease
B. Case-control study of a rare risk factor
C. Crossover trial of a new antibiotic
D. Cross-sectional study of stroke incidence
E. Placebo-controlled trial of a new antibiotic in meningitis

18. Clinical trials
A. A systematic review is one that accurately reflects current thinking
B. All systematic reviews should include a meta-analysis
C. Meta-analysis is a way of combining data from different sorts of trial
D. Evidence from single trials may be better than that from meta-analysis
E. Positive publication bias favours type I errors

19. The following drugs are matched with the cytochrome P450 enzymes responsible for their metabolism:
A. Cyclosporin and CYP3A4
B. Haloperidol and CYP2D6
C. Phenytoin and CYP2C9
D. Paracetamol and CYP2E1
E. Lithium and CYP3A4

20. The oral bioavailability of the following drugs is augmented by grapefruit juice:
A. Lithium
B. Penicillin
C. Terfenadine
D. Saquinavir
E. Felodipine

THERAPEUTICS

21. Prolongation of the QT interval
A. May be caused by bradycardia
B. May be caused by hyperkalaemia
C. May be caused by acquired heart disease
D. Predisposes to torsade de pointes
E. Predisposes to sudden death

22. The following drugs prolong the QT interval:
A. Cisapride
B. Salmeterol
C. Sertindole
D. Astemizole
E. Erythromycin

23. Inhaled beclomethasone dipropionate

A. Has a linear dose–response curve up to 5000 μg per day
B. Is a prodrug
C. Has greater systemic absorption in individuals with severe asthma
D. Prolonged high-dose therapy may cause growth suppression in children
E. Is not associated with the formation of cataracts

24. Cyclo-oxygenase (COX)

A. Is the enzyme responsible for converting arachidonic acid to prostaglandins
B. COX-1 is the inducible form of the enzyme
C. COX-2 is the isoform that regulates renal blood flow
D. Meloxicam is a selective COX-1 inhibitor
E. Aspirin is an irreversible COX inhibitor

25. Sildenafil

A. Is a selective inhibitor of phosphodiesterase isoenzyme 3 (PDE3)
B. Prolongs cyclic adenosine monophosphate (cAMP) activity in erectile tissue
C. Is metabolized by cytochrome P450 3A4
D. Plasma levels peak 20 minutes after oral administration
E. Therapy may be complicated by a green/blue discoloration of vision

26. The new epilepsy drugs

A. Lamotrigine is licensed as monotherapy for generalized tonic–clonic seizures
B. Lamotrigine should be started at lower doses in patients already taking phenytoin
C. The most serious side effect associated with vigabatrin is an allergic skin reaction
D. Gabapentin is the treatment of choice for infantile spasms
E. Tiagabine's mode of action is through sodium channel blockade

27. Drug treatments for depression

A. Tricyclic antidepressants may cause diarrhoea and weight loss
B. Selective serotonin reuptake inhibitors are less sedative than tricyclics
C. Mirtazapine has noradrenergic and selective 5-hydroxytryptamine (5-HT) 2 activity
D. Sexual dysfunction is a recognized adverse effect of treatment with selective serotonin reuptake inhibitors
E. Cognitive behavioural therapy is as effective as standard drug treatment for mild to moderate depression

28. Drug treatment of Alzheimer's disease

A. Tacrine is associated with hepatotoxicity
B. Donezepil is an acetylcholine agonist
C. Donezepil may cause cardiac conduction abnormalities
D. Donezepil has been shown to improve scores on quality of life scales in patients with Alzheimer's disease
E. Donezepil is metabolised by enzymes of the cytochrome P450 system

29. 5-Fluorouracil (5FU)

A. Inhibits thymidylate kinase
B. Folinic acid can potentiate the effect of 5FU
C. Causes less bone marrow suppression if given as a continuous infusion
D. Desquamation of the palms and soles often occurs following bolus administration
E. Can be used as a radiation sensitizer

30. Paclitaxel (Taxol)

A. Paclitaxel is used in the adjuvant treatment of breast carcinoma
B. Paclitaxel has a role as first-line therapy for advanced ovarian carcinoma
C. Paclitaxel inhibits spindle formation
D. Paclitaxel results in alopecia
E. Hypersensitivity reactions are common

31. Doxorubicin-induced cardiomyopathy

A. Is more likely after mediastinal radiotherapy
B. Is more frequent following continuous infusions of doxorubicin
C. Cardiac damage is mediated via free radicals
D. Electrocardiographic changes are diagnostic
E. The incidence of cardiomyopathy is decreased when dexrazone is given with doxorubicin

32. 'Ecstasy'

A. Ecstasy is a cannabinoid
B. Ecstasy commonly causes paranoid and aggressive behaviour
C. Deaths from hyperthermia are common
D. Water intoxication is partly the result of reduced secretion of antidiuretic hormone
E. There is evidence of neurotoxicity in frequent users

33. Cannabis

A. The source is the male plant of *Cannabis sativa*
B. The active moiety is δ-9-tetrahydrocannabinol
C. Is not associated with an increased risk of using other illicit drugs
D. Causes panic attacks in occasional users
E. Chronic use is associated with the development of schizophrenia

34. In carbon monoxide poisoning

A. Carbon monoxide is excreted by the kidneys
B. Blood carboxyhaemoglobin levels commonly exceed 10% in smokers
C. Solvents in paint remover are a source of carbon monoxide
D. The commonest symptom of carbon monoxide poisoning is nausea
E. Normobaric oxygen therapy is indicated for comatose patients with carbon monoxide poisoning

35. The following statements regarding drug-induced hypokalaemia are true:

A. Carbenoxolone causes hypokalaemia by inhibiting the Na/K ATPase pump
B. Thiazide diuretics block chloride-associated sodium reabsorption
C. High-dose intravenous penicillin causes hypokalaemia by inhibiting phosphodiesterase activity
D. Aminoglycosides cause hypokalaemia through magnesium depletion
E. Liquorice causes hypokalaemia by inhibiting 11B-hydroxysteroid dehydrogenase

36. Treating a patient with glucocorticoids

A. Increases serum 25-hydroxycholecalciferol levels
B. Reduces calcium absorption from the gastrointestinal tract
C. Reduces calcium excretion in the kidney
D. Results in more trabecular than cortical bone loss
E. Results in the most rapid rate of bone loss during the first 6 months of therapy

NEUROLOGY

37. Haematological causes of acute stroke

A. Anticardiolipin antibodies are a specific marker of systemic lupus erythematosus
B. Protein C deficiency is the hallmark of Leiden factor V mutation
C. Leiden factor V mutation is the most commonly inherited prothrombotic state
D. Thrombocytosis is a feature of the antiphospholipid syndrome
E. 50% of all strokes in women aged 20–44 are attributable to the oral contraceptive pill

38. Status epilepticus

A. Is defined as any seizure lasting more than 5 minutes
B. Despite appropriate treatment there is a 10% mortality associated with convulsive status
C. If intravenous access cannot be established, benzodiazepines should be given intramuscularly
D. Hypoglycaemia is a recognized cause
E. A normal electroencephalogram recording is incompatible with the diagnosis

39. In Friedreich's ataxia

A. The genetic mutation is an abnormally expanded CAG trinucleotide repeat in a gene on chromosome 9
B. Patients frequently present in childhood with difficulty walking
C. Diabetes mellitus is a recognized association
D. Retinitis pigmentosa is a recognized feature of the disease
E. There is no association with epilepsy

40. The following are true of diabetic peripheral neuropathy:

A. Alcohol is the commonest cause of neuropathy in the UK
B. Adult-onset diabetes commonly presents with a peripheral neuropathy
C. Diabetic amyotrophy commonly presents with painful wasting of the small muscles of the hand
D. Nerve compression palsies are an uncommon neuropathy in diabetes mellitus
E. The pain of diabetic peripheral neuropathy responds well to simple analgesics

41.   In the treatment of Parkinson's disease

A. L-dopa was first used in the 1970s for the treatment of Parkinson's disease
B. Ropinirole is one of a new class of dopa agonists
C. The adverse effects of the new dopa agonists include hallucinations and confusion
D. L-dopa is broken down by a single enzyme pathway which is inhibited by dopa decarboxylase inhibitors
E. Entacapone may cause dyskinesia

42.   Neurosurgical treatments for Parkinson's disease (PD)

A. Neurosurgical lesions for the treatment of PD were first performed in the 1990s
B. Lesions in the thalamus improve contralateral tremor
C. Low-frequency electrical stimulation has the same therapeutic effect as ablative lesions
D. During surgery stimulating electrodes are used to identify the correct site for a lesion
E. Bilateral pallidal ablative lesions have been associated with cognitive deficits

43.   In trinucleotide repeat disorders

A. The genetic mutation in myotonic dystrophy is an expanded CTG repeat in a gene on chromosome 9
B. Hypothyroidism and diabetes are associated with myotonic dystrophy
C. Fragile X syndrome is an X-linked recessive disorder
D. Machado–Joseph disease presents with ataxia
E. Kennedy's disease is autosomal dominant

44.   In the diagnosis and management of migraine

A. Migraine with aurae accounts for 75% of cases of migraine
B. There is an association between migraine and epilepsy
C. In acute migraine there is delayed gastric emptying
D. Sumatriptan has good oral bioavailability
E. The 5-hydroxytryptamine$_{1B/D}$ agonists are contraindicated in patients over 65 years of age

45.   In the pathophysiology of migraine

A. Migraine headache is thought to be due to vasoconstriction
B. The aurae of migraine typically progress over a few seconds
C. Negative scotomata precede positive scintillating phenomena
D. Half of all cases of familial hemiplegic migraine have a CAG repeat expansion in a gene on chromosome 19
E. Disruption of calcium channel function has been implicated in the pathogenesis of migraine

46.   In the management of headache

A. Headache occuring daily is typical of analgesia-induced headache
B. Tension headache is typically unilateral and pulsating
C. Cluster headache is six times more common in men than in women
D. Cluster-like headaches may be associated with posterior fossa lesions
E. Trigeminal neuralgia typically involves pain in the distribution of the ophthalmic branch of the trigeminal nerve

RESPIRATORY MEDICINE

47.   Brittle asthma

A. Is the same as steroid-resistant asthma
B. Is more common in females
C. May be associated with premenstrual improvement
D. Is characteristically associated with a persistently low peak flow
E. Patients are not usually atopic

48.   With regard to bronchial asthma

A. Leukotriene D_4 (LTD_4) is less potent than histamine at inducing smooth muscle cell contraction
B. Leukotrienes C_4 / D_4 / E_4 are components of the slow relaxing substance of anaphylaxis
C. Zileuton is a leukotriene D_4 receptor antagonist
D. Montelukast is a 5-lipoxygenase inhibitor
E. Leukotriene antagonists reduce both early- and late-phase asthmatic responses

49. α_1–Antitrypsin (AAT)

A. AAT deficiency has an autosomal dominant pattern of inheritance
B. The proteinase MZ phenotype is not associated with emphysema
C. AAT deficiency is associated with bronchiectasis
D. Can be administered orally as replacement therapy
E. Replacement therapy clearly reduces mortality in affected individuals

50.   With respect to pulmonary fibrosis

A. Steroid therapy produces a persistent clinical improvement in over 80% of patients
B. Transforming growth factor (TGF)-β lung levels are characteristically reduced
C. Human T-cell lymphotrophic virus (HTLV)-1 has been implicated in the pathogenesis of pulmonary fibrosis
D. Smokers are at an increased risk
E. Most commonly occurs in patients less than 40 years of age

51. In pulmonary fibrosis

A. There is excess accumulation of collagen in the lung
B. Men are more frequently affected than women
C. Median survival from diagnosis is greater than 10 years
D. There is no animal model
E. There is an inheritable form

52. With respect to nebulizer therapy

A. The ideal particle size is between 5μm and 10μm
B. Nasal deposition increases with age
C. Particles of 1–3μm are usually cleared by phagocytosis
D. Up to 20% of a dose is exhaled
E. Deposition in smaller airways produces more coughing than deposition in larger airways

53. Primary pulmonary hypertension

A. Is associated with HIV infection
B. Is associated with phentermine therapy
C. Affects approximately 1 in 10 000 people
D. Prostacyclin therapy has not been shown to improve survival
E. The majority of cases are familial

54. Lung volume reduction surgery

A. Cannot be performed by video-assisted thoracoscopy (VATS)
B. Is contraindicated in those with a 6-minute walking distance of <100 m
C. Is indicated in patients with a residual lung volume >150% predicted
D. The early improvement in lung function post procedure is due to an increase in elastic recoil
E. Improves exercise capacity

55. With respect to lung transplantation

A. It is contraindicated in smokers
B. Post procedure immunosuppression is usually with azathioprine only
C. Chronic lung rejection occurs in <10% of patients
D. Early mortality is due principally to acute lung rejection
E. Disease recurrence is often seen in those transplanted for primary pulmonary hypertension

ENDOCRINOLOGY

56. The following are causes of hirsutism in women:

A. Cyclosporin
B. Phenytoin
C. Cyproterone acetate
D. Spironolactone
E. 5α-reductase deficiency

57. Polycystic ovary syndrome

A. Is an autosomal dominant disorder
B. All patients have elevated serum luteinizing hormone (LH) and testosterone levels
C. The risk of developing non-insulin dependent diabetes mellitus (NIDDM) in late life is 20 times that of the normal population
D. Is associated with dyslipidaemia
E. Is the most common cause of hirsutism

58. Endocrine hypertension

A. Underlying endocrine disorders are found in 2% of patients with hypertension
B. Most patients with primary hyperaldosteronism are symptomatic
C. 30% of patients with primary hyperaldosteronism have normal serum potassium
D. Adrenal adenomas are a common incidental finding on CT or MRI scans in non-hypertensive patients
E. Glucocorticoid-suppressible hyperaldosteronism (GSM) is an autosomal recessive condition

59. Phaeochromocytoma

A. Is the underlying diagnosis in 5% of patients with hypertension
B. Does not occur in the bladder
C. 60% of patients have sustained hypertension
D. α-Blocker therapy should be initiated only after β-blockade has been established
E. The 5-year survival rate is 95%

60. Multiple endocrine neoplasia (MEN)

A. MEN-2 is an autosomal recessive disorder
B. The genetic abnormality in MEN-2 lies within the *RET* oncogene on chromosome 11
C. Parathyroid tumours occur in less than 50% of MEN-1 patients
D. The gene associated with MEN-1 is located on chromosome 11
E. Patients with MEN-2 may develop megacolon

61.   Type 2 diabetes mellitus
A. The incidence is decreasing
B. Tight diabetic control results in a 25% risk reduction of microvascular disease
C. The addition of metformin to sulphonylurea therapy has a higher risk of mortality than sulphonylurea therapy alone in hyperglycaemic patients
D. Tight diabetic control has been shown to significantly reduce the frequency of myocardial infarction
E. Insulin therapy produces a greater reduction in microvascular disease than sulphonylurea therapy

62.   In type 2 diabetes mellitus
A. A fasting plasma glucose of greater than 7.0 mmol/l confirms the diagnosis
B. Tight blood pressure control reduces the risk of stroke
C. Mortality is reduced when angiotension-converting enzyme inhibitors rather than β-blockers are used to treat hypertension
D. Microvascular complications are significantly reduced in patients with tight blood pressure control
E. Following myocardial infarction, tight blood glucose control using insulin reduces mortality at 3.5 years by 11%

63.   Hypothyroidism
A. The prevalence of hypothyroidism in males is 1 per 100 population
B. Non-thyroid illness can result in a reduction in free and total thyroxine and a serum thyroid stimulating hormone (TSH) level within or below the normal range
C. 10% of patients on amiodarone have clinically significant changes in thyroid function
D. A decreased serum TSH in association with normal serum thyroxine (T_4) is termed subclinical hypothyroidism
E. Thyroxine replacement corrects the hypercholesterolaemia of hypothyroidism

64.   The following are common causes of primary hypothyroidism:
A. Congenital thyroid dysgenesis
B. Hashimoto's autoimmune thyroiditis
C. Grave's disease
D. Follicular cell carcinoma
E. Pituitary insufficiency

65. The following are features associated with primary hyperparathyroidism:

A. Adrenal insufficiency
B. Hypocalcaemia
C. Nephrocalcinosis
D. Mucocutaneous candidiasis
E. Osteitis fibrosa cystica

66. Adult growth hormone deficiency (GHD)

A. The commonest cause of adult-onset GHD is a pituitary macroadenoma
B. A low serum insulin growth factor-1 (IGF-1) is diagnostic
C. Patients with adult GHD have a twofold increase in cardiovascular and cerebrovascular mortality
D. There is an increased incidence of impaired glucose tolerance
E. There is no difference clinically or diagnostically between GHD of childhood onset or adult onset

67. Carcinoid tumours

A. Most commonly present with flushing and diarrhoea
B. Are associated with the Zollinger–Ellison syndrome
C. Are associated with colonic adenocarcinoma
D. Are diagnosed by a low urinary excretion of 5-hydroxyindoleacetic acid
E. Are most commonly found in the colon

CARDIOLOGY

68. Cardiac physiology

A. Diastole involves energy-dependent ventricular relaxation
B. Diastolic dysfunction is associated with a decreased isovolumetric relaxation time on Doppler echocardiogram
C. Symptoms of heart failure may develop with normal systolic function
D. β-Blockers improve left ventricular (LV) function by increasing the length of diastole
E. Constrictive pericarditis results in diastolic dysfunction

69. In unstable angina and non-Q wave myocardial infarction

A. Plaque fissuring results in thrombin generation
B. The 30-day mortality is approximately 10%
C. Low molecular weight heparin (LMWH) has not been shown to be superior to unfractionated heparin in preventing myocardial infarction (MI)
D. Thrombolysis has been shown to reduce mortality
E. Coronary revascularization rates are lower when LMWH is used rather than unfractionated heparin

70. In ventricular fibrillation (VF)

A. Adrenaline increases aortic diastolic blood flow
B. Amiodarone reduces the defibrillation threshold
C. Lignocaine should be administered after 12 DC shocks
D. Bretylium induces spontaneous defibrillation
E. Sodium bicarbonate should be administered when VF is associated with tricyclic antidepressant overdose

71. In chronic heart failure

A. There is a 50% down-regulation of β_1 adrenoceptors
B. Plasma catecholamine levels are a poor predictor of mortality
C. Mortality is reduced by treatment with β-blockers
D. β-Blockers have no effect on left ventricular ejection fraction
E. β-Blockers are well tolerated

72. In chronic heart failure

A. Digoxin reduces mortality
B. In patients in sinus rhythm, digoxin has no effect on worsening cardiac failure
C. Withdrawing digoxin increases left ventricular ejection fraction
D. The angiotensin II receptor antagonist losartan has a licence for treatment
E. Losartan has been shown to reduce mortality by 46%

73. In ischaemic heart disease (IHD)

A. Triglyceride levels are not an independent risk factor
B. Pravastatin does not reduce the risk of stroke post myocardial infarction
C. Early reduction in mortality in patients taking statins is due to low-density lipoprotein (LDL) reduction alone
D. The NCEP (National Cholesterol Education Programme) recommends lowering LDL cholesterol to 2.6 mmol/l in patients with manifest IHD
E. Statins result in plaque regression

74. Antiplatelet agents in coronary artery disease

A. Aspirin as primary prevention for myocardial infarction (MI) has been shown to confer a 44% risk reduction in low-risk groups
B. Aspirin is associated with fewer gastrointestinal adverse reactions than clopidrogel
C. When given at the time of percutaneous transarterial coronary angioplasty (PTCA), the glycoprotein IIb/IIIa antagonist abciximab has been shown to reduce the rate of MI by 50%
D. Activated glycoprotein IIb/IIIa receptor binds to fibrinogen with high affinity
E. Glycoprotein IIb/IIIa inhibitors do not confer any additional benefit over heparin with aspirin in unstable angina

75. Arrhythmogenic right ventricular dysplasia (ARVD)

A. May present with sudden death
B. Is characterized by fibrofatty replacement of myocytes
C. Can result in left ventricular failure
D. May be diagnosed by magnetic resonance imaging
E. Requires insertion of an internal cardioverter defibrillator (ICD)

76. Right ventricular infarction

A. May occur with inferior myocardial infarction
B. Is associated with a good prognosis
C. Causes a low-output state
D. May be treated with inotropic support and volume loading
E. Can be improved by angioplasty to the left circumflex artery

GASTROENTEROLOGY

77. Primary biliary cirrhosis

A. Pruritus is the commonest presenting symptom
B. Vitiligo is frequently associated with primary biliary cirrhosis
C. Patients with xanthelasma have an increased incidence of coronary artery disease
D. Ursodeoxycholic acid is the treatment of choice for asymptomatic disease
E. The characteristic histological lesion is an onion-skin lesion surrounding the portal tract, with fibrosis around small bile ducts

78. Acute pancreatitis

A. Carries an overall mortality of 5%
B. Is complicated by organ failure or local complications in 20% of cases
C. Is associated with pentamidine treatment
D. Pregnancy is protective
E. Ranson's criteria will predict the severity of an attack within 24 hours of presentation

79. In Barrett's oesophagus

A. The risk of developing oesophageal adenocarcinoma is twice that of the general population
B. The incidence of oesophageal adenocarcinoma is decreasing
C. Proton pump inhibitors are curative
D. The commonest metaplastic change is from squamous epithelium to junctional-type columnar epithelium
E. The risk of adenocarcinoma increases with the length of Barrett's segment

80. In the management of obesity

A. The body mass index (BMI) is a more important determinant of morbidity than the distribution of body fat in obese individuals
B. Orlistat therapy needs to be supplemented with vitamins D and E to prevent deficiency
C. Dexfenfluramine treatment of obesity is recommended for patients with a BMI greater than 28
D. Prader–Willi syndrome is a multiple gene abnormality associated with obesity
E. Vitamin B_{12} injections are needed in the postoperative management of gastric bypass surgery

81. Hepatitis A infection

A. Is caused by a double-stranded DNA virus
B. Intravenous drug users are at increased risk compared to the general population
C. Persistent cholestasis is common in adults following acute infection
D. Is associated with an increase in chronic liver disease
E. Is often complicated by mononeuritis multiplex

82. Haemochromatosis

A. Is an autosomal recessive disease
B. Occurs with equal incidence in men and women
C. Invariably leads to death from end-stage liver disease
D. Phlebotomy is the treatment of choice
E. Is caused by a mutation on chromosome 17

83.   In the assessment of nutritional status

A. Body mass index (BMI) is calculated by dividing height by surface area
B. There is increased mortality in patients with a BMI of less than 15
C. Normal BMI is between 18 and 22
D. Albumin has a plasma half-life of 2 days
E. Anthropomorphic measurements allow adjustment of BMI for body build

84.   Nutritional supplementation

A. Elemental formulae consist of free amino acids, triglycerides and glucose
B. Most routinely used commercial liquid supplements contain approximately10 kcal/ml
C. The reintroduction of oral feeds following surgery should be delayed until bowel sounds return
D. Enteral nutrition reduces septic complications following surgery
E. Oral supplements can lead to an increased consumption of standard hospital food

85.   In a patient presenting to casualty with general malaise as a result of the short bowel syndrome

A. Rehydration with large volumes of oral hypotonic saline should be instituted immediately
B. A low serum potassium level is usually seen
C. Serum creatinine is a good indicator of fluid and electrolyte depletion
D. Convulsions most commonly result from hypotension
E. Octreotide can be beneficial

86.   In the management of gastro-oesophageal reflux disease

A. Cisapride is a dompaminergic antagonist
B. Cisapride delays gastric emptying
C. Elevating the head of the bed has been shown to be beneficial
D. Adding H_2 receptor antagonist therapy to proton pump inhibitor (PPI) therapy can be more effective than increasing the dose of PPI
E. PPI therapy causes hypergastrinaemia

87. In coeliac disease

A. The prevalence in northern Europe is approximately 1 in 5000
B. First-degree relatives have a 50% chance of developing the disease
C. It is as common in the USA as in Europe
D. It is four times as common in women than in men
E. There is an association with HLA DR3, DR7 and DQ2

88. In coeliac disease

A. Diagnosis requires the demonstration of histological relapse on gluten challenge
B. IgA antibody tests are more reliable because of selective IgG deficiency
C. Antigliadin antibodies are the most useful in detecting relapse
D. There is an increased risk of carcinoma of the oesophagus
E. The risk of malignancy is unaffected by adherence to a gluten-free diet

NEPHROLOGY

89. The nephrotic syndrome

A. Is defined by a 24-hour urinary protein loss exceeding 1.0 g/1.73 m^2 body surface area
B. In adults is often caused by IgA glomerulonephritis
C. Is a rare presentation of HIV nephropathy
D. Is associated with elevated levels of circulating atrial natriuretic peptide
E. May be associated with prolongation of the partial thromboplastin time

90. Following solid organ transplantation

A. Patterns of infection are variable depending on the organ transplanted
B. Opportunistic infections commonly occur within the first month
C. Infection with CMV can be diagnosed by viral culture within a few days
D. The coadministration of erythromycin increases blood levels of cyclosporin and tacrolimus
E. The risk of developing non-Hodgkin's lymphoma declines after the first year

91. In solid organ transplantation

A. Concordant treatment with allopurinol and azathioprine may lead to decreased levels of immunosuppression
B. Mycophenylate mofetil may be used instead of azathioprine for maintenance immunosuppression
C. Cyclosporin is excreted via the kidneys
D. Diabetes mellitus is a recognized complication of cyclosporin administration
E. Tacrolimus (FK506) is less nephrotoxic than cyclosporin

92. Atheromatous renovascular disease

A. Is the single most common cause of chronic renal failure in patients over 60
B. Often causes heavy proteinuria
C. Renal artery stenosis is usually located in the proximal 2–3 cm of the renal artery
D. Associated with hypertension causes an exaggerated diurnal blood pressure pattern
E. Stenoses are usually corrected in elderly patients in order to improve blood pressure control

93. During pregnancy

A. Glomerular filtration rate (GFR) increases mainly during the first trimester
B. Pre-eclampsia is associated with an increase in plasma volume
C. Antiphospholipid antibody syndrome increases the risk of developing pre-eclampsia
D. The HELLP syndrome is a severe form of pre-eclampsia
E. The relative risk of developing pre-eclampsia in women with chronic renal disease is 5:1

94. Kidney stones

A. Are more likely to form in patients with hypocitraturia
B. Hypercalciuria is found in only 20% of patients with calcium-containing stones
C. Loop diuretics are used to treat patients with hypercalciuria
D. Dietary protein restriction is often part of conservative management
E. Uric acid stones are usually diagnosed incidentally on plain abdominal X-ray

95.   Acute renal failure

A. Has been demonstrated to have a shorter duration if dopamine is administered early
B. Is more likely to be caused by ibuprofen than other NSAIDs
C. In myeloma may be treated by plasmapheresis
D. In ethylene glycol poisoning is caused by oxalic acid precipitation in the kidney
E. In lithium overdose can be prevented by haemodialysis

96.   In end-stage renal failure

A. Hypotension during haemodialysis is usually due to volume depletion
B. Cellulose haemodialysis membranes are generally tolerated better than other types of membrane
C. Sepsis is the most common single cause of death
D. The average serum creatinine is the laboratory test most correlated with risk of death
E. In patients on continuous ambulatory peritoneal dialysis (CAPD) yeast peritonitis usually requires removal of the peritoneal catheter

97.   In the management of rhabdomyolysis

A. Myoglobinuria without haematuria tests negative for blood on dipstick urinalysis
B. Loss of peripheral pulses is usual in the presence of a compartment syndrome
C. Hypocalcaemia should be treated promptly with intravenous calcium
D. Unlike frusemide, mannitol does not acidify the urine
E. Plasmapheresis is of no proven benefit

98.   IgA nephropathy

A. Is the most common cause of glomerulonephritis in adults
B. Is more common in women
C. Is part of a clinical spectrum involving Henoch–Schönlein purpura
D. Is usually cured with immunosuppressive therapy
E. Almost always progresses to end-stage renal failure

INFECTIOUS DISEASES

99. The following are true of leprosy:

A. BCG vaccination is highly protective
B. HIV increases the risks of leprosy transmission
C. Multibacillary cases should be isolated throughout treatment
D. Tuberculoid and lepromatous leprosy are caused by different strains
E. Thalidomide is an important drug in managing complications

100. The following parasites commonly first present several years after exposure:

A. *Plasmodium falciparum*
B. *Strongyloides stercoralis*
C. *Leishmania donovani*
D. *Entamoeba dispar*
E. *Entamoeba histolytica*

101. The pathology of the following is mediated by exotoxins:

A. Cholera
B. Gram-negative septic shock
C. Tetanus
D. Diphtheria myocarditis
E. *Entamoeba histolytica*

102. The following are nematodes that migrate through the lung:

A. *Ascaris lumbricoides*
B. *Schistosoma haematobium*
C. *Paragonimus westermani*
D. Hookworm
E. *Onchocerca volvulus*

103. Diseases transmitted by specific vectors include

A. Malaria by culex mosquitoes
B. Yellow fever by aedes mosquitoes
C. *Trypanosoma cruzi* by tsetse flies
D. *Chlamydia trachomatis* by houseflies
E. HIV by anopheles mosquitoes

104. Relative contraindications to the use of the following antimalarial drugs include

A. Primaquine in glucose-6-phosphate dehydrogenase (G6PD) deficiency
B. Chloroquine and psoriasis
C. Quinine and diabetes
D. Mefloquine and epilepsy
E. Proguanil and pregnancy

105. The following are the clinical diagnostic methods of choice:

A. Polymerase chain reaction (PCR) in pulmonary tuberculosis
B. Widal test in typhoid
C. The leishmanin skin test in visceral leishmaniasis
D. Blood microscopy in malaria
E. Blood culture in secondary syphilis

106. In infection the following are true:

A. CD4 cells are central in developing immunity to malaria
B. Nitric oxide is important in septic shock
C. Eosinophils protect against worm infections
D. Corticosteroids should be used in severe typhoid infection
E. Anti-tumour necrosis factor (TNF) drugs reduce mortality in severe sepsis

107. The following antimicrobials are an appropriate treatment for the associated infections:

A. Artemether in severe malaria
B. Norfloxacin in typhoid disease
C. Amphotericin B in leishmaniasis
D. Azithromycin in legionella
E. Rifampicin in brucellosis

HIV

108. Clinical features of acute HIV-1 infection

A. A seroconversion illness that is prolonged is associated with more rapid disease progression
B. Mucosal ulceration is characteristic
C. A vesicular rash occurs in more than 40% of patients
D. Lymphopenia is common
E. A negative viral RNA assay excludes the diagnosis

109. In the pathogenesis of acute HIV-1 infection

A. Transmission of HIV-1 has not been reported following genital–oral sex
B. Breaks in the genital mucosal barrier increase the risks of acquiring HIV-1 infection
C. The time from genital mucosal HIV-1 infection to viraemia varies from 4 to 11 days
D. High titres of HIV-1 are found in the genital tract during acute infection
E. The decrease in the initial burst of viraemia is due to the production of neutralizing antibodies

110. The effect of HIV infection on the immune system is characterized by

A. Progressive depletion of CD4+ cells from the circulation and lymphoid tissue
B. Chronic immune activation in CD4+ cells, CD8+ cells and circulating monocytes
C. Reduction in numbers of circulating CD8+ cells in early infection
D. Selective loss of naive CD4+ cells in early infection
E. Defects in CD4+ cell-dependent antigen responsiveness

111. Immune reconstitution in HIV-positive patients treated with highly active antiretroviral therapy (HAART)

A. Phase 1 is characterized by increases in circulating naive and memory CD4+ cells, CD8+ cells and B lymphocytes
B. Phase 1 lasts approximately 3 months in individuals with advanced HIV disease
C. Phase 1 is characterized by large increases in natural killer cells
D. Phase 2 is characterized by increases primarily in memory CD4+ and CD8+ cells
E. Delayed-type hypersensitivity to skin test antigens improve over the first year of HAART

112. British HIV Association (BHIVA) guidelines for the treatment of HIV-1 infection recommend

A. Initiating antiretroviral therapy before the CD4 lymphocyte count falls below 350 cells/ml
B. Initiating antiretroviral therapy with three drugs for the majority of patients
C. Aiming for a plasma HIV RNA viral load below the limit of detection of standard assays
D. Including a protease inhibitor in initial therapy for patients with a plasma HIV RNA viral load greater than 50 000 copies/ml
E. That dual therapy should never be used

113. Treatment of HIV-infected patients with highly active antiretroviral therapy (HAART)

A. Treatment with three antiretroviral agents confers no survival benefit over dual therapy
B. Lamivudine is a non-nucleoside analogue reverse transcriptase inhibitor
C. Protease inhibitors prevent entry of HIV RNA into CD4-positive T lymphocytes
D. Valaciclovir is a protease inhibitor
E. Nevirapine inhibits reverse transcriptase

114. Reservoirs of HIV-1 in patients receiving highly active antiretroviral therapy (HAART)

A. Treatment with HAART for 3 years has been demonstrated to eradicate HIV-1 from the body
B. P-glycoprotein transports protease inhibitors out of macrophages
C. Resting CD4+ T cells act as reservoirs of HIV-1
D. The central nervous system contains predominately T-tropic HIV-1
E. Levels of lamivudine in the cerebrospinal fluid are 90% of plasma levels

115. Adverse effects of antiretroviral therapy

A. Saquinavir is associated with renal stone formation
B. The dose-limiting toxicity of protease inhibitors is peripheral neuropathy
C. Zidovudine has been reported to cause hepatic steatosis
D. Ritonavir may precipitate diabetes mellitus
E. Lipodystrophy is associated with an increase in intra-abdominal fat

116. Resistance to antiretroviral drugs

A. Antiretroviral-resistant HIV variants may exist before the initiation of antiretroviral therapy
B. Antiretroviral-resistant HIV variants may be selected for during incompletely suppressive antiretroviral therapy
C. Resistance to HIV protease inhibitors has not been described
D. Cross-resistance between individual drugs does not occur
E. Antiretroviral-resistant HIV variants are replication incompetent and cannot be sexually transmitted

ONCOLOGY

117. Radiotherapy

A. Following surgery, the most common way of delivering radiation to the tumour bed is by implanting radioactive sources
B. Kills cells by causing double-strand DNA breaks
C. Well oxygenated tumours are more radioresistant
D. Late effects may occur many years after irradiation
E. The acute side effects of radiotherapy are irreversible

118. Radiotherapy

A. Is the primary curative treatment in 5% of patients with cancer
B. Radical (curative) radiotherapy consists of 1–5 fractions of external beam irradiation
C. Single fractions of radiotherapy are an effective way of palliating bone metastases
D. Radiotherapy is given in multiple small fractions to reduce normal tissue damage
E. Radiation beams can be shaped using lead blocks

119. Adjuvant chemotherapy (chemotherapy given after curative surgery in an attempt to eradicate micrometastases)

A. Is indicated in Dukes' B colorectal carcinoma
B. Results in a 25% improvement in survival in Dukes' C colorectal carcinoma
C. Is indicated in all premenopausal women with breast cancer
D. Results in infertility in premenopausal women with breast cancer
E. High-dose adjuvant chemotherapy with peripheral stem cell transplantation is offered to women with breast cancer who have more than four positive axillary lymph nodes at diagnosis

120. Immunotherapy

A. Is used as adjuvant therapy in melanoma
B. Has been shown to improve survival when given as adjuvant therapy in colorectal cancer
C. Bacille Calmette–Guérin (BCG) is used in the treatment of superficial bladder cancer
D. Antibody-delivered radiation has been shown to be effective in the treatment of follicular lymphoma
E. MART-1, gp100 and tyrosinase are colorectal tumor antigens that can be used as targets for immunotherapy

121. Tamoxifen

A. Is given to all patients with localized oestrogen receptor-positive breast cancer for 2 years (adjuvant therapy)
B. Given adjuvantly for localized breast cancer reduces the risk of cancer in the contralateral breast
C. Has the same side effect profile as raloxifene
D. Should be given prophylactically to BRCA1 carriers
E. Increases the risk of endometrial cancer

122. Screening

A. In prostate cancer, has been shown to be of no benefit in a randomized control trial
B. Prostate-specific antigen (PSA) has a 95% specificity as a screening test
C. There is no evidence to support screening of unselected women below 50 years of age for breast cancer
D. Two-yearly mammograms are currently recommended in the UK breast cancer screening programme
E. With fecal occult bloods has been shown to decrease mortality by 40% in colorectal cancer

123. In non-small cell lung cancer

A. Radical radiotherapy gives equivalent results to surgery in stage 1 non-small cell cancer
B. CHART (continuous hyperfractionated accelerated radiotherapy) has been shown to improve survival in locally advanced non-small cell cancer
C. Response rates of 80% are obtained with combination chemotherapy
D. Prophylactic cranial irradiation reduces the chances of developing cerebral metastases and results in a survival advantage
E. Radiotherapy should be given after radical surgery

124. High-grade B-cell non-Hodgkin's lymphoma

A. In stage 1 and 2 disease combination radiotherapy and chemotherapy has been shown to be more effective than chemotherapy alone
B. Is associated with human T-cell leukaemia virus I (HTLV I)
C. Stage 2 disease should be treated with high-dose chemotherapy
D. Localized to the stomach may respond to antibiotics
E. Young age, raised lactate dehydrogenase (LDH) and raised ESR are poor prognostic factors

125. Control of cancer pain

A. When converting from oral morphine to subcutaneous diamorphine the dose of diamorphine is two-thirds of the dose of oral morphine
B. Dehydration exacerbates opiate toxicity
C. Fentanyl can be given transcutaneously to control severe pain
D. Antiarrhythmics such as mexiletine are of use in uncontrolled neuropathic pain
E. Bisphosphonates have been shown to reduce the incidence of bone pain and pathological fractures in metastatic breast cancer

HAEMATOLOGY

126. In patients with multiple myeloma

A. A raised β_2-microglobulin is an important prognostic factor
B. Human herpesvirus 8 (HHV-8) is found with increased frequency
C. Hypercalcaemia is associated with high tumour load
D. Current treatment regimens can result in 50% 5-year survival
E. Tumour contamination of graft can complicate autologous bone marrow transplantation (BMT)

127. In patients with sickle cell disease

A. Median survival in the west is 24 years
B. Preoperative prophylactic exchange transfusion is mandatory
C. Fetal haemoglobin (HbF) inhibits polymerization of HbS
D. Short-chain fatty acids increase fetal haemoglobin
E. Hydroxyurea reduces the frequency of vaso-occlusive events

128. Heparin-induced thrombocytopenia (type 2)

A. Typically occurs 1 day after starting heparin
B. Is associated with thromboembolic complications
C. Is optimally treated with low molecular weight heparin
D. Is an immunological phenomenon
E. Should be confirmed in the laboratory before commencing treatment

129. High homocysteine levels

A. Are an independent risk factor for coronary artery disease
B. Occur in situations of cobalamin excess
C. Are typically found in vitamin B_1 deficiency
D. May occur after prolonged nitrous oxide exposure
E. Can be lowered by supplementary folic acid

130. Chronic myeloid leukaemia (CML)

A. 5-year survival following allogeneic bone marrow transplantation for CML is 15%
B. The BCR-ABL fusion gene encodes a protein tyrosine kinase
C. Cytomegalovirus (CMV)-positive recipients have a superior outcome post allogeneic bone marrow transplantation compared to CMV-negative recipients
D. Response rate to donor lymphocyte infusion is higher in patients with haematogical relapse than in those with molecular relapse
E. Cytogenetic response to α-interferon is associated with prolonged survival

131. In essential thrombocythaemia the following statements are true:

A. Essential thrombocythaemia (ET) is characterized by clonal thrombocytosis
B. Decreased thrombopoietin concentrations are diagnostic of ET
C. ET is associated with a significantly reduced life expectancy
D. Anegralide causes thrombocytopenia in humans
E. Cardiovascular side effects have been reported with the use of anegralide

132. In severe haemophilia A

A. Spontaneous mutations account for one-third of cases
B. Inversion mutations are a rare cause
C. Intracranial haemorrhage is the most frequent cause of death in the UK
D. Parvovirus B19 infection can be transmitted by virally inactivated high-purity factor VIII concentrates
E. Increased frequency and severity of bleeding episodes has been described in HIV-positive patients treated with protease inhibitors

133. Human T-cell leukaemia (HTLV) viruses

A. HTLV is a single-stranded DNA virus
B. *Tax* is a transcriptional regulatory gene
C. Breastfeeding is an important route of viral transmission
D. Median survival of patients affected by adult T-cell leukaemia/lymphoma is 2 years
E. HTLV-I associated myelopathy predominantly affects the spinal cord

134. In acute myeloid leukaemia (AML)

A. Myelodysplasia often precedes the presentation of therapy-induced leukaemia
B. Increased incidence of AML has been described after exposure to the epipodophyllotoxin drugs (etoposide)
C. Autologous bone marrow transplantation plays no role in the treatment of AML
D. All-*trans* retinoic acid (ATRA) induces terminal differentiation of blasts
E. P-glycoprotein expression is associated with a good response to chemotherapy

RHEUMATOLOGY

135. Antineutrophil cytoplasmic antibodies (ANCA)

A. Indirect immunofluorescence is used to identify the specific target antigen for ANCA
B. Typically recognize serine proteinase 3 as the target antigen in vasculitis
C. Are found in the majority of new patients with polyarteritis nodosa
D. Are rarely seen in HIV-positive patients
E. May persist in high titres in patients with Wegener's granulomatosis despite clinical remission

136. Scleroderma

A. Is usually associated with low levels of factor VIII–von Willebrand factor
B. There is an association with benzene exposure
C. Of limited cutaneous type (CREST) may be complicated by isolated pulmonary hypertension
D. Renal crises are associated with a microangiopathic haemolytic anaemia
E. Prognosis in patients in renal crisis is improved with high-dose prednisolone (more than 20 mg)

137. Compared to the normal population, HIV infection is associated with an increased incidence of

A. The presence of antinuclear antibodies
B. A Sjögren's-like syndrome characterized by the presence of anti-Ro and anti-La antibodies
C. Rheumatoid arthritis
D. Reiter's disease
E. Myositis

138. Mixed cryoglobulinaemia

A. Typically IgG rheumatoid factors are present
B. Hepatitis C is the most commonly identified infectious cause
C. There is an association with cutaneous leucocytoclastic vasculitis
D. Erosive arthritis is a common feature
E. Low C4 complement levels are present

139. Poor prognostic markers in patients presenting with rheumatoid arthritis include

A High socioeconomic status
B Absence of rheumatoid factor
C. Presence of rheumatoid nodules
D. Early development of erosions
E. Presence of rheumatoid 'shared' epitope in caucasians

140. Bone mineral density (BMD)

A. More than 1 standard deviation below the young adult mean value on DEXA scanning defines osteoporosis
B. Is lower in female caucasian than Afro-Caribbean healthy populations
C. Is lower in patients with polycystic ovary syndrome than in healthy controls
D. Is lower in rheumatoid arthritis than in healthy controls
E. Is increased with raloxifene treatment given to postmenopausal women with low BMD

DERMATOLOGY

141. Acne vulgaris

A. The primary lesion in the pathogenesis of acne vulgaris is the papule
B. Corticosteroid-induced acne resembles typical polymorphic acne vulgaris
C. Oral minocycline can rarely precipitate autoimmune disease
D. Following a single course of oral isotretinoin around 60% of patients achieve cure or significant improvement in their acne
E. Acne is a recognized feature of Apert's syndrome

142. Alopecia

A. Drugs that inhibit type one (I) 5_α-reductase can be used in the treatment of male androgenetic alopecia
B. Alopecia areata is associated with onycholysis
C. The prognosis of alopecia areata in atopic individuals is generally good
D. In lupus erythematosus destruction of the hair follicles can occur, producing permanent scarring
E. Overdose of vitamin E commonly gives rise to diffuse hair loss

143. Atopic eczema

A. Cutaneous poxvirus infection is a recognized complication of atopic eczema
B. Adult-onset atopic eczema can mimic cutaneous T-cell lymphoma
C. *Staphylococcus aureus* isolated from the lesional skin of patients with eczema can release exotoxins which have the ability to non-specifically activate T cells
D. Raised serum IgE is an essential diagnostic feature of atopic eczema
E. In the treatment of severe eczema analysis of serum thiopurine methyltransferase levels can be used to assess the risk of hepatotoxicity when considering treatment with azathioprine

144. Pyoderma gangrenosum

A. Surgical debridement of the cutaneous ulceration may result in clinical deterioration of the lesion
B. An underlying carcinoma is found in association with the majority of cases
C. The acute lesions are regularly accompanied by a neutrophil leucocytosis
D. Associated benign monoclonal gammopathy is most commonly IgA class
E. The ulcers typically heal without scarring

145. Mycosis fungoides

A. Is a cutaneous B-cell lymphoma
B. Incidence is more common in females
C. Patients may present with erythroderma
D. The initial patch stage may last for several years without disease progression
E. PUVA (oral Psoralen plus UVA irradiation) is a well recognized treatment modality

146. Psoriasis

A. Psoriasis is genetically linked to the HLA-B locus
B. Withdrawal of systemic steroids can lead to a deterioration of psoriasis
C. High-output cardiac failure is a rare complication of psoriasis
D. Nail changes are present in almost all cases of psoriasis
E. The pustules of generalized pustular psoriasis are generally secondary to cutaneous *Staphylococcus aureus* infection

147. Effects of ultraviolet radiation (UVR) on the skin

A. UVR does not penetrate into the dermis as it is completely absorbed by the epidermis
B. UVR suppresses the number and function of antigen-presenting cells within the skin
C. Cigarette smoking can induce a cutaneous ageing effect which is most pronounced in UV-exposed areas
D. UVR induced DNA damage produces mutations which are common to a number of other mutagens
E. p53 levels within the skin typically fall following UVR-induced DNA damage

148. Skin cancer in organ transplant recipients

A. Non-melanoma skin carcinoma (NMSC) is a relatively uncommon carcinoma in this group of patients
B. The ratio of basal cell to squamous cell carcinomas reflects that seen in the general population
C. Human papillomavirus has a putative role in the pathogenesis of NMSCs in the transplant population
D. The lip is more commonly affected by NMSC compared to the normal population
E. A single course of oral retinoids will provide long-term benefits in preventing the development of new skin tumours

149. Neurocutaneous disorders

A. Axillary freckling is found more commonly in neurofibromatosis type 2 (NF-2) than NF-1
B. Up to five café-au-lait macules can be found in up to 40% of normal schoolchildren
C. The periungual fibromas in tuberous sclerosis are present soon after birth
D. In tuberous sclerosis shagreen patches can be detected by Wood's light examination
E. In xeroderma pigmentosum skin carcinomas on sun-exposed sites can occur before the age of 20

150. Bullous pemphigoid

A. The clinical appearance can mimic a severe reaction to insect bites
B. On histopathological examination of the lesions the blister roof is composed of full-thickness epidermis
C. Circulating IgA antibodies to the basement membrane zone are found in 70% of patients
D. Associated oral lesions are rare
E. Intralesional steroids can be used to treat localized lesions

Part 2:
Answers

BASIC SCIENCE, IMMUNOLOGY AND GENETICS

1. Cell death
A.F B.F C.F D.F E.T

Apoptosis, necrosis and cytotoxicity are all mechanisms of cell death. Apoptosis and necrosis have very different characteristics and occur in different situations. Cytotoxicity refers to the cell-killing ability of a chemical or a cell, and is mediated through apoptosis or necrosis or both.

Apoptosis is the process of 'programmed cell death'. In health, unwanted or useless cells are destroyed by apoptosis. It plays an important role in normal physiological processes, including development, ageing, the immune system, the menstrual cycle and gastrointestinal tract cell turnover. Abnormal rates of apoptosis are seen in a wide variety of diseases, with increased rates in some neurodegenerative conditions such as Alzheimer's disease and Parkinson's disease. Neoplastic cells show decreased rates of apoptosis. Improved understanding of apoptotic pathways may lead to the development of new therapies for many diseases.

It is important to distinguish between apoptosis and necrosis. Cell necrosis occurs after exposure to a chemical or physical insult and is not 'planned' for the benefit of the organism.

The first stage in cell necrosis is a failure of the cell's normal homoeostatic control of water and electrolyte balance. An influx of water and electrolytes causes cell swelling and membrane rupture. Intracellular contents are released into the extracellular space and an intense inflammatory response is seen in the surrounding area. Microscopically, swelling of cellular organelles, particularly the mitochondria, occurs early, with nuclear destruction occurring late in the process. In necrosis cell energy demands fall and protein synthesis is halted.

Apoptosis can be contrasted with necrosis in several ways. First, the cell's mitochondrial morphology is preserved, whereas nuclear changes are seen early. Chromatin condensation is followed by DNA fragmentation. Secondly, the cell does not swell. The cell volume shrinks and cell blebbing occurs. Thirdly, cell fragmentation is characterized by the development of apoptotic bodies which have intact cell membranes. Fourthly, apoptotic bodies are phagocytosed by macrophages and epithelial cells and an inflammatory process is avoided. Finally, apoptosis, unlike necrosis, is an energy-dependent process.

Reference

Kinloch RA, Treherne JM, Furness LM, Hajimohamadreza I 1999 The pharmacology of apoptosis. Trends in Pharmacological Sciences 20: 35–42

---

2.   T-cell activation
A.T   B.F   C.T   D.T   E.T

Lymphocytes can be divided into T cells and B cells. T cells have their origin in the thymus, whereas B cells originate in the bone marrow. T cells are important in cell-mediated immunity. B cells are important in the humoral immune response, producing antibodies. T cells may be subdivided into helper T cells, which carry the cluster differentiation molecule CD4, and cytotoxic T cells which express CD8. All T cells express the CD3 molecule closely complexed with the T-cell receptor.

Antigen-presenting cells present antigen to the T-cell receptor in the context of their major histocompatibility complex. The T-cell receptor has both antigen- and MHC-binding sites. The majority of cells express MHC class 1 molecules, whereas only certain cells, such as B cells and dendritic cells, also express class 2 molecules on their surface. In certain conditions MHC class 1 expression is downregulated, for example in many tumour cells. As cytotoxic T cells recognize antigen presented in conjunction with the class 1 molecule this may be one method by which tumour antigens evade immune surveillance.

T cells may be further subdivided according to the type of cytokines they secrete. Initially this subdivision was defined for mouse helper T cells, hence the nomenclature Th1 and Th2 responses. Th1 responses tend to activate cytotoxic and inflammatory mechanisms. The predominant mouse Th1 cytokines are γ-interferon, which activates cytotoxic T cells, and interleukin 2. Interleukin 2 is produced by activated T cells and initiates clonal T-cell proliferation. Mouse Th2 responses tend to activate the humoral arm of the immune system, particularly IgE production, and enhance eosinophil function. This response is involved in the pathogenesis of allergy. Important cytokines in this group include interleukins 4, 5, 6, 9, 10 and 13. Interleukin 10 inhibits cytokine synthesis by activated Th1 cells. This effect is mediated through macrophages. Human Th1 and Th2 cells produce similar cytokine profiles, although the synthesis of IL-2, IL-6 and IL-13 is not as tightly restricted to T cells alone.

References

Male D, Cooke A, Owen M, Trowsdale J, Champion B 1996 Advanced immunology, 3rd edn. Times Mirror International, London

Mosman TR, Sad S 1996 The expanding universe of T cell subsets: Th1, Th2 and more. Immunology Today 17: 138–146

3. Th2 cells

A.F   B.F   C.T   D.F   E.T

Activated T helper (Th) cells secrete a number of different cytokines. There are two subdivisions of helper T cell commonly referred to in immunology. Th1 and Th2 cells differ in their cytokine profiles and in their role in different immune responses.

The type of cytokine produced depends on the signals that naïve precursor T helper cells receive. For example, interleukin 12 (IL-12) derived from antigen-presenting cells promotes differentiation towards the Th1 subset, whereas interleukin 4 (IL-4) derived from mast cells favours Th2 differentiation.

Th1 cells secrete IL2 and γ-interferon, whereas Th2 cells secrete IL-4, IL-5 and IL-10. Th1 cytokines are involved in inflammatory responses favouring T-cell mediated cellular immunity and cytotoxicity, delayed-type hypersensitivity and monocyte activation. Th2 cytokines favour B-cell mediated humoral immunity, induce IgE production, activate eosinophils and deactivate monocytes.

Initial studies in rheumatoid arthritis identified a predominance of Th1 cells. This is consistent with the inflammatory nature of this disease. Similar conclusions were reached for insulin-dependent diabetes mellitus, autoimmune thyroid disease and multiple sclerosis. In contrast, diseases where the Th2 response is implicated in their pathogenesis include asthma and other allergic conditions, consistent with the high levels of IgE found in these conditions.

Increasing work in humans is revealing that the division of T helper cells into Th1 and Th2 subsets is an oversimplification of the true effect of cytokine interactions: as new cytokines are being investigated further T helper subsets are being suggested (e.g. Th3). T helper cells secreting an intermediate cytokine profile are termed T0.

Debate continues in rheumatoid arthritis as to whether the T cell is the key cell in the pathophysiology of the disease. Although the T cells are predominantly Th1, the cytokines found in the synovium of joints affected by rheumatoid arthritis are those secreted by monocytes, not T cells. This apparent discrepancy between in vitro studies and in vivo findings is the subject of much active research at present.

References

Dudley J, Kai-Lik So A 1998 T cells and related cytokines. Current Opinion in Rheumatology 10: 207–211

Miossec P, Van den Berg W 1997 Th1/Th2 cytokine balance in arthritis. Arthritis and Rheumatism 40: 2105–2115

Muraille E, Leo O 1998. Revisiting the Th1/Th2 paradigm. Scandinavian Journal of Immunology 47: 1–9

4.   Chemokines

A.T   B.T   C.F   D.T   E.T

Chemokines are chemoattractant cytokines. They are low molecular weight proteins which are structurally related, with 20–70% amino acid sequence homology. There are four classes of chemokine. α-Chemokines have two cysteine residues separated by a different amino acid designated X (CXC), whereas β-chemokines do not contain the separating amino acid (CC). The other two classes have not been well differentiated.

The prototype for the α or CXC chemokines is interleukin 8. This chemokine attracts cells expressing the CXC receptors 1 and 2 and is chemoattractant for neutrophils. IP-10 (interferon inducible protein-10) and MIG (monokine induced by γ-interferon) are CXC chemokines that lack a glutamic acid–leucine–arginine sequence and act on cells expressing CXC receptor 3. These are chemoattractant for activated T lymphocytes. Other CXC chemokines include stromal cell-derived factor and I-TAC.

The prototype for the β or CC chemokines is MCP-1 (monocyte chemotactic protein-1). This acts on basophils, lymphocytes, monocytes and mast cells through its CC receptor 2 (CCR2). Biological functions of MCP-1 on monocytes include chemotaxis, endothelial adhesion and induction of phagocytosis. MCP-1 on mast cells induces histamine release as well as chemotaxis. Other CC chemokines include RANTES, MCP2–4 and MIP-1α (macrophage inflammatory protein). The latter enhances the tumour cytotoxicity of T cells and natural killer cells in vitro.

Chemokines have many important functions. They are important mediators of leukocyte recruitment to sites of inflammation, and highly increased levels of chemokines are found at such sites. They play an important role in the adhesion of leucocytes and other inflammatory cells to vascular endothelium and in their migration through the endothelium to the extravascular space. They also increase leucocyte activation, enhancing effector function. In tissue healing a balance of angiogenesis-promoting chemokines and angiogenesis-inhibitory chemokines may be important in the regulation of angiogenesis. Increased chemokine expression has been reported in several chronic inflammatory diseases, such as rheumatoid arthritis and psoriasis and also in allergic responses and asthma. Antichemokine therapies may have a role to play in the treatment of these conditions in the future.

CC chemokines are strongly expressed in the lymph nodes of patients with HIV, and research in this field may lead to novel therapeutic approaches to the management of the disease.

References

Adams DH, Lloyd AR 1997 Chemokines: leukocyte recruitment and activation cytokines. Lancet 349: 490–495

Baggiolini M 1998 Chemokines and leukocyte traffic. Nature 392: 565–568

Luster AD 1998 Chemokines – chemotactic cytokines that mediate inflammation. New England Journal of Medicine 338: 436–445

---

5.   Chemokines and HIV-1 receptors

A.T   B.T   C.T   D.T   E.F

In 1996 it was discovered that certain chemokines could suppress HIV-1 replication. HIV-1 infection is initiated by interaction of the viral envelope glycoprotein GP120 with at least two cellular receptors, the CD4 molecule and a seven-transmembrane domain G-protein coupled chemokine receptor. Macrophage-tropic (M-tropic) strains of HIV-1 replicate in macrophages and CD4+ T lymphocytes and use the chemokine receptor CCR5. These HIV-1 viruses have been classified R5 on the basis of their receptor usage. The CCR5 receptor is also used by almost all primary (infecting) HIV-1 isolates. T lymphocyte-tropic (T-tropic) isolates of HIV-1 replicate in CD4+ T lymphocytes, as well as macrophages. T-tropic viruses use the chemokine receptor CXCR4 as a coreceptor with the CD4 molecule.

M-tropic (R5) HIV-1 is the main type of virus involved in the transmission of infection. HIV-1 negative individuals have been identified who have had high exposure to the virus but appear resistant to infection. These individuals lacked CCR5 because of homozygosity for a 32 base-pair deletion (δ-32 allele), which inhibits the expression of the receptor on the cell surface. Although homozygotes are rare, heterozygotes make up 10–15% of caucasian populations. Being heterozygous for this mutation may afford limited protection from infection. Infected heterozygotes progress to disease more slowly, exhibit lower viral loads and slower rates of CD4+ T cell decline, and have a higher likelihood of being long-term non-progressors than do homozygous wild-type individuals.

Other genetic polymorphisms in CCR5 have been described which may also confer resistance to infection and slow the progression of disease. More recently it has been found that individuals homozygous for a polymorphism in the SDF-1 gene, the ligand for CXCR4, experience delayed disease progression.

Understanding the naturally occurring variation in chemokines and their receptors offers hope that strategies designed to affect levels of these molecules may have therapeutic application in the future. Various strategies are under investigation. Gene therapy may result in the production of modified chemokines which cannot be secreted and bind the CCR5 and CXCR4 receptors intracellularly, leading to their destruction. Ribozymes and antisense RNA which bind to, and cleave or inactivate, specific sequences of mRNA, preventing translation of the chemokine receptors, are being investigated. Monoclonal antibodies which block the receptors are being developed and may be of use in preventing materno-fetal transmission or as post exposure prophylaxis. Therapeutic use of the natural or modified chemokines as competitive receptor antagonists is also being studied. The most hopeful strategy, however, is the development of small molecules (i.e. not peptides like the chemokines) which could block the receptors or prevent membrane fusion.

References

Cairns JS, D'Souza MP 1998 Chemokines and HIV-1 second receptors: the therapeutic connection. Nature Medicine 4: 563–568

Garred P 1998 Chemokine-receptor polymorphisms: clarity or confusion for HIV-1 prognosis? Lancet 351: 2–3

6.   IgE in asthma

A.T   B.T   C.F   D.T   E.T

IgE is an important inflammatory mediator in a number of allergic diseases, including allergic rhinitis and asthma. Serum levels of IgE are known to correlate very closely with the severity of asthma. IgE activates a number of different cell types that are involved in both allergic and inflammatory diseases. These cell types are activated by cell surface receptors, of which two types are recognized. The FεSR1 receptor is predominantly located on mast cells but is also found on other cell types, including basophils and eosinophils. The lower affinity FεSR2 receptor is found on lymphocytes. Activation of these cells leads to the production of mediators that are involved in both the early and the late asthmatic response.

Monoclonal antibodies that block these receptors have been developed as possible therapies for asthma. They are directed against the Fc portion of IgE. Clinical studies of these antibodies in asthma have demonstrated a reduction in circulating IgE levels. This reduction correlated well with symptomatic improvement in both the acute and the late stages of asthma responses. These antibodies require further evaluation as new therapies for asthma.

References

Boulet LP, Chapman KR, Cole J et al. 1997 Inhibitory effects of an anti-IgE antibody E25 on allergen-induced early asthmatic response. American Journal of Respiratory and Critical Care Medicine 155: 1835–1840

Fahy JV, Fleming HE, Wong HH et al. 1997 The effect of an anti-IgE monoclonal antibody on the early and late phase responses to allergen inhalation in asthmatic subjects. American Journal of Respiratory and Critical Care Medicine 155: 1828–1834

7. Allergen immunotherapy

A.T   B.F   C.T   D.F   E.T

Allergen immunotherapy involves the administration of a gradually increasing dose of allergen to patients with specific allergies. The aim is to reduce symptoms following exposure to the allergen. The practice of immunotherapy can be dangerous and a number of deaths from anaphylaxis have been attributed to it. Guidelines have been introduced to ensure safe practice. This technique should only be performed in specialist centres with good resuscitation facilities.

Despite these problems, it is well recognized that immunotherapy can be highly effective in selected patients with known IgE-mediated disease. These include patients suffering from severe allergic rhinitis, wasp and bee venom reactions, allergic conjunctivitis and allergic asthma. In severe asthma the risk of severe reactions is increased and the chance of successful immunotherapy greatly reduced. Several trials have shown a benefit in mild asthma, particularly that due to house dust mite sensitivity. Immunotherapy against cat allergens is less successful. It is also recognised that the age of the patient is important: younger patients can be more successfully treated than older ones. Younger subjects are more at risk of adverse reactions. There is also evidence suggesting that children who are sensitive to one allergen and who receive immunotherapy tend to develop fewer new sensitivities as they grow older.

The mechanism by which immunotherapy is successful is not yet known. It does not appear to correlate with the serum immunogloblin levels of either IgG or IgE. IgE levels to a particular allergen are elevated at the start of treatment and increase as the allergen is administered. As immunotherapy progresses specific IgE levels fall, but rarely get below starting levels. Possible mechanisms include the production of IgG antibodies that block IgE antibody binding, and a switch in lymphocyte subsets with an increase in Th1 and a decrease in Th2 lymphocytes. Th2 cells are characteristically proinflammatory, whereas Th1 cells suppress allergic reactions.

Immunotherapy is a promising technique that may provide an alternative treatment for allergic individuals. It is likely to be successful in younger patients with an isolated allergy, where it can be life-saving. More research is needed to elucidate the exact mechanism of action and to improve safety.

References

Bousquet J, Michel FB 1994 Specific immunotherapy in asthma; is it effective? Journal of Allergy and Clinical Immunology 94: 1–11

Report of a WHO/IUIS Working Group 1989 The current status of allergen immunotherapy (hyposensitisation). Allergy 44: 369–379

Secrist H, Chelen CJ, Wen Y, Marshall JD, Umetsu DT 1993 Allergen immunotherapy decreases interleukin-4 production in CD4+ T cells from allergic individuals. Journal of Experimental Medicine 178: 2123–2130

8.   HBV vaccination

A.T   B.T   C.F   D.F   E.F

Hepatitis B virus (HBV) is a DNA virus which causes a spectrum of clinical disease. Infection may be asymptomatic or symptomatic. Acute hepatitis occasionally leads to fulminant liver failure. Although the disease is self-limiting in over 90% of patients, in the remainder it produces chronic infection leading to liver cirrhosis or hepatocellular carcinoma. In the UK and USA HBV infection is largely limited to defined high-risk groups, but in many parts of the world it is endemic and chronic disease in particular has huge implications for public health in these areas. In endemic areas such as Africa and many parts of Asia, vertical transmission from mother to infant and horizontal transmission between children contribute to the high prevalence of the disease as well as the well recognized parenteral routes of infection. Vaccination recommendations and national vaccination policies therefore vary around the world.

In low-prevalence areas candidates for vaccination are those likely to be at high risk of exposure to the virus. These include homosexual men, intravenous drug users, patients with clotting disorders or chronic renal failure patients on haemodialysis, and individuals exposed at work, such as healthcare workers. In addition, people with partners who are infectious (i.e. carrying the hepatitis B surface (s) or envelope (e) antigens) or who have multiple sexual partners are candidates for vaccination. Infants born to hepatitis B surface antigen (HbsAg)-positive mothers should be vaccinated at birth.

Recombinant HBV vaccines are made using HBsAg expressed by recombinant DNA in the yeast *Saccharomyces cerevisiae*. The only contraindications to use of this vaccine are allergies to yeast or to components of the vaccine. The vaccine is given as a series of three intramuscular injections, with the second and third doses separated by at least 2 months. Adverse effects are uncommon, but include injection site reactions (most commonly), fever and systemic effects (uncommonly) and anaphylaxis (rarely). Intradermal injections will produce antibodies, but not at sufficient titres and subcutaneous injection is ineffective. Gluteal injection results in poor immunogenicity, probably owing to failure to achieve intramuscular delivery at this site. It can be given safely and without loss of efficacy with HBV immunoglobulin (HBIG) or with other vaccines. Neutralizing antibodies to HBsAg are produced in 95–99% of cases and, in 50% of cases where protective antibody titres are not reached, immunity can be achieved by giving further doses. HBV infection rates in infants born to HBsAg mothers are decreased by vaccination, but the first dose must be given at birth and HBIG must be administered at the same time for this result.

Certain individuals are at risk of not developing protective titres and in these people postimmunization testing is recommended. These include smokers, those over 40 years of age, patients on haemodialysis and the immunocompromised.

HBV vaccination is highly efficacious. The incidence of HBV infection is reduced by 90–95% in cohort studies of homosexual men and in healthcare workers. A policy in Taiwan to immunize all infants at birth resulted in a greatly reduced rate of chronic disease over 10 years, reflecting the potential importance of such programmes in endemic areas. Epidemiological data show a strong association between HBV infection and hepatocellular carcinoma.

Existing vaccines may not protect against rare HBV variants with mutations in the s protein, part of which includes the HBsAg, such as those seen in patients transplanted for HBV disease who are also treated with HBIG and lamivudine.

Refrence

Lemon SM, Thomas DL 1997 Vaccines to prevent viral hepatitis. New England Journal of Medicine 336: 196–204

9.   Flow cytometry

A.**T**   B.**T**   C.**F**   D.**T**   E.**F**

Flow cytometry is widely used in scientific research and clinical centres to measure the properties of individual cells. Flow cytometers are used routinely in the fields of haematology, immunology and pathology. A number of properties of cells can be measured, including cell viability, proliferation, surface antigen expression and intracellular enzyme activity.

Flow cytometers are designed to deliver cells in single file past a detector, which then measures the variable of interest. As a consequence, information about cell morphology and spatial relationships to other cells in a tissue is lost using this technique.

A basic flow cytometer has a source of light, a flow cell, a means to focus light of different colours on to a detector, electronics to amplify the signal and a computer. The flow cell delivers cells singly to the point of focus of the light source. To do this it injects a sample into a stream of fluid. The light source is usually a laser, which focuses light into a small concentrated beam to maximally excite a single cell. The techniques used to identify properties of a cell rely on labelling with fluorescent markers. The number of fluorescent markers flow cytometers can detect is determined by the range of laser wavelengths available. For example, the commonly used fluorochromes fluoroscein and phycoerythrin are detected by lasers with a major line at 488 nm. The light emitted by each cell is electronically amplified and data are displayed as a histogram, which can then be analysed.

The commonest application of flow cytometry is cell-surface antigen detection. An example of this in clinical use is in counting CD4 cells in the blood of patients with HIV infection. After isolating the lymphocytes, the CD4 antigen is labelled with a monoclonal antibody tagged to a fluorescent marker. Flow cytometry detects cells bearing that marker. If further information is required these cells can be labelled with monoclonal antibodies to other surface antigens tagged to different fluorescent markers. The flow cytometer is then programmed to detect all the other fluorescent markers. Similar techniques are used in haematological malignancies to identify cell markers in various leukaemias and lymphomas. Cells from solid tissue can be isolated and studied in the same way.

The second most common application of flow cytometry is the measurement of cellular DNA. This provides information on the cell cycle, cell ploidy and cell viability. This is useful in the study of cytotoxic drugs whose mechanism of action relies upon interruption of the cell cycle. The most widely used dye for staining DNA is propidium iodide. Cells are prepared for this method by membrane permeabilization so that the dye can enter the cell. Non-dividing cells in the G0 phase of the cell cycle will not take up as much propidium iodide as those in the DNA synthetic (S) phase or those in the G2 phase, where DNA has doubled prior to mitosis. Labelling cells with 5-bromodeoxyuridine (BrdU) provides further information about cell proliferation, as it is incorporated into proliferating cells instead of thymidine. Measurements of cell viability are also possible. If cells have not been prepared by permeabilization, propidium iodide is only taken up by non-viable cells.

Reference

Ormerod MG 1994 Flow cytometry. BIOS Scientific Publishers, Oxford

10. The Human Genome Project
A.F   B.F   C.F   D.T   E.F

For the clinician the four main promises of molecular genetics are the mapping of the approximate location of genes; the identification and characterization of mutations of those genes; the elucidation of the pathophysiological consequences of these mutations and the development of rational treatment strategies for these genetic disorders.

The Human Genome Project set itself three major scientific goals: the creation of genetic maps, the development of physical maps, and the determination of the complete sequence of human DNA. There are 3 000 000 000 (3 billion) nucleotides in haploid human DNA, but only 3% of these contribute to the genetic code. The project plans to define the functional importance and structure of the estimated 80 000 genes contained within the genome. 30 000 genes are thought to be involved in encoding the human nervous system, of which 20 000 are exclusively expressed in the brain. Currently detailed information is available for only a few thousand structural and regulatory genes known to be active in the central nervous system (CNS).

The density of genetic maps is now sufficient to map any Mendelian human trait given sufficient sized families. Once a disorder is mapped, genetic linkage analysis can be used to identify family members at increased risk. The density of the current maps is also sufficient to support the analysis of some common polygenic traits, such as multiple sclerosis and Tourette's syndrome. One of the new genetic maps consists of short tandem repeats of two or more nucleotides. The number of these repeats varies from individual to individual. The advantage of these markers over previous types of marker, such as restriction fragment length polymorphisms, is that they can be assayed by the polymerase chain reaction under uniform conditions.

Genetic markers need to have high heterozygosity, i.e. a high likelihood that a marker will be different in any two copies of a chromosome. Another important characteristic of a genetic map is that it should have a high density of coverage. The current maps have a marker every 0.7 centimorgans, or 700 000 base pairs. One centimorgan is equal to a 1% chance that two markers will be separated during meiosis by recombination.

The physical map of the human genome consists of 30 000 sequence-tagged-site (STS) markers distributed at intervals of approximately 100 000 bases along the entire genome. Physical maps of several chromosomes have now been completed.

The biggest impact of gene identification has been in its application to individuals at risk of disease, negating the need for family linkage studies. A number of diseases, including Duchenne and Becker muscular dystrophies, Charcot–Marie–Tooth type Ia, the triplet repeat disorders, and diseases resulting from gross structural changes in DNA, such as deletions and replications, can now be detected routinely in the laboratory. In some diseases single point mutations can be detected using DNA-based diagnosis. A small number of point mutations are found to result in the majority of cases of certain diseases, such as myoclonic epilepsy associated with ragged red fibres, Leber's hereditary optic neuropathy and Gaucher's disease. In many other disorders, however, non-recurring private point mutations occur anywhere among thousands of nucleotides within a given gene, making screening extremely expensive and time-consuming.

Sequencing of a mutant gene and decoding the structure of its protein product is only one step in understanding the protein's function in health and disease. Until this final step is tackled, translating new understanding of molecular genetics into treatments will be difficult. Nevertheless, delineation of the molecular defects of a few diseases have directed pharmaceutical investigations. An example of this is the increased understanding of the role of neuronal nicotinic acetylcholine receptors in the rare heritable epilepsies.

References

Allen KM, Walsh C 1996 Shaking down new epilepsy genes. Nature Medicine 2: 516–518

Jordan E, Collins FS 1996 A march of genetic maps. Nature 380: 111–112

Steinlein OK et al. 1995. A missense mutation in the neuronal nicotinic acetylcholine receptor alpha4 subunit is associated with autosomal dominant nocturnal frontal lobe epilepsy. Nature Genetics 11: 201–203

11.   Neurogenetics
A.F   B.F   C.F   D.T   E.F

Many of the highlights of human molecular genetics involve neurological disorders. Huntington's disease was the first autosomal disorder to be mapped exclusively using DNA markers (1983). The first pathogenic human gene to be identified by positional cloning was that for dystrophin, the absence of which is responsible for Duchenne muscular dystrophy (1986). In addition, several novel genetic mechanisms have been elucidated which do not fit with classic Mendelian genetics.

Genetic imprinting describes the differential expression of autosomal genes of different parental origin and is seen in two disparate neurogenetic disorders. In Angelman syndrome cerebellar ataxia and mental retardation results from dysfunction of maternally inherited genes in 15q11–13. Disruption of the same region in the paternally inherited chromosome results in Prader–Willi syndrome, characterized by hypotonia, hypogonadism, hyperphagia and hypopigmentation.

Anticipation describes a tendency for a disease to manifest at an earlier age and follow a more aggressive course in consecutive generations. Originally observed in Huntington's disease and myotonic dystrophy, it was dismissed as bias until the discovery of the underlying pathogenetic mechanism, an unstable trinucleotide repeat sequence. This form of genetic mutation was first identified in spinal muscular atrophy or Kennedy's disease, but has since been identified in different genes, resulting in a diverse group of neurodegenerative disorders including Huntington's disease, olivopontocerebellar atrophy, dentatorubropallidoluysian atrophy, a number of the spinocerebellar ataxias (SCAs 1, 2, 3, 6 and 7 to date), myotonic dystrophy, fragile X and Friedreich's ataxia. Many of these disorders involve CAG repeats which encode expanded polyglutamine tracts in the gene's protein product, but other trinucleotide repeat sequences are also pathogenic. The common genetic mutation and similar age of onset of the CAG repeat disorders, as well as the observed dose effect between CAG repeat length and age of onset of symptoms, has led researchers to postulate a common pathogenic mechanism for these different disorders. Intranuclear inclusions have been identified in SCA1, SCA3 and Huntington's disease. It has been proposed that proteins containing expanded polyglutamine tracts are cleaved and the expanded polyglutamine tract forms high molecular weight complexes, which trigger the formation of intranuclear inclusions and may eventually result in cell death.

References

Brice A 1998 Unstable mutations and neurodegenerative disorders. Journal of Neurology 245: 505–510

Hardy J, Gwinn-Hardy K 1998 Genetic classification of primary neurodegenerative disease. Science 282: 1075–1079

Keverne EB 1997 Genomic imprinting in the brain. Current Opinion in Neurobiology 7: 463–468

12.   The mitochondrial genome
A.T   B.F   C.F   D.F   E.T

The circular double-stranded human mitochondrial genome consists of 16 569 nucleotides. It is maternally inherited. The 37 mitochondrial genes encode structural RNA (22 transfer and two ribosomal) and 13 proteins. Complexes I, III, IV and V of the respiratory chain contain subunits encoded by both nuclear DNA and mitochondrial DNA, whereas complex II consists entirely of nuclear DNA-encoded subunits. Nearly all tissues in the human body are partially dependent on oxidative metabolism.

Leber's hereditary optic neuropathy (LHON) was the first human disease to be pathogenetically linked to mitochondrial DNA. It presents with painless subacute bilateral visual loss with central field defects, abnormal colour vision and optic atrophy. The mean age of onset is 23 years and it is three to four times more common in men than in women. It demonstrates a maternal inheritance pattern. The pathophysiology of the visual loss, however, involves both genetic and epigenetic factors. The male preponderance is postulated to result from an X-linked nuclear DNA factor, and alcohol and tobacco consumption are important epigenetic factors in its clinical expression. The inherited mitochondrial DNA mutations implicated in LHON are heterogeneous, with mutations in at least eight genes which encode three biochemical complexes. Those studied to date result in subtle complex-specific impairments of oxidative phosphorylation; however, many of the characteristic features of LHON, such as long latency, the acute nature of visual loss and the clinical involvement of the optic nerve, are not explained by such a mechanism.

Tissue-specific accumulation of somatic (non-inherited) mitochondrial DNA mutations may result in late-onset neurodegenerative diseases. Both the high mutation rate and the poor repair capacity of mitochondrial DNA contribute to the accummulation of mitochondrial mutations in post-mitotic tissues. Environmental factors also affect mitochondrial DNA; the antiretroviral agent zidovudine (AZT) depletes muscle mitochondrial DNA and causes an acquired mitochondrial DNA myopathy. The accumulation of mitochondrial DNA mutations and the consequent deficit in ATP production below a critical threshold in subpopulations of neurons may contribute to the pathogenesis of neurodegenerative disorders such as Alzheimer's and Parkinson's diseases. Mitochondrial energy deficits have been postulated to contribute to neuronal injury via an excitotoxic mechanism. Oxygen free radicals, glutamate and nitric oxide may mediate neuronal cell injury and death, in part via these mechanisms. These mechanisms may also play a role in ageing.

Reference

Johns DR 1996 The other human genome: mitochondrial DNA and disease. Nature Medicine 2(10): 1065–1068

13. Prothrombin-gene G20210A mutation

A.T   B.F   C.T   D.F   E.T

A prothrombotic mutation that has recently been described involves a guanine-to-adenine transition at nucleotide 20210 of the gene encoding prothrombin. The mutation occurs in the 3′ untranslated region of the prothrombin gene. Higher prothrombin levels are noted in individuals with the mutation. Prothrombin is the precursor of the serine protease thrombin, which is the end product of the coagulation cascade. The mechanism(s) by which the G20210A allele contributes to higher prothrombin levels is not clear, but suggestions include higher translation efficacy or increased stability of the transcribed mRNA.

The mutation is present in 1–2% of the population and in 18% of families with a history of venous thromboembolic disease. Heterozygous carriers are known to have a risk of deep vein thrombosis that is three to six times that of the general population. After the mutation in the factor V gene (factor V Leiden), the prothrombin-gene mutation is the most common genetic determinant of deep vein thrombosis of the lower extremities.

Recently the prothrombin-gene mutation G20210A has been identified as an important risk factor for cerebral vein thrombosis. The presence of the prothrombin mutation increases the risk of the disorder by a factor of 10. The use of oral contraceptives appears also to be a strong risk factor for cerebral vein thrombosis, with a relative risk of approximately 13–20 reported. Women who are both carriers of the G2010A prothrombin gene allele and current users of oral contraceptives appear to have a risk of cerebral vein thrombosis (odds ratio = 149.3) that far exceeds the sum of the separate risks associated with these two factors. Cerebral vein thrombosis, however, is a rare condition and screening for the prothrombin-gene mutation prior to prescribing oral contraceptives has not been recommended.

References

Martinelli I, Sacchi E, Landi G et al. 1998 High risk of cerebral vein thrombosis in carriers of a prothrombin-gene mutation and in users of oral contraceptives. New England Journal of Medicine 338: 1793–1797

Poort SR, Rosenthal FR, Reitsma PH et al. 1996 A common genetic variant in the 3′-untranslated region of the prothrombin gene is associated with elevated prothrombin levels and an increase in venous thrombosis. Blood 88: 3698–3707

Vandenbroucke JP 1998 Cerebral sinus thrombosis and oral contraceptives. British Medical Journal 317: 483–484

14. Nutritional requirements

A.F B.F C.T D.T E.F

In order to determine the nutritional requirements of an individual patient it is important to be aware of their energy requirements. Total daily energy expenditure (TEE) can be divided into several components. Basal metabolic rate (BMR) is the minimal expenditure of an individual 12–18 hours after a meal, while at complete rest. Resting energy expenditure (REE) is the energy expenditure while resting several hours after a meal or physical activity. Thermic effect of muscle (TEW) varies with activity but usually represents 15–20% of TEE. The thermic effect of food is influenced by diet, but usually makes up about 10% of TEE. BMR makes up approximately 65% of TEE and 90% of REE, and REE about 75% of TEE.

REE can be derived experimentally by measuring the carbon dioxide and oxygen content in a hood placed over the patient's head for 2 hours. REE can also be estimated using equations such as the Harris–Benedict:

For males: REE (kcal/day) = 66.5 + (13.8 × W) + (5 × H) − (6.8xA)
For females: REE (kcal/day) = 65.5 + (9.6 × W) + (1.8 × H) − (4.7 × A)
    where   W = weight in kg, H = height in cm, and A = age in years.

From this estimate of REE an estimate of TEE can be determined by multiplying by two factors, one for the thermic effects of food and physical activity (1.1–1.3) and the other for the disease state (1.0–1.6). Fever also influences energy expenditure (1.0 + 0.13 per °C).

Nutritional management plans aim to give adequate calories for each patient depending on their condition. Protein provides approximately 4.0 kcal/g of energy, compared to 9–10 kcal/g for fats and about 3.5 kcal/g for carbohydrates.

Protein requirements tend to increase with disease severity. In mild disease 0.8–1.0 g/kg/day is required, but in severe disease this can rise to 1.5 g/kg/day or more. Nitrogen makes up 16% of the mass of most proteins. The nitrogen requirements are therefore equivalent to the protein requirements divided by 6.25. A 70 kg man with mild disease will require about 70 g of protein per day, which is equivalent to 11.2 g of nitrogen.

References

Anon 1996 Malnourished inpatients: overlooked and undertreated. Drug and Therapeutics Bulletin. 34: 57–59

Payne-James JJ 1995 Enteral nutrition. European Journal of Gastroenterology and Hepatology 7: 501–506

Silk D 1995 Nutrition for gastroenterologists: when, how and for how long? European Journal of Gastroenterology and Hepatology 7: 491–500

PHARMACOLOGY AND DRUG DEVELOPMENT

15. Drug development
A.F   B.F   C.F   D.F   E.F

The development of a new medicine from a newly synthesized chemical compound, a chemical extracted from a naturally occurring source or a compound produced by biotechnology is a complex process. Of every 10 000 molecules extracted, synthesized or tested, usually only one will become a licensed medicine. The entire process from discovery to licensing takes about 8–10 years for treatments for acute conditions and up to 12 years for treatments for chronic illnesses. It has been estimated that the cost of the development process is approximately £350 million per new chemical entity.

Chemists in the pharmaceutical industry produce thousands of compounds each year. All initial studies on a new compound are carried out in vitro. A comprehensive profile of the new chemical is built up, including examination of its chemical stability and its ability to be prepared in various dosage forms (pharmaceutical development). Initial in vivo studies then examine its effects and kinetics (absorption, distribution, metabolism and excretion) in animals. If initial pharmacological screening proves promising, i.e. the compound has some or all of the pharmacological effects that might have been predicted from its chemical structure, compounds with minor variations of the chemical structure are also prepared and investigated. There is always a possibility that such structural changes may improve the pharmacological profile (e.g. a minor change in the chemical structure may produce higher blood levels). Screening will also take place for unexpected effects that a chemical might have.

One of the major growth areas within the past 15 years has been the development of compounds derived from biotechnological processes. More than 50 new medicines have already been produced using such methods. Agents classed as biotechnology medicines include proteins, enzymes, antibodies, genetic materials and other naturally occurring substances that fight infection and disease. The production of biotechnological medicines is assisted by other living organisms: plant and animal cells, viruses and yeasts.

Before any drug candidate is administered to humans, extensive toxicopharmacological testing in animals is undertaken to assess harmful as well as beneficial effects of the drug. Long-term toxicological testing, including reproductive testing, continues long after a potential drug has been tested in humans.

Phase I clinical studies are the first studies to be conducted in humans and are performed on small numbers of healthy volunteers (who have neither the condition under investigation nor any other illness). Initial doses are as low as possible to produce an expected effect. Doses are then gradually increased and physiological parameters and pharmacokinetic data collected.

Phase II clinical studies are the first time the drug is given to patients with the actual condition it is intended to treat. In order to ascertain the correct dosage levels for therapeutic effects and unwanted side effects, the drug is given to different groups of patients at different dosages. The number of patients treated in such studies is still relatively small, numbering between 200 and 400.

After satisfactory completion of phase II studies, major clinical trials are initiated which will determine the fate of the drug. These phase III studies are designed to measure whether the effect of a medicine is statistically significant compared to either placebo or an established treatment. Typically more than 3000 patients will be included in phase III studies. The double-blind placebo-controlled trial remains the gold standard for phase III studies. However, comparisons with established treatments are also commonly performed. This is particularly important for conditions where it would be unethical not to treat the patient.

Of the medicines that are successfully taken through all these stages of development, one important hurdle remains before marketing: the approval or licensing process. Regulatory authorities, such as the Medicines Control Agency (MCA) in the UK and Food and Drug Administration (FDA) in the USA, are responsible for ensuring that all marketed medicines are of demonstrated safety, quality and efficacy. Only once a medicine has gained a licence can it be marketed.

Reference

Harman RJ 1999 The drug development process – introduction and overview. Pharmaceutical Journal 262: 334–337

---

16. The Yellow Card Scheme

A.T   B.T   C.T   D.F   E.F

Adverse drug reactions (ADRs) are an important cause of morbidity and mortality. A meta-analysis of prospective studies of the incidence of ADRs in hospital inpatients estimated that 6.7% of patients had a serious ADR and 0.32% a fatal ADR. The UK Yellow Card Scheme for reporting suspected ADRs was established in 1964 following the thalidomide disaster. The scheme invites reports of suspected ADRs to be sent to the Medicines Control Agency and the Committee of Safety on Medicines for analysis.

The quality and efficacy of a medicine are fairly well defined at the time of licensing. However, information on the adverse effect profile of medicines from clinical trials is limited by the number of patients included in such trials, their duration, the selection criteria used and the somewhat artificial conditions under which they are conducted. Therefore, safety in normal conditions of use can only be fully assessed after marketing. It is well recognized that safety hazards may emerge at any time during the life of a product, hence the need to continually monitor all medicines. Spontaneous reporting schemes such as the Yellow Card Scheme underpin such monitoring.

Important drug safety issues identified through spontaneous ADR reporting schemes have included the following: selective serotonin reuptake inhibitors (SSRIs) and withdrawal symptoms; high lipase pancreatins and colonic strictures in children; rifabutin and uveitis; tramadol and psychiatric reactions; quinolone antibiotics and tendonitis; troglitazone and hepatitis; and HIV protease inhibitors and diabetes mellitus.

The Yellow Card Scheme invites reports from UK doctors, dentists, coroners and pharmacists. Newly introduced drugs are designated by a black triangle in the *British National Formulary* (*BNF*). For these drugs, all suspected ADRs should be reported to the Scheme. For older, more established drugs (non-black triangle) only serious suspected ADRs should be reported.

Yellow Cards reported to the MCA/CSM are individually analysed by scientists, pharmacists and doctors and used to identify previously unrecognized drug safety hazards, as well as changes in the profile of established safety hazards. Yellow Card reports remain one of the key sources of data on which decisions about the balance of risks and benefits of an individual medicine are taken.

References

Bates DW 1998 Drugs and adverse drug reactions – how worried should we be? Journal of the American Medical Association 279: 1216–1217

Lazarou J, Pomeranz BH, Corey PN 1998 Incidence of adverse drug reactions in hospitalised patients; a meta-analysis of prospective studies. Journal of the American Medical Association 279: 1200–1205

Routledge P 1998 150 years of pharmacovigilance. Lancet 351: 1200–1201

17. Study designs
A.F   B.F   C.F   D.F   E.F

There are three commonly used observational study designs in epidemiology. Case-control studies involve selecting patients with a disease and comparing them with controls without the disease. Such studies are particularly appropriate for studying common risk factors for a relatively rare disease. An example might be alcohol as a risk factor for leukaemia. If the risk factor is rare neither cases nor controls will have been exposed, so it is usually impossible to draw any conclusions.

Cohort studies take subjects with one risk factor and follow them over time to see if they develop a disease. It is therefore appropriate for studying rare exposures causing a common disease, for example veganism as a risk for heart disease. Clinical trials are a form of cohort study.

Cross-sectional studies study a large number of people at a particular point in time. They are appropriate for the study of common chronic conditions such as diabetes or rheumatoid arthritis. With rare conditions too few cases will be detected. Cross-sectional studies give a prevalence, that is, the proportion of the population with a disease. The correct measurement for any acute condition such as infections, stroke, heart attack or road traffic accidents, is incidence, which is prevalence over time. Only prospective or retrospective cohort studies can provide this information. Prevalence is an unhelpful measure in acute disease.

Usually clinical trials are placebo controlled only when there is no current effective treatment. It may be unacceptable to ethics committees to use placebo if proven treatments are already available. This can depend on the disease under study. Trials are often designed to compare differences between a new treatment and the best currently available treatment, or with both arms of the study receiving the best currently available treatment in addition to the new agent or placebo. It would, for example, be reasonable to perform a trial of ceftazidime plus steroid against ceftazidime plus placebo for bacterial meningitis.

Crossover trials are difficult to perform. They are only appropriate in the long-term management of chronic conditions, for example different analgesics in rheumatoid arthritis. They have no place in studying acute conditions.

References

Barker DJP, Rose G 1990 Epidemiology in medical practice, 4th edn. Churchill Livingstone, Edinburgh

Coggon D 1995 Statistics in clinical practice. BMJ publishing, London

---

18. Clinical trials

A.F   B.F   C.F   D.T   E.T

A systematic review is one written after an attempt to obtain data from all sources and assess it in an unbiased way. As a minimum this means a full electronic and hand search of the literature. However, it should ideally mean an attempt also to obtain data from unpublished trials. This is to circumvent the serious problem in medical publishing of positive publication bias. A 'positive' result is much more likely to be published in a mainstream journal than one which finds no significant difference. As one trial in 20 will achieve statistical significance ($P<0.05$) by chance alone, many trials which find a chance effect are published and the follow-up trials that find no effect are not. This means that the literature always tends to exaggerate the effectiveness of any treatment. A systematic review should inform current thinking rather than reflect it. Traditional reviews tend to try to reflect current opinion.

Type I errors are where the null hypothesis is falsely rejected, i.e. a difference which has occurred by chance alone is accepted and enters practice. The opposite problem is type II error, where the null hypothesis is falsely accepted. This is also common in reporting of clinical trials. To get their 'negative' trial published authors who found no difference between treatment A and treatment B will say this proves there is no difference between the two treatments. Trials that claim this are seldom large enough to have the statistical power to make this claim.

Meta-analysis is a powerful statistical technique. However, it should be handled with caution. It is used to combine data from several trials to give the data more power to detect differences. It is only appropriate where there are similar trial methodologies (statistical and methodological homogeneity). If a systematic review reveals trials that are very different it is inappropriate to combine them into a meta-analysis. This rule is often broken. A meta-analysis is only as good as the trials that make it up. Half a dozen indifferently conducted small trials with different endpoints and methods lumped together may provide less good evidence than a single, large, well conducted trial, even if the P- numbers are very small.

Reference

Naylor CD 1997 Meta-analysis and the meta-epidemiology of clinical research. British Medical Journal 315: 617–619

---

19. Cytochrome P450 enzymes
A.T   B.T   C.T   D.T   E.F

Knowledge of the cytochrome P450 drug oxidation system has expanded rapidly and increased our understanding of adverse drug reactions related to drug metabolism. These enzymes primarily catalyse oxidizing reactions. They are present in greatest amounts in the endoplasmic reticulum of the liver, but are also found in other organs, such as lung, intestinal wall and kidney.

The standard nomenclature of enzymes of the cytochrome P450 (CYP) group designates the family by a number, the subfamily by a letter, and the specific enzyme by another number, e.g. CYP3A4.

The corresponding gene which encodes the enzyme is indicated in italics, e.g. *CYP3A4*. Each P450 enzyme has a unique but sometimes overlapping range of drug substrates. In addition, different factors regulate the expression and activity of each individual P450 enzyme. As knowledge of the substrates of each enzyme has expanded and the influence of environmental and genetic factors has become better defined, the important role of CYP450-mediated metabolism in adverse drug reactions has become apparent. The enzyme-inducing effect of alcohol, tobacco and other drugs has been known for many years, but more recently attention has focused on genetic control, even though it has only been fully characterized for a few enzymes.

A number of the P450 enzymes are under polymorphic genetic control. The most extensively investigated is CYP2D6. Over 50 drugs are metabolized by this one enzyme alone. Other polymorphic enzymes include 2C9, 2C19, 2A6 and 2E1. Molecular biology techniques have identified the genes encoding these enzymes, establishing the normal or wild-type genotype and a number of mutations, of which some reduce or abolish enzyme activity whereas others are silent. All enzymes are encoded by two alleles of the relevant gene, and homozygotes with two normal alleles can metabolize the substrate drugs efficiently. Individuals with this genotype are known as extensive metabolizers. Individuals who inherit two alleles resulting in an enzyme of reduced or absent activity are poor metabolizers of substrate drugs. Heterozygotes who inherit one normal and one mutant allelle may have lower metabolic activity than individuals with two normal genes, an observation known as the 'gene dose effect'. Some individuals inherit multiple copies of drug-metabolizing genes and display increased rates of drug metabolism. These individuals are termed ultrarapid metabolizers. One example is with CYP2D6. Ultrarapid metabolizers have been identified who require large doses of drug substrates to achieve therapeutic efficacy, and who have been shown to possess two or more copies of the *CYP2D6* gene.

The frequency of genetic polymorphisms in CYP450 enzymes differs in populations of different ethnic backgrounds. This may account for some of the differential drug responses reported among ethnic groups. For example, poor metabolizers of CYP2D6 have a frequency of 6% in caucasian populations, but less than 1% in Asian groups. In contrast, poor metabolizers for CYP2C19 have a frequency of up to 19% in some Asian populations but are rare in caucasian populations. Molecular biological techniques can be utilized to genotype P450 alleles in an individual, enabling metabolic capacity to be predicted. Alternatively, phenotyping can be performed using a marker drug known to be metabolized predominantly by one enzyme.

Type A adverse drug reactions (augmented pharmacological reactions) depend on drug concentration. Poor metabolizers who have higher than usual plasma or tissue concentrations of the parent drug are at increased risk of these reactions. Inhibition of a CYP450 enzyme will also increase the risk of a type A reaction to another drug metabolized by the same enzyme. Ultrarapid metabolizers might theoretically experience more adverse reactions due to toxic metabolites. They may also suffer therapeutic inefficacy and need higher than normal doses of the relevant drug. Phenformin was removed from the market in the 1970s because of an unacceptable incidence of lactic acidosis. It has subsequently been found to be metabolized by CYP2D6. It is likely that the poor metabolizers had the most severe lactic acidosis, which is related to plasma drug concentrations. Conversely, the therapeutic effects of codeine are in part due to its metabolic conversion to morphine. This is catalysed by CYP2D6. For this reason poor metabolizers do not produce significant amounts of morphine and therefore do not experience an analgesic effect from codeine.

CYP3A4 is the most abundant cytochrome P450 enzyme. More than half of all drugs are completely or partially metabolized by this enzyme and it is present in the gut as well as the liver. The activity of CYP3A4 depends on its concentration, which varies greatly among individuals. Those at the lower end of the activity spectrum are more likely to be at risk of adverse reactions from unmetabolized drug or induction interactions, and those with greater enzyme activity are more likely to have significant effects from inhibitory interactions. The most common cause of adverse drug reactions related to CYP450 is inhibitory interactions. A drug which inhibits a P450 enzyme will reduce the extent of metabolism of other drugs metabolized by that enzyme. The elimination of the other drug metabolized by this pathway will be reduced, its half-life prolonged and increased plasma concentrations can result. For example, cimetidine is a non-specific P450 inhibitor and causes significant increases in plasma concentrations of propranolol, with an associated decrease in heart rate, and of warfarin with elevations of INR. Ketoconazole, itraconazole and HIV protease inhibitors are potent inhibitors of CYP3A4. Serious and fatal reactions can result from inhibition of terfenadine metabolism, elevating plasma concentrations and resultant torsade de pointes.

In the case of genetic polymorphisms, inhibition interactions will affect poor metabolizers more than extensive metabolizers. Inhibition interactions may convert extensive metabolizers to phenotypic poor metabolizers. Many antipsychotic drugs and tricyclic antidepressants are metabolized by CYP2D6. Inhibition of this enzyme, e.g. by selective serotonin reuptake inhibitors (SSRIs), may produce phenotypic poor metabolizers, resulting in more adverse reactions to these drugs. The toxicity of paracetamol is due to its active metabolite. Induction of paracetamol metabolism by chronic ethanol use can increase paracetamol-induced hepatotoxicity. Ultrarapid metabolizers of paracetamol are also at high risk. Enzyme induction can reduce the plasma concentration of drugs metabolized by CYP450 enzymes and cause significant clinical problems. For example, rifampicin reduces plasma phenytoin concentrations and epileptic fits can occur.

References

Shenfield G, Gross A 1999 The cytochrome P450 system and adverse drug reactions. Adverse Drug Reaction Bulletin 194: 739–742

Tanaka E 1998 Clinically important pharmacokinetic drug–drug interactions: role of cytochrome P450 enzymes. Journal of Clinical Pharmacology and Therapeutics 23: 403–416

20. Oral bioavailability of drugs
A.F   B.F   C.T   D.T   E.T

Grapefruit juice selectivity downregulates cytochrome P4503A4 in the intestinal wall. Many drugs are broken down in the intestinal wall by this isoenzyme, and its downregulation can therefore lead to increased oral bioavaibility. As the duration of effect of grapefruit juice lasts up to 24 hours, repeated consumption may result in a cumulative increase in the blood levels of such drugs. The size of this effect of grapefruit juice varies widely among individuals and appears to be dependent on inherent differences in intestinal P4503A4 protein expression. Thus individuals with the highest baseline levels have the highest potential for enhanced drug absorption following grapefruit juice consumption.

At least 20 drugs have been shown to interact with grapefruit juice. Drugs with an innately low oral bioavailability due to substantial P4503A4-mediated metabolism are most affected. Clinically relevant interactions occur with dihydropyridines, terfenadine, saquinavir, cyclosporin, midazolam and verapamil.

Reference

Bailey DG, Malcolm J, Arnold O, Spence J D 1998 Grapefruit–drug interactions. British Journal of Clinical Pharmacology 46: 101–110

THERAPEUTICS

21. Prolongation of the QT interval
A.T B.F C.T D.T E.T

22. Drug prolongation of QT interval
A.T B.F C.T D.T E.T

The QT interval on the electrocardiogram (ECG) is measured from the beginning of the Q wave to the end of the T wave. As QT interval varies with heart rate, various formulae have been derived to correct the QT interval for heart rate (QTc). The QT interval consists of two components: (1) the QRS duration, which reflects the conduction velocity of the wave of depolarization in the bundle of His and ventricles; (2) the JT interval, which is a measure of the duration of ventricular repolarization. It is therefore an indirect measure of the duration of the ventricular action potential and ventricular repolarization. Prolongation of ventricular repolarization results in an increase in the absolute refractory period, and this is the mechanism by which antiarrhythmic drugs with this property prevent or terminate ventricular tachyarrhythmias. However, prolonging repolarization can also cause arrhythmias. The most characteristic is a form of ventricular tachycardia known as torsade de pointes. This can sometimes degenerate into ventricular fibrillation and cause sudden death.

Causes of a prolonged QT interval include bradycardia, certain inherited disorders, biochemical disturbances such as hypokalaemia, and acquired heart disease. Drugs are an important remediable cause. Drugs that slow His–Purkinje conduction velocity, such as flecainide, can result in minor QT interval prolongation even if the JT interval is unchanged. However, in the majority of cases abnormal prolongation of the QT interval is caused by factors that delay ventricular repolarization and prolong the JT interval.

Ventricular repolarization occurs by outward movement of potassium through specific channels in myocardial cell membranes. The T wave on the ECG is generated by a wave of repolarization spreading from the apex to the base of the ventricles. Drugs are thought to prolong ventricular repolarization either by blocking potassium channels and thus delaying the outward movement of potassium, or by affecting inward sodium or calcium currents. All drugs that delay repolarization will prolong the QT interval, and then may produce either T- or U-wave abnormalities. The effects on repolarization may be the intended action of an antiarrhythmic drug or an unintended effect of a drug used to treat non-cardiac disease.

Class IA antiarrhythmic drugs (Vaughan Williams classification) block fast sodium entry into myocardial cells, delay ventricular repolarization, and prolong the refractory period and QT interval. Examples include quinidine, procainamide and disopyramide. Therapy with all these agents may be complicated by torsade de pointes.

QT prolongation may also occur with class III antiarrhythmic drugs, which delay repolarization by blocking potassium channels, particularly at slow heart rates. Examples include amiodarone, sotalol and bretylium.

Antipsychotic drugs which prolong the QT interval include thioridazine, chlorpromazine, haloperidol, pimozide and sertindole. Antidepressants, including tricyclic antidepressants and lithium, can prolong the QT interval, and this is particularly a problem when these drugs are taken in overdose.

The non-sedating antihistamines terfenadine and astemizole can rarely cause QT interval prolongation and torsade de pointes. Terfenadine prolongs the action potential by inhibiting potassium efflux. It is rapidly metabolized by cytochrome P4503A4 to fexofenadine, a histamine H_1 antagonist which does not prolong the QT interval. Arrhythmias occur when the metabolism of terfenadine is impaired, for example by drug interactions with CYP3A4 inhibitors such as ketoconazole, itraconazole, erythromycin, grapefruit juice, HIV protease inhibitors, or in the presence of liver disease. Excessive terfenadine doses can also provoke arrhythmia. Recently, fexofenadine has been developed as a non-sedating antihistamine without electrophysiological effects. Astemizole can also provoke arrhythmias. This has usually been reported in the context of overdose or pre-existing prolonged QT intervals in affected patients. Other agents reported to cause QT prolongation include erythromycin, quinine, cisapride and tacrolimus.

The most important way of preventing arrhythmias is to avoid using drugs that prolong the QT interval in patients at high risk of arrhythmia. These include patients with prior QT interval prolongation, underlying heart disease and previous ventricular arrhythmias. Patients receiving digoxin, drugs which affect electrolyte balance such as diuretics, other QT-prolonging drugs, or drugs likely to interact are also at increased risk. Patients at high risk who are prescribed arrhythmogenic drugs should have an ECG prior to starting treatment. This should be repeated shortly after starting therapy. If the QT interval is prolonged either prior to or during therapy, the risks and benefits of treatment should be reconsidered.

Drugs that prolong the QT interval should be stopped immediately in patients developing symptoms of arrhythmia, such as palpitations, dizziness or syncope, and an ECG recorded. Torsade de pointes should be managed by withdrawing the offending drug. The arrhythmia must be controlled until the drug and its active metabolites have been eliminated. This can be achieved by increasing the heart rate by atrial pacing or isoprenaline infusion.

Electrolyte abnormalities should be corrected. Magnesium infusion may terminate torsade de pointes even if the plasma magnesium concentration is normal. Antiarrhythmic drugs, especially class IA and III agents, may worsen the arrhythmia and should be avoided.

References

Bonn D 1997 Getting to the heart of the long QT syndrome. Lancet 349: 408

Thomas SHL 1997 Drugs and the QT interval. Adverse Drug Reaction Bulletin 182: 691–694

Woosley RL 1996 Cardiac actions of antihistamines. Annual Review of Pharmcological Toxicology 36: 233–252

23. Inhaled beclomethasone dipropionate
A.F   B.T   C.F   D.T   E.F

The prevalence of asthma has increased in recent years, with 15% of 5–11-year-olds in the UK now diagnosed with asthma. Inhaled corticosteroids were introduced in the early 1970s and have revolutionized the management of asthma. Inhaled corticosteroids may be delivered to the airways by a metered dose inhaler with or without a spacer device, as a dry powder or in a nebulizer. With a metered dose inhaler 80% of the dose impacts in the mouth and oropharynx and is swallowed. Use of a spacer device can increase lung delivery by 20%. Inhaled corticosteroids, including beclomethasone dipropionate, budesonide and fluticasone propionate, are absorbed by three routes: through the alveoli of the lung, directly across the oral mucosa, and via the gastrointestinal (GI) tract. The swallowed portion of the dose is absorbed by the GI tract and is then extensively metabolized by cytochrome P450 enzymes (predominantly CYP3A4). Inhibitors of CYP3A4, such as erythromycin and azole antifungals, may increase plasma levels.

A clear dose–response relationship has been established for inhaled corticosteroids at low doses (less than $1000 \mu g$ beclomethasone dipropionate daily). At higher doses, however, the dose–response curve plateaus. As the dose–response curve levels out, the dose–adverse effect curve increases exponentially, so that the balance of risk and benefit of high doses of inhaled corticosteroids is far less favourable than the balance at lower doses.

It is well established that inhaled corticosteroids cause important systemic adverse effects. These are dependent on the dose and duration of use, inhaler technique, inhaler device and the severity of underlying disease. As a significant proportion of the active drug reaching the alveoli is absorbed directly into the systemic circulation and bypasses liver metabolism, patients with mild asthma, who have better drug delivery to the alveoli, may suffer higher plasma levels of corticosteroid than patients with more severe disease. Various systemic adverse effects have been established as being causally related to inhaled corticosteroids; hypothalamo–pituitary–adrenal (HPA)–axis suppression, changes in bone mineral density, growth inhibition in children, cataract and glaucoma. At high doses, all well designed studies have shown that inhaled corticosteroids cause depression of HPA-axis function. This suppression is dose dependent. Osteoporosis is an important cause of fractures, particularly of the vertebral column, wrist and hip. One study of 81 asthmatic patients used X-ray absorptiometry to measure bone mineral density, and showed a 0.11 standard deviation reduction in bone mineral density per 1000 µg per day of beclomethasone dipropionate used per year. If this relationship between inhaled corticosteroids and reduction in bone mineral density is linear, then women using 1000 µg a day of beclomethasone dipropionate would suffer a three standard deviation reduction in bone mineral density over 30 years. This would correspond to an eightfold increase in risk of fractures.

Systemic corticosteroids cause a profound inhibition of linear growth. These drugs reduce growth hormone production, androgen secretion, osteoblast function, mineral and nitrogen retention, and increase the inhibitory effect of somatostatin on the pituitary. Interpreting clinical studies of growth suppression with inhaled corticosteroids is difficult because asthma may delay puberty and reduce growth rate. Furthermore, few studies have studied final adult height, and most studies are short term. Despite this, numerous studies have shown that, in the short term, high-dose inhaled corticosteroid use leads to slowing of lower leg growth. Studying the effect of nasal corticosteroids is helpful in this respect as studies are not confounded by the underlying disease (i.e. asthma inhibiting growth). A 12-month randomized double-blind placebo-controlled study in 100 children with perennial allergic rhinitis showed that children treated with beclomethasone dipropionate grew 0.9 cm less than those treated with placebo over 12 months.

Cataract is responsible for 20–25% of all blindness in the UK. Systemic corticosteroids, as well as ophthalmic corticosteroids, have clearly been shown to increase the risk of cataract. The mechanism is complex but may include altered glutathione and glucose metabolism in the lens, altered electrolyte transport, sodium/potassium pump inhibition and water accumulation. A recent cross-sectional study of 3654 adults revealed a statistically significant association between long-term high-dose inhaled corticosteroid use and the formation of cataract. Furthermore, a separate study showed a significant association between cataract extraction and inhaled corticosteroid use in elderly patients.

Topical ophthalmic corticosteroids cause ocular hypertension, which is thought to be due to resistance to aqueous humour outflow. A recent case-controlled study of 9793 patients with glaucoma aged 65 years and 39 325 controls showed a statistically significant association between glaucoma and long-term high-dose inhaled corticosteroid use.

Inhaled corticosteroids remain the prophylactic treatment of choice for asthma. Their benefits far outweigh their risks. Despite this, systemic adverse effects may occur, particularly with high-dose, prolonged use. For this reason the dose should be titrated to the lowest dose at which effective control of asthma is maintained.

References

Cave A, Arlett P, Lee E 1999 An assessment of the potential for inhaled and nasal corticosteroids to cause systemic adverse effects. Pharmacology and Therapeutics 83: 153–179

Cumming RG, Mitchell P, Leeder SR 1997 Use of inhaled corticosteroids and the risk of cataracts. New England Journal of Medicine 337: 8–14

Garbe E, LeLorier J, Boivin JF, Suissa S 1997 Inhaled and nasal glucocorticoids and the risk of ocular hypertension or open angle glaucoma. Journal of American Medical Association 277: 722–727

MCA/CSM 1998 The safety of inhaled and nasal corticosteroids. Current Problems in Pharmacovigilance 24: 8

24. Cyclo-oxygenase (COX)

A.T   B.F   C.F   D.F   E.T

Although often effective in the relief of inflammation and pain, non-steroidal anti-inflammatory drugs (NSAIDs) are associated with a high incidence of adverse reactions. NSAIDs have anti-inflammatory, analgesic and antipyretic actions. Their main site of action is the enzyme cyclo-oxygenase (COX). This converts arachidonic acid to prostaglandins and exists in two isoforms, COX-1 and COX-2. COX-1 is the physiological form involved with homeostatic functions, such as protection of the gastric mucosa and control of renal blood flow. Unlike the COX-1 form, COX-2 is almost undetectable in normal healthy tissue, but is inducible locally at sites of inflammation. It has been suggested that preferential inhibition of COX-2 enzyme would result in an anti-inflammatory effect, while reducing the risk of adverse reactions, particularly gastrointestinal (GI) damage. Although there is some correlation between the COX-2 selectivity of NSAIDs and their risk of causing adverse reactions, the reduction in risk is not directly proportional to the degree of COX-2 inhibition. Characteristics other than COX-2 selectivity are probably important in determining the degree of GI toxicity of NSAIDs. These include non-acidity, short half-life, absence of biliary excretion and lack of effect on mitochondrial oxidative phosphorylation.

NSAIDs are reported to be responsible for between 500 and 4000 deaths per year in the UK. The most commonly reported serious reactions involve the upper GI tract. The risk of an upper GI bleed in NSAID users is up to three times that of non-users. Other serious reactions include kidney, liver and blood disorders and allergic reactions. Various epidemiological studies and spontaneous reports to the Committee of Safety of Medicines suggest that there may be important differences in the risk of GI toxicity associated with different NSAIDs. Azapropazone is associated with the highest risk; piroxicam, ketoprofen, diclofenac, naproxen and indomethacin with intermediate risk; and ibuprofen with the lowest risk. These adverse reactions are thought to be dose related.

Meloxicam is structurally related to piroxicam. In vitro work shows that it inhibits COX-2 to a greater extent than COX-1. Evidence suggests that meloxicam has similar efficacy to other NSAIDs. Limited short-term clinical data suggest that it may be associated with fewer adverse reactions than some other NSAIDs at comparable doses. Despite this, GI adverse reactions still commonly occur with meloxicam.

References

Hawkey CJ 1999 COX-2 inhibitors. Lancet 353: 307–314

Yeomans ND, Cook GA, Giraud AS 1998 Selective COX-2 inhibitors: are they safe for the stomach? Gastroenterology 115: 227–229

25. Sildenafil

A.**F**   B.**F**   C.**T**   D.**F**   E.**T**

In the UK 10% of men are unable to achieve or maintain an erection sufficient for satisfactory sexual activity (erectile dysfunction). Organic factors are implicated in about 80% of cases. These include cardiovascular disease, diabetes mellitus, multiple sclerosis, Alzheimer's disease, Parkinson's disease, surgery (e.g. prostatectomy) and spinal cord injury. About 25% of cases are due to adverse reactions to medicines, including β-blockers, thiazide diuretics, digoxin, antidepressants, antipsychotics or benzodiazepines. Alcohol and heavy smoking are also risk factors. Psychological factors are the primary cause in about 14% of cases. However, psychological factors frequently exacerbate pre-existing organic problems. In all patients with erectile dysfunction the cause needs to be sought and, where possible treated.

The erectile response to sexual stimulation is mediated by the release of nitric oxide from nerves supplying local vessels in the corpora cavernosa of the penis. The nitric oxide increases intracellular levels of cyclic guanosine monophosphate (cGMP), which acts on vascular smooth muscle, causing vasodilatation. The effects of cGMP are terminated by the isoenzyme phosphodiesterase type 5 (PDE5), which converts cGMP to inactive non-cyclic GMP. Sildenafil is an orally active selective inhibitor of isoenzyme PDE5. It is at least 70 times more selective for PDE5 then for PDE1, 2, 3 and 4. It is about nine times more selective for PDE5 than isoenzyme PDE6. By inhibiting PDE5, sildenafil prolongs cGMP activity in erectile tissue amplifying the natural vasodilatory actions of nitric oxide and thereby enhancing the erectile response to sexual stimulation.

Sildenafil reaches peak plasma concentrations 30–120 minutes after oral dosing although its absorption is delayed when taken with food. The drug is metabolized predominantly by cytochrome P4503A4. Clearance is reduced in patients with renal or hepatic impairment and in the elderly. Inhibitors of cytochrome P4503A4, such as cimetidine, erythromycin, azole antifungals and HIV protease inhibitors, will increase sildenafil blood levels. Sildenafil has a pharmacodynamic interaction with organic nitrate (GTN, sodium nitroprusside or amyl nitrite). Sildenafil should not be used by patients with severe hepatic impairment, blood pressure below 90/50 mmHg, recent stroke or myocardial infarction, or hereditary retinal disorders such as retinitis pigmentosa. Caution is also advised in patients with penile deformity, conditions predisposing to priapism (such as sickle cell anaemia, leukaemia or multiple myeloma), and in those with bleeding disorders or active peptic ulcer disease.

In double-blinded, randomized placebo-controlled multicentre trials, sildenafil resulted in a greater proportion of men achieving erections than did placebo. The mean number of successful attempts at sexual intercourse per month was also greater in the sildenafil groups than in the placebo groups. The most commonly reported adverse reactions to sildenafil are headache, flushing, dyspepsia and nasal congestion. All these reactions are dose related and usually transient. In randomized trials rates of myocardial infarction and other serious cardiovascular events were not significantly higher in patients taking sildenafil than in those taking placebo. In about 3% of patients a mild transient green/blue tingeing of vision occurs, probably due to weak inhibition of isoenzyme PDE6 in the retina. Cases of priapism have also been reported since sildenafil was marketed.

No comparative trials of sildenafil with other treatments for erectile dysfunction have been published. However, the convenience of administration and the fact that sildenafil's effects are stimulation dependent are likely to make it a more popular choice then alternatives such as intracavernosal injection or intraurethral application of alprostadil, implantable semirigid rods, hydraulic devices or vacuum constriction devices.

References

Anon 1998 Sildenafil for erectile dysfunction. Drug and Therapeutics Bulletin 36: 81–84

Goldstein I, Lew TS, Padma-Nathan H, Rosen RC, Steers WD, Wicker PA 1998 Oral sildenafil in the treatment of erectile dysfunction. New England Journal of Medicine. 338: 1397–1404

Rendell MS, Rajfer J, Wicker PA, Smith MD 1999 Sildenafil for treatment of erectile dysfunction in men with diabetes Journal of American Medical Association 281: 421–426

26.   The new epilepsy drugs

A.T   B.F   C.F   D.F   E.F

In treating epilepsy the choice of drug regimen must be matched to the individual patient and the type of epilepsy. New drugs for epilepsy have been licensed in recent years. All were initially licensed as add-on treatments for poorly controlled partial seizures with or without generalization.

Lamotrigine is now also licensed as monotherapy for partial seizures and generalized tonic–clonic seizures. It causes little cognitive impairment or overt sedation compared to other treatments, and may even result in unwanted agitation in the elderly. Lamotrigine can cause an allergic skin rash (3%), which rarely can be severe (Stevens–Johnson syndrome) and life-threatening. For this reason lamotrigine must be introduced at a low dose with a gradual increase over many weeks, as detailed in the *British National Formulary*. Special care must be taken when prescribing lamotrigine to someone already taking sodium valproate, as this drug inhibits lamotrigine metabolism and hence a lower starting dose is required.

Vigabatrin has been used as add-on therapy for epilepsy not adequately controlled by other drugs. It is indicated as monotherapy for infantile spasms (West syndrome). Adverse reactions are predominantly neurological or psychiatric. Most importantly it has been associated with the development of visual field defects, which can develop at any time, from within a month to several years of treatment. In most reported cases the field defect persisted despite stopping treatment. Visual field testing should be performed before treatment and during follow-up.

Gabapentin has a low incidence of unpleasant side effects but may be less efficacious in poorly responsive epilepsy. Like vigabatrin, gabapentin is not metabolized and is excreted unchanged in the urine. Topiramate, on the other hand seems to be effective but many patients are unabe to tolerate the side effects, which include cognitive problems and weight loss. The dose should be increased slowly to minimize these. A recent report details two cases of transient hemiparesis with topiramate which resolved on withdrawal of the drug. Topiramate is thought to act through sodium channel blockade, attenuating the responses induced by kainate and enhancing the inhibition mediated by γ-aminobutyric acid.

Tiagabine is a γ-aminobutyric acid (GABA) uptake inhibitor. It specifically increases the amount of the inhibitory neurotransmitter GABA only at the GABAergic synapse. Dizziness, headaches and somnolence are the commonest side effects.

Surgical removal of an epileptic lesion in the temporal lobe has been shown to be highly effective in selected patients who are refractory to drug treatment. Before surgery is considered, however, the diagnosis of epilepsy must be beyond doubt, the seizures must have proved refractory to anti epileptic drugs, a single epileptic focus must be identified and located, and the epileptic focus must be deemed amenable to surgery.

References

Feely M 1999 Drug treatment of epilepsy. British Medical Journal 318: 106–109

Leach JP, Brodie MJ 1998 Tiagabine. The Lancet. 351: 203–207

Marson AG, Kadir ZA, Chadwick DW 1996 New antiepileptic drugs: a systematic review of their efficacy and tolerability. British Medical Journal 313: 1169–1173

MCA/CSM 1999 Vigabatrin (Sabril): visual field defects. Current Problems in Pharmacovigilance. 25: 13

Stephen LJ, Maxwell JE, Brodie MJ 1999 Transient hemiparesis with topiramate, British Medical Journal 318: 845

27. Drug treatments for depression

A.F   B.T   C.F   D.T   E.T

In the past decade at least 10 new antidepressant drugs have become available. These have been rationally developed to try and reduce the unwanted adverse effects of some of the older drugs. Because of adverse effects many patients are prescribed subtherapeutic doses or are poorly compliant. Clinical studies have demonstrated much higher non-compliance rates in patients taking drugs with more adverse effects.

Tricyclic antidepressants have been prescribed for depression since the 1950s. They are effective and cheap, but all have dose-related anticholinergic effects that limit compliance. Antimuscarinic effects (constipation, dry mouth, blurred vision), cardiovascular effects (tachycardia, palpitations) and unwanted central nervous system effects (tremor and vertigo), as well as sedation, increased appetite and weight gain, are well recognized adverse effects of this class of drugs. Postural hypotension may cause falls in elderly patients. Many drugs in this class are fatal in overdose. Lofepramine, one of the newer tricyclics, is relatively safe in overdose and almost free of anticholinergic adverse effects.

Selective serotonin reuptake inhibitors (SSRIs) such as paroxetine and fluoxetine are free from sedative and anticholinergic effects. Compliance is better than with the older tricyclics. The SSRIs are safer in overdose. Serotonin-related adverse effects include insomnia, nausea and diarrhoea, and sexual dysfunction; withdrawal symptoms are also recognized.

Monoamine oxidase inhibitors are unpopular because of the rare incidence of fatalities from hypertension when taken with tyramine-containing foods.

Nefazadone is a mixed SSRI and 5-hydroxytryptamine (5-HT)2 receptor antagonist. It causes fewer gastrointestinal adverse effects and sexual dysfunction than other selective serotonin reuptake inhibitors and is more sedative, and so is useful for patients with sleep disturbance. Postural hypotension can be problematic.

Venlafaxine was the first mixed serotonin and noradrenaline reuptake inhibitor. It results in fewer anticholinergic and cardiovascular adverse effects and causes less weight gain than tricyclics.

Reboxetine is a selective noradrenaline reuptake inhibitor. Some of the older tricyclics such as desipramine do have some selectivity for noradrenaline (as opposed to 5-HT) reuptake, but share the antimuscarinic, sedative and cardiovascular adverse effects of other tricyclic antidepressants. Despite its low affinity for muscarinic receptors in vitro, reboxetine causes dry mouth, constipation, urinary hesitancy, increased sweating and impotence more frequently than placebo, but less frequently than desipramine. Reboxetine has not yet been compared with newer, better tolerated tricyclics such as lofepramine or with SSRIs.

Mirtazapine was the first noradrenergic and specific serotonergic antidepressant. Its action involves the blocking of central presynaptic α-adrenoceptors which results in increased release of noradrenaline and serotonin. In addition it blocks postsynaptic 5-HT2 and 5-HT3 receptors but not 5-HT1A receptors. Thus there is increased central noradrenergic and serotinergic 5HT1A transmission, both of which are thought to be important for antidepressant activity. Blockade of 5HT2 and 5HT3 receptors should mean that the typical unwanted adverse effects of unselective serotonergic stimulation (insomnia, agitation, sexual dysfunction and nausea) are minimized. Mirtazapine has low affinity for muscarinic, dopaminergic and α_1-adrenergic receptors but blocks histamine H_1 receptors. Studies comparing mirtazapine and amitryptiline have shown similar antidepressant efficacy and time of onset of effect, but fewer adverse effects. Mirtazapine should not be prescribed with or within 14 days of stopping a monoamine oxidase inhibitor because of the risk of precipitating the serotonin syndrome (agitation, tremor, myoclonus and hyperthermia). As yet mirtazapine has not been compared with the newer, better tolerated tricyclics.

Virtually all antidepressants are equally effective if given at an adequate dose for a sufficient period of time. Clinically the choice is a balance of safety and tolerability in individual patients.

For mild to moderate depression cognitive behavioural therapy and antidepressants are equally effective. Cognitive behavioural therapy is brief focused psychotherapy requiring between 6 and 20 sessions. For more severe depression, however, antidepressant drugs have been shown to be more effective.

References

Anon 1998 Reboxetine – another new antidepressant. Drug and Therapeutics Bulletin 36(11): 86–88

Anon 1999 Mirtazapine – another new class of antidepressant. Drug and Therapeutics Bulletin 37(1): 1–3

Hale AS 1997 Depression (ABC of mental health). British Medical Journal 315: 43–45

28. Drug treatment of Alzheimer's disease
A.T   B.F   C.T   D.F   E.T

5% of people aged 65 years and over have dementia and in the majority of cases the cause is Alzheimer's disease (AD). AD is the fourth commonest cause of death in the USA. Several neurotransmitter abnormalities have been described in AD, with a consistent finding being a reduction in acetylcholine production secondary to a decrease in choline acetyltransferase. Traditionally the mainstay of AD treatment has been supportive care, but recent drug research and development has focused on increasing acetylcholine within the brain. These novel treatments have symptomatic benefits but no effect on the underlying disease process.

The first drug in this class to show beneficial results was tacrine, an acridine acetylcholinesterase inhibitor. Early reports of hepatotoxicity, however, have curtailed its use.

Donepezil is a piperidine-based selective inhibitor of acetylcholinesterase. It was licensed in the UK in 1997 for the symptomatic treatment of mild to moderate AD. Donepezil may cause bladder outflow obstruction and should be prescribed with care in patients with asthma or obstructive pulmonary disease, and in patients with a history of peptic ulcer disease. Donepezil can cause sick sinus syndrome and other cardiac conduction abnormalities. Other adverse reactions include headache, diarrhoea, nausea, vomiting and other gastrointestinal disturbances, muscle cramps, fatigue, insomnia, dizziness and increases in muscle creatinine kinase. Hallucinations, agitation and aggressive behaviour have been reported.

Donepezil is metabolized in the liver by enzymes of the cytochrome P450 system, and thus inhibitors of these enzymes, such as ketoconazole, erythromycin and fluoxetine, may lead to increased plasma concentrations of donepezil. Enzyme inducers such as rifampacin, phenytoin, carbamazepine and alcohol may reduce blood levels of donepezil.

Donepezil has been shown to improve the cognitive subscale in the Alzheimer's Disease Assessment Scale (ADAS-cog) by 2.6 points over a 12–24 week treatment period in patients with mild to moderate AD, and cause some improvement in the Clinician's Global Rating Scores of overall dementia. There were no improvements in patient- or carer-rated quality of life scales and no proven effect on activities of daily living. It is recommended that treatment with donepezil should be initiated by a physician experienced in the diagnosis and management of AD, and should only be started if there is a carer who can monitor drug intake. The effects of the drug should be assessed by the clinician after 12 weeks of treatment and donepezil should only be continued if there is clear evidence of benefit.

Rivastigmine is the latest of this class of drugs and has also been shown to improve cognitive function on the ADAS-cog scale after 26 weeks of treatment.

Trials of these drugs to date have focused on patients with mild to moderate disease. Concerns have been raised about how the modest improvements seen in cognition and global impression scales translate into clinical effects.

References

Anon 1997 Donepezil for Alzheimer's disease? Drug and Therapeutics Bulletin 35 (10): 75–76

Anon 1998 Donepezil update. Drug and Therapeutics Bulletin 36 (8): 60–61

Flicker L 1999 Acetylcholinesterase inhibitors for Alzheimer's disease. British Medical Journal 318: 615–616

MCA/CSM 1999 In focus: Donepezil. Current Problems in Pharmacovigilance 25: 7

Rogers SL, Farlow MR, Doody RS, Mohs R, Friedhoff LT and the Donepezil Study Group 1998 A 24-week, double-blind, placebo-controlled trial of donepezil in patients with Alzheimer's disease. Neurology 50: 136–145

Rosler M, Anand R, Cicin-Sain A, et al. 1999 Efficacy and safety of rivastigmine in patients with Alzheimer's disease: international, randomised controlled trial. British Medical Journal 318: 633–640

29.   5-Fluorouracil (5FU)

A.F   B.T   C.T   D.F   E.T

5-fluorouracil (5FU) is widely used in the treatment of colorectal, breast and head and neck cancer. It is an antimetabolite and requires intracellular activation. 5FU enters cells via the facilitated uracil transport mechanism, where it is phosphorylated to its active form (5-fluoro 2´ deoxyuridine monophosphate, FdUMP) by thymidine phosphorylase and thymidine kinase. In the presence of a reduced folate cofactor the active substrate forms a stable complex with thymidylate synthase. This enzyme catalyses the formation of thymidine 5´ monophosphate (dTMP) from 2-deoxyuridine 5´ monophosphate (dUMP), which is necessary for DNA synthesis and repair. The addition of pharmacological concentrations of folinic acid enhances the cytotoxicity of 5FU by expanding intracellular pools of folate and increasing the stability of the thymidylate synthase–FdUMP complex. 5FU is also extensively incorporated into RNA and interferes with normal RNA processing.

5FU can be given as an intravenous bolus or a continuous infusion. Its primary effects are exerted on rapidly dividing tissues such as gastrointestinal mucosa and bone marrow. The toxicity spectrum depends on dose and schedule and includes mucositis, pharyngitis, dysphagia, gastritis and colitis. Myelosuppression is greatest with bolus administration. With continuous infusion stomatitis and diarrhoea are the dose-limiting toxicities. Subacute toxicity from hand and foot syndrome (desquamation of the hands and feet) may eventually become dose-limiting with this schedule. Other skin reactions include alopecia, fingernail changes, dermatitis, photosensitivity, increased pigmentation over veins into which 5FU has been injected and enhanced toxicity of radiotherapy. Neurotoxicity and cardiac toxicity (myocardial infarction secondary to vasospasm) have also been reported.

5FU enhances the cytotoxicity of ionizing radiation. The underlying mechanism may include increased DNA damage, inhibition of repair, and the accumulation of cells in S phase. Infusional 5FU is given synchronously with pelvic radiotherapy in the treatment of rectal carcinoma.

Tomudex is a quinazdine antifolate that is a potent and specific inhibitor of thymidylate synthase and has been shown to be as effective as 5FU in metastatic colorectal cancer. It has the advantage of being given as a single monthly injection rather than the 4–5 bolus injections that are required when giving bolus 5FU.

Irinotecan (CPT-11) is an inhibitor of topoisomerase 1 and has been shown to be effective in patients with metastatic colorectal cancer resistant to 5FU. Its side effects include neutropenia and delayed diarrhoea. Its administration is associated with an early cholingergic syndrome (diaphoresis, diarrhoea, abdominal

cramps), which can be prevented or reduced by giving atropine
sulfate intravenously.

References

Cunningham D, Pyrhonen S, James RD et al. 1998 Randomised trial of
irinotecan plus supportive care versus supportive care alone after
fluorouracil failure for patients with metastatic colorectal cancer.
Lancet 352: 1413–1418

Devita VT, Hellman S, Rosenberg SA 1997 Cancer, principles and
practice of oncology. 5th edn. Lippincott-Raven, Philadelphia

Rougier P, Van Cutsem E, Bajetta E et al. 1998 Randomised trial of
irinotecan versus fluorouracil by continuous infusion after fluorouracil
failure in patients with metastatic colorectal cancer. Lancet 352:
1407–1412

---

30. Paclitaxel (Taxol)

A.F   B.T   C.F   D.T   E.T

Paclitaxel (Taxol) is extracted from the Pacific yew tree and has
cytotoxic activity against many tumours, particularly breast and
ovarian. It promotes polymerization of tubulin and prevents
disassembly of the microtubules, thus disrupting cell division.
Neutropenia is the principal haematological toxicity, which occurs
8–10 days after treatment. Hypersensitivity reactions are common
and include bronchospasm, urticaria and hypotension. These
reactions are reduced by routinely giving high-dose
dexamethasone as a premedication, together with
diphenhydramine. The other dose-limiting side effect is peripheral
neuropathy. Cardiac effects are most commonly transient
bradycardia. Second- and third-degree heart block has also been
reported. Other side effects include alopecia and mild vomiting.
The drug is excreted by the liver and dose reductions are required
in patients with raised bilirubin or aminotransferases.

Recently paclitaxel has been recommended by the Joint Council
for Clinical Oncology as first-line treatment of ovarian carcinoma in
combination with a platinum compound. This recommendation is
based on the results of two large, well designed and closely
audited trials comparing standard chemotherapy of
cyclophosphamide and cisplatin with paclitaxel and cisplatin as
first-line therapy. Both trials showed higher response rates,
prolonged progression-free survival and an increase in overall
survival in the paclitaxel arm. Both paclitaxel and a synthetic
taxane, docetaxel, have been used extensively in metastatic breast
cancer resistant to anthracyclines, with response rates of 48%.
However, at present they are not used for adjuvant therapy.

References

Anon 1997 Paclitaxel and docetaxel in breast and ovarian cancer Drug and Therapeutics Bulletin 35: 43–46

Joint Council for Clinical Oncology 1998 The current role of paclitaxel in the first-line chemotherapy of ovarian cancer: Royal College of Physicians, London

31. Doxorubicin-induced cardiomyopathy

A.T   B.F   C.T   D.F   E.T

Doxorubicin (adriamycin) is an anthracycline. It has an important role in the treatment of non-Hodgkin's lymphoma, breast cancer and sarcoma.

Doxorubicin-induced cardiac damage includes acute reactions such as arrhythmias, myocarditis and pericarditis, which occur within days of treatment. Subacute damage involves the development of cardiomyopathy up to 230 days after treatment. Cardiomyopathy presents as right-sided heart failure and has a mortality of 30–60%. In some patients a late cardiomyopathy develops 4–20 years after treatment. The development of cardiomyopathy is dose dependent with an incidence of over 30% with cumulative doses of over 550 mg/m^2. It is thought to be caused by free radical damage to the cardiac muscle myofibrils and disruption of sarcoplasmic reticulum. Elderly patients and patients receiving combination therapy, or who have had mediastinal radiotherapy or whole body hyperthermia, or have a history of previous cardiac disease, hypertension or liver disease, are at increased risk of developing cardiomyopathy following doxorubicin.

Prior to starting chemotherapy with this agent patients should have an electrocardiogram (ECG) and an echocardiogram or MUGA (multigate acquistion) scan. Serial measurements of ejection fraction are a sensitive non-invasive tool for the primary detection and follow-up of doxorubicin-induced cardiomyopathy. Typical but non-specific ECG changes are flattening of T waves, prolongation of the QT interval and loss of voltage of the R wave. The diagnostic test with the greatest specificity and sensitivity is endomyocardial biopsy, which shows typical histological changes, including loss of myofibrils, distension of the sarcoplasmic reticulum and vacuolization of the cytoplasm. These changes can be used to grade the injury and indicate when therapy should be stopped.

Doxorubicin is normally given as a rapid infusion. Continuous infusion reduces cardiotoxicity but has other side effects, such as mucositis. Studies using liposomal doxorubicin have been disappointing. An iron chelating agent, dexrazone, has been shown to reduce cardiac toxicity but its use with doxorubicin can result in fatal myelosuppression.

Doxorubicin-induced cardiomyopathy tends to be refractory to conventional therapy. β-Blockers have been reported to be beneficial, but the only successful treatment for severe cardiomyopathy is heart transplantation.

Reference

Singal PW, Iliskovic N 1998 Doxorubicin induced cardiomyopathy. New England Journal of Medicine 339: 900–905

32. 'Ecstasy'

A.F   B.F   C.F   D.F   E.T

Ecstasy is the popular name for the drug 3,4-methylenedioxy-methamphetamine (MDMA), although the term is also used to cover a group of related compounds which are all phenethylamines. Amphetamine is also a phenethylamine, its name being derived from α-methylphenethylamine. All of these drugs are class A drugs and were made illegal in the UK in 1977.

Ecstasy use is common in the UK especially in the dance scene, where up to 90% of young adults admit to using it. MDMA alters mood through its effects on dopaminergic and serotoninergic pathways. Its action on noradrenergic pathways may explain its effect on thermoregulation. The mood-altering effects are said to make users feel relaxed, happy and warm towards each other. Aggression is reduced and users feel less fearful and defensive. Sensory, visual and time perceptions are altered. The physical effects cause nausea, sweating, jaw clenching and muscle aches. Hypertension, tachycardia and cardiac arrhythmias may occur. Sleep becomes disordered and appetite may be reduced for up to a week. Midweek blues following weekend use are commonly reported. Physical and mental tasks may be more difficult to perform and there is a lack of motivation. The development of complications following ecstasy use is unpredictable. Most people who use Ecstasy experience no short-term side effects and fatal complications are rare.

A number of deaths have been reported following Ecstasy use. Of seven deaths in the UK in 1990 and 1991 all had been admitted to hospital with raised body temperature. Five had disseminated intravascular coagulation and three rhabdomyolysis and acute renal failure. One developed liver failure and had a liver transplant, but died from graft rejection. Although hyperpyrexia has been the main cause of death from Ecstasy in the UK, other mechanisms have been implicated.

After the deaths from heatstroke, users were advised to take time out from dancing and to drink plenty of fluid. In 1993 deaths from water intoxication were reported. These were caused by the impulsive drinking of large amounts of plain water and the inappropriate secretion of antidiuretic hormone.

In addition to fatal heatstroke and water intoxication, reported complications include convulsions, cardiac arrhythmias, renal failure, hepatitis and fulminant liver failure, pneumomediastinum, aplastic anaemia, cerebral infarction, cerebral haemorrhage and cerebral venous sinus thrombosis.

Amphetamines have long been recognized to cause psychiatric disorders and MDMA has been reported to cause psychosis, flashbacks, hallucinations and depersonalization and derealization phenomena. Depression, panic attacks and anxiety have been reported. CSF examination in regular users has shown reductions in 5-hydroxyindoleacetic acid (5-HIAA), the major metabolite of serotonin, and reductions in homovanillic acid, the main metabolite of dopamine, suggesting neurotoxic damage. This, and data from animal studies, raises the possibility of long-term neurotoxicity.

Reference

Milroy CM 1999 Ten years of 'Ecstasy'. Journal of the Royal Society of Medicine 92: 68–72

---

33. Cannabis:

A.F   B.T   C.F   D.T   E.T

Cannabis is a widely used drug in western society and there has been much discussion regarding its legalization in the UK, both in the popular press and in medical journals. Its use is common in Europe, Australia and the USA and is probably underreported. It is most commonly used by teenagers and those in their early to mid-20s. Use tends to be intermittent and most users stop in their late 20s. Only about 10% become daily users. Heavy use is generally defined as daily use, but this reflects a wide range of exposures because of the differing strengths of preparations. Daily cannabis users tend to be male, less educated, and to use tobacco, alcohol and other illicit drugs, compared to occasional users. A study into the potential benefits of cannabinoids as analgesic agents is currently ongoing. There is much conflicting evidence regarding the adverse effects of cannabis.

Cannabis preparations are made from the female plant of *Cannabis sativa*. The main active moiety responsible for its psychoactive effects is δ-9-tetrahydrocannabinol, or THC. This is found in greatest concentration in the flowering tops of the plants and less so in the leaves and stems. The commonest preparations are marijuana, derived from dried flowers and leaves, and the more potent hashish, derived from compressed flowers and dried cannabis resin. Cannabis is usually smoked either alone or with tobacco. It can be smoked through a water pipe or eaten.

THC acts on receptors widely distributed throughout the brain. The natural endogenous agonist for these receptors, anandamide, is much shorter acting and less potent than cannabis. The receptors are located in areas of the brain governing memory, cognition, pain perception and motor coordination.

The acute effects of cannabis are euphoria, relaxation, intensified sensory experience, distorted perception and cognition and impaired short-term memory. Motor skills and reaction times are impaired during intoxication. This has particular implications for machine operators and car drivers. Anxiety and panic attacks are the most common unpleasant effects of cannabis use, and occur in naïve and occasional users or in experienced users with higher than usual doses. The heart rate is increased, sedentary blood pressure increased and standing blood pressure decreased. Acute toxicity is very uncommon and there is no confirmed mortality accountable to acute cannabis toxicity.

The chronic effects of cannabis include respiratory side effects. Bronchitis and premalignant histological change in the lung tissue of chronic users have been reported. This effect is independent of but additive to the respiratory effects of tobacco use. There is a theoretical risk of adverse immune effects of cannabis based on evidence from rat studies, but this has not been proved in humans. It has been difficult to asses the effects of chronic cannabis use in pregnancy, but it seems likely that it is associated with low-birthweight infants. Cannabis does not appear to be teratogenic. Children exposed to cannabis in utero may have sustained attention, memory and cognitive deficits. These effects are, however, much smaller than the effect of maternal tobacco smoking. The most alarming in utero effect of maternal cannabis use during pregnancy is the reported increased risk of various childhood malignancies including lymphoblastic leukaemia and astrocytoma. However, these reports were incidental findings in studies not designed to study the associations of cannabis with childhood diseases and need further assessment.

The mental health effects of chronic cannabis use give cause for concern. Heavy cannabis users tend to be those with poor school performance, and subsequently these users experience poor job stability. In adolescence cannabis use precedes progression to hard drugs such as opioids. This may be a direct relationship, but the association is mostly interpreted as reflecting the selective recruitment into cannabis use of adolescents who are non-conforming and have poor school records. These individuals then have greater access to illicit drugs through interaction with drug-using peers. There is a recognized cannabis dependence syndrome, with features similar to alcohol dependency. The long-term cognitive effects of cannabis are subtle and may not be significant for normal everyday functioning. In high doses cannabis can cause acute anxiety, hallucinations and psychosis. These are rare reactions and usually reversible with cessation of the drug. There is, however, an association between cannabis use and schizophrenia. The incidence of schizophrenia has not increased despite increasing cannabis use in populations, leading to the hypothesis that cannabis use may precipitate schizophrenia in vulnerable individuals, rather than being a causative factor.

References

Hall W, Solowij N 1998 Adverse effects of cannabis. Lancet
352: 1611–1616

---

34. Carbon monoxide poisoning
A.F   B.T   C.T   D.F   E.F

Carbon monoxide poisoning occurs both accidentally and intentionally. Carbon monoxide concentrations in air are usually around 0.001% and normal levels in blood reach 1–3%.

Important exogenous sources of carbon monoxide are exhaust fumes, poorly functioning heating systems and tobacco smoke. Blood levels of carbon monoxide in smokers are commonly 10% and higher. Methylene chloride, found in paint removers and other solvents, is another source of carbon monoxide. Methylene chloride is easily absorbed through the skin and metabolized in the liver, generating carbon monoxide.

Carbon monoxide is absorbed through the lungs. It binds to haemoglobin, competing for the oxygen-binding site and creating carboxyhaemoglobin. The oxygen–haemoglobin dissociation curve is shifted to the left and tissue hypoxia results. It has an even greater affinity for fetal haemoglobin, and carbon monoxide poisoning in pregnancy can be fatal to the fetus. The gas is excreted unchanged by the lungs.

The commonest symptom of carbon monoxide poisoning is headache. Dizziness, nausea, vomiting and tachypnoea are also common presenting features. However, the classic triad of cherry-red lips, cyanosis and retinal haemorrhage is rare. In severe acute poisoning a patient may present in coma. A delayed neuropsychiatric syndrome has also been described, particularly in the elderly, where personality and cognitive changes occur several days or even months after exposure.

Carbon monoxide can be detected in the blood as carboxyhaemoglobin. Pulse oximetry cannot distinguish between oxyhaemoglogin and carboxyhaemoglobin, therefore formal measurement of levels by spectrophotometry is required. Levels do not always correlate with clinical symptoms, as the duration of exposure and minute respiratory volume also influence toxicity. Therefore, detection of carbon monoxide in exhaled breath can be useful.

Patients poisoned by carbon monoxide should be removed from the source and high-flow, 100% normobaric oxygen administered immediately. The half-life of carbon monoxide is 4–6 hours in air, 40–80 minutes in 100% oxygen and 15–30 minutes in hyperbaric oxygen. Indications for hyperbaric oxygen are coma or any period of unconsciousness, carboxyhaemoglobin levels greater than 40%, carboxyhaemoglobin levels greater than 15% in pregnant women, signs of cardiac arrhythmia or ischaemia, or symptoms not resolving on normobaric oxygen within 4–6 hours.

References

Ernst A, Zibrak JD 1998 Carbon monoxide poisoning. New England Journal of Medicine 339: 1603–1608

Tibbles PM, Edelsberg JS 1996 Hyperbaric oxygen therapy. New England Journal of Medicine 334: 1642–1648

35. Drug-induced hypokalaemia

A.**F** B.**T** C.**F** D.**T** E.**T**

Hypokalaemia is defined as a serum potassium concentration of less than 3.6 mmol/l. It can be due to decreased potassium intake or increased potassium losses. Mechanisms of potassium loss include excess loss in diarrhoea or hyperchloraemic loss through vomiting. Long-term regulation of potassium excretion takes place in the kidney, and abnormalities of renal potassium excretion can cause either hypokalaemia or hyperkalaemia.

Hypokalaemia can be well tolerated in otherwise healthy people, and in the absence of heart disease cardiac arrhythmias are uncommon. However, in the presence of cardiac ischaemia, heart failure or left ventricular hypertrophy even mild hypokalaemia can have severe cardiac consequences. Hypokalaemia will also exacerbate digoxin toxicity.

The commonest cause of hypokalaemia is drug use. Both insulin and β-agonists act as endogenous potassium regulators and their therapeutic use can cause hypokalaemia. 98% of total body potassium is intracellular, and this homoeostasis is maintained by the active transport of cations out of the cell by the Na/K-ATPase channel, which exports three sodium cations in exchange for two potassium cations. This creates a voltage gradient across cell membranes known as the resting membrane potential, and this holds potassium ions within the cell. β-Adrenergic agents activate the Na/K-ATPase pump, thus promoting the transport of potassium intracellularly. Aldosterone, acting on sodium reabsorbtion in the collecting ducts of the kidney, promotes the excretion of potassium in the urine. Normal urinary excretion of potassium is between 60 and 80 mmol in 24 hours.

Bronchodilators, decongestants such as pseudoephedrine, caffeine, theophylline and chloroquine cause hypokalaemia through a transcellular potassium shift. Theophylline and caffeine probably do this by inhibiting intracellular phosphodiesterase and thereby increasing Na/K-ATPase activity. Chloroquine prevents potassium from exiting cells.

Many drugs cause increased renal potassium loss. The commonest cause of hypokalaemia is diuretic therapy. Thiazide and loop diuretics block chloride-associated sodium reabsorption. With the exception of acetazolamide-induced hypokalaemia, diuretic-induced hypokalaemia is associated with a mild metabolic alkalosis. Acetazolamide causes hypokalaemia with a mild acidosis because it inhibits hydrogen-linked sodium reabsorption, whereby sodium is exchanged for intracellular hydrogen ions. Carbenoxolone and liquorice cause a syndrome of apparent mineralocorticoid excess by inhibiting 11β-hydroxysteroid dehydrogenase, whereas fludrocortisone causes hypokalaemia by actual mineralocorticoid excess, promoting renal potassium excretion. High-dose intravenous penicillin increases sodium delivery to the distal tubules in the kidney, which promotes increased potassium loss and can cause hypokalaemia. Aminoglycosides, on the other hand, cause potassium loss due to magnesium depletion. Other drugs causing hypokalaemia in this way are cisplatin, amphotericin B and foscarnet. Amphotericin B also causes hypokalaemia through inhibition of hydrogen ion secretion.

A third way in which drugs can affect potassium loss and cause hypokalaemia is through losses in the faeces. The concentration of potassium in stool is normally 80–90 mmol/l, but actual potassium loss is relatively low because of the low water volume of normal faeces. Although the concentration of potassium decreases in the watery stool of diarrhoeal states, the volume can be greatly increased and this can greatly increase the amount of potassium excreted in this way. Laxative agents such as phenol phthalein can cause hypokalaemia.

References

Gennari J 1998 Hypokalaemia. New England Journal of Medicine 339: 451–458

Halperin ML, Kamel KS 1998 Potassium. Lancet 352: 135–140

36. Treating a patient with glucocorticoids
A.F   B.T   C.F   D.T   E.T

Glucocorticoids enhance bone resorption and decrease bone formation in a dose-dependent (particularly above 7.5 mg prednisolone daily) and duration-dependent manner. This results in significant loss of bone and increased fracture risk. Bone loss occurs more at trabecular (e.g. vertebrae) than cortical (e.g. radius) sites.

Mechanisms of glucocorticoid-induced bone loss are incompletely understood but include disturbed calcium homoeostasis, inhibition of bone formation and sex hormone effects. Calcium absorption from the gut is decreased and urinary calcium excretion is increased. This may result in secondary hyperparathyroidism. Glucocorticoid treatment does not affect serum vitamin D levels. Decreases in osteoblast proliferation and synthesis of collagen and non-collagen matrix proteins contribute to inhibition of bone formation. There is a rapid phase of bone loss in the first 6 months of treatment followed by a continuous slower decline in bone density. Glucocorticoids decrease pituitary hormone levels and adrenal androgen secretion, leading to a decrease in both male and female sex hormones.

Guidelines for preventing and managing corticosteroid-induced osteoporosis are constantly evolving. General advice applies particularly to patients who are expected to receive more than 7.5 mg prednisolone daily for 6 months or longer. The dose of steroid should be kept to a minimum and local routes of administration should be used where possible, e.g. enemas and inhalers. Lifestyle advice includes recommending weightbearing exercise, avoiding smoking and moderating alcohol intake. Dietary intake of calcium and vitamin D should be adequate. Poor eyesight and mobility could compound the fracture risk.

Specific measures to protect against osteoporosis are needed in certain patient subgroups. Early menopause, personal or family history of osteoporotic fractures, amenorrhoea, poor mobility and low body weight are all risk factors for osteoporosis. A low T score on DEXA scanning is also a risk factor (below −1.5). Hormone replacement therapy should be considered for all postmenopausal women and testosterone for all hypogonadal men in any of these risk groups.

Bisphosphonates have been shown in prospective randomized controlled trials to reduce bone loss and the incidence of vertebral fracture in patients recently commenced on corticosteroid treatment. It is less certain that hormone replacement alone can achieve this same benefit.

References

Adachi JD, Benson WA, Brown J et al. 1997 Intermittent cyclical etidronate therapy in the prevention and treatment of corticosteroid induced osteoporosis. New England Journal of Medicine 337: 382–387

American College of Rheumatology Task Force on Osteoporosis Guidelines 1996 Recommendations for the prevention and treatment of glucocorticoid induced osteoporosis. Arthritis and Rheumatism 39: 1791–1801

Canalis E 1996 Mechanisms of glucocorticoid action in bone: implications for glucocorticoid induced osteoporosis. Journal of Endocrinology and Metabolism 81: 3441–3447

NEUROLOGY

37. Haematological causes of acute stroke

A.F   B.F   C.T   D.F   E.F

Stroke in patients under 55 years of age is uncommon. Possible haematological causes need to be investigated. In all patients with stroke a full blood count (FBC) and measurement of erythrocyte sedimentation rate (ESR) and plasma viscosity are mandatory. In addition, in young stroke patients specific causes of a coagulopathy should be investigated. Blood tests should include proteins S and C, antithrombin III, lupus anticoagulant, anticardiolipin antibodies, activated protein C resistance/Leiden factor V mutation, and haemoglobin electrophoresis (for patients of African and Mediterranean origin).

Lupus anticoagulant and anticardiolipin antibodies react with proteins associated with phospholipid. These antibodies are found in patients with systemic lupus erythematosus and the antiphospholipid syndrome. However, anticardiolipin antibodies are not specific to these disorders, being found in healthy subjects, patients with other autoimmune disorders, patients with malignancy or HIV infection, and in patients treated with phenytoin, sodium valproate, procainamide, hydralazine and quinidine. The antiphospholipid syndrome is characterized by recurrent miscarriages, arterial and venous thromboses, livedo reticularis, cardiac valve vegetations and thrombocytopenia. Leiden factor V mutation is the most commonly inherited prothrombotic state so far identified. It results in a functional resistance to activated protein C.

Acquired disorders of coagulation and fibrin include disseminated intravascular coagulation, pregnancy and the puerperium, oral contraceptive pill use and paraproteinaemias. 13% of all strokes in women aged 20–44 in Europe are attributable to the oral contraceptive pill (OCP). The risk of stroke in women on the OCP significantly increases with age, smoking and hypertension. Other haematological disorders associated with ischaemic stroke include myeloproliferative disorders, polycythaemia rubra vera, essential thrombocythaemia, sickle cell disease, paroxysmal nocturnal haemoglobinuria, thrombocytopenia, leukaemia and intravascular lymphoma.

Other inherited causes of stroke include familial hypercholesterolaemia, pseudoxanthoma elasticum, Ehlers–Danlos syndrome, Marfans' syndrome, homocystinuria, Fabry's disease, mitochondrial cytopathy and migraine.

Reference

Markus HS, Hambley H 1998 Neurology and the blood: haematological abnormalities in ischaemic stroke. Journal of Neurology, Neurosurgery and Psychiatry 64: 150–159

38. Status epilepticus

A.**F**   B.**T**   C.**F**   D.**T**   E.**T**

Status epilepticus is defined as two or more epileptic seizures (convulsive or non-convulsive) occurring without the patient regaining consciousness between attacks, or any seizure lasting more than 30 minutes. Despite appropriate management about 10% of patients die during convulsive status, frequently of the underlying brain condition. Without appropriate management there is a 60% mortality. Benzodiazepines must not be given intramuscularly as absorption is erratic. Instead they should be given intravenously or rectally. A normal electroencephalogram (EEG) recording during a seizure should strongly suggest a diagnosis of pseudoseizure. Absence status and complex partial seizure status are characterized by a confused state where the patient intermittently partially rouses. They can last for several days and can be terminated at once with injection of a fast acting benzodiazepine.

Initial intervention should involve removing the patient from any potential danger and immediate resuscitation (airways, breathing and circulation). This includes securing an airway and administering oxygen.

During the first hour there should be regular neurological and cardiovascular observations, plus temperature measurements. Blood glucose testing is mandatory. Monitoring of blood biochemistry, full blood count, clotting and blood gas measurements should be repeated regularly. Specific investigations aimed at identifying the underlying cause of the seizure should be initiated.

Within the first few minutes of seeing the patient a single intravenous bolus injection of a fast-acting benzodiazepine should be given. This will abolish seizure activity in 80% of cases. Patients must be monitored for adverse effects such as respiratory depression and hypotension. Hypoglycaemia is an easily reversible cause of status epilepticus. If there is any doubt 50 ml 50% glucose should be given intravenously. Intravenous thiamine should be given to patients at risk of vitamin B_1 defiency and acidosis should be treated if severe. If the patient continues to fit despite treatment with a benzodiazepine a second antiepileptic agent should be given such as phenytoin. This must be given through a separate giving set because of the possibility of crystallization. Phenytoin supresses seizure spread without causing cortical or respiratory depression. It must be given as a slow infusion with cardiac monitoring as rapid infusion can cause cardiac dysrhythmias and hypotension. Once status is controlled long-term maintenance antiepileptic treatment should be started.

Within the first 90 minutes the underlying aetiology should have been established and the appropriate treatment initiated. The medical complications of status should be addressed and pressor therapy given when appropriate. All patients who have been in status from between 30 and 90 minutes should be transferred to an intensive care unit (ITU). At this stage it is important to exclude pseudostatus and to check that all drugs and doses have been given according to protocol. On ITU, EEG monitoring can be started, with intracranial pressure monitoring where appropriate. If status epilepticus persists a general anaesthetic should be given (thiopentone or propofol are commonly used) and ventilation, haemodynamic and organ support provided.

The complications of status epilepticus include cerebral anoxia, respiratory aspiration or obstruction, physical injury, hyperpyrexia, pneumoperitoneum and brain damage.

References

Anon 1996 Stopping status epilepticus. Drug and Therapeutics Bulletin. 34(10): 73–75

Delanty N, Vaughan CJ, French JA 1998 Medical causes of seizures (seminar). Lancet 352: 383–390

Hughes RAC 1994 Neurological emergencies. BMJ publishing, London

Lowenstein DH, Alldredge BK 1998 Status epilepticus (review). New England Journal of Medicine 338: 970–978

---

39. Friedreich's ataxia

A.F   B.T   C.T   D.T   E.T

Friedreich's ataxia is an autosomal recessive inherited spinocerebellar degenerative disorder with an incidence of 2 per 100 000 in the UK. The disease has been mapped to a gene on chromosome 9 which encodes a protein, frataxin. In patients with Friedreich's ataxia this gene contains an abnormally expanded and unstable GAA trinucleotide repeat. Pathologically there is degeneration of the posterior and lateral columns of the spinal cord and dorsal roots. Degeneration of the brain stem and cerebellum is also seen, but is less extensive.

Patients present with progressive neurological deterioration through childhood and adolescence, with most becoming wheelchair bound in the fourth decade. The signs include pes cavus, scoliosis and a high arched palate. There is ataxia of all four limbs and trunk, an intention tremor, nystagmus and dysarthria. It is one of a number of disorders in which the deep tendon reflexes are lost but there are upgoing plantars. Position and vibration sense are diminished in the feet. There is optic and retinal atrophy, retinitis pigmentosa, sensorineural deafness and commonly mild cognitive impairment.

Epilepsy is not a feature. A cardiomyopathy can occur and the electrocardiogram typically shows inverted T waves and evidence of left ventricular hypertrophy. 20% of patients develop diabetes mellitus.

Reference

Brice A 1998 Unstable mutations and neurodegenerative disorders. Journal of Neurology 245 (8): 505–510

---

40. Diabetic peripheral neuropathy
A.F   B.T   C.F   D.F   E.F

Diabetes mellitus may be complicated by a number of different peripheral neuropathies. It is the most common cause of neuropathy in the developed world, with 50% of patients with diabetes for over 20 years having symptoms of a peripheral neuropathy. Diabetic neuropathy is more common in men than women.

Neuropathy is a common presenting feature of adult-onset diabetes but not of juvenile-onset disease, and diabetes mellitus should be excluded in any patient presenting with a neuropathy.

The peripheral neuropathies that complicate diabetes mellitus include mild peripheral sensory neuropathy, sensorimotor neuropathy, autonomic neuropathy, mononeuritis multiplex, radiculopathy including diabetic amyotrophy, entrapment neuropathies and vascular nerve lesions.

Peripheral sensorimotor neuropathy with loss of sensation to all modalities is commonly accompanied by pain which is refractory to treatment. Amitriptyline, phenytoin and carbamazepine are sometimes helpful.

Diabetic amyotrophy presents with excruciating pain in the front of the thigh, with rapidly progressive weakness and wasting of the quadriceps and loss of the knee jerk. The pain and progression of symptoms lasts 5–10 days and recovery usually occurs over 6–18 months. The cause is a lumbar plexopathy affecting L2, 3, 4.

Carpal tunnel syndrome and ulnar and femoral compression neuropathies are examples of entrapment neuropathies. They are common and may occur in sequence, causing a mononeuritis multiplex. Other causes of a mononeuritis multiplex include polyarteritis nodosa, Churg–Strauss syndrome, rheumatoid arthritis, systemic lupus erythematosus, Wegener's granulomatosis, sarcoid, Behçet's disease, paraneoplastic disease, amyloidosis and leprosy.

References

Boulton AJ 1998 Guidelines for diagnosis and outpatient management of diabetic peripheral neuropathy. European Association for the Study of Diabetes, Neurodiabetes, Diabetes Metabolism. 94 (3): 55–65

Thomas PK 1997 Clinical features and investigation of diabetic somatic peripheral neuropathy. Clinical Neuroscience 4 (6): 341–345

Younger DS, Rosoklija G, Hays AP 1998. Diabetic peripheral neuropathy. Seminars in Neurology 18 (1): 95–104

41. Parkinson's disease
A.F   B.T   C.T   D.F   E.T

In 1957 the discovery that the dopamine precursor L-dihydroxy phenylalanine (L-dopa) could alleviate reserpine-induced akinesia in rodents paved the way for its widespread use as a symptomatic treatment for Parkinson's disease. However, treatment with L-dopa results in a spectrum of adverse effects, including motor response fluctuations and treatment-related dyskinesias, which typically begin 3–6 years into treatment.

Two new types of medical treatments have recently been introduced. Pramipexole, ropinirole and cabergoline are second-generation dopa agonists. Direct-acting dopa agonists have been available for some years, but evidence suggests that the newer agonists have better efficacy and are associated with fewer adverse effects. Compared to placebo they significantly improve the motor and activities of daily living (ADL) scores of the Unified Parkinson's Disease Rating Scores (UPDRS) when used as monotherapy in early disease. Ropinirole has been shown to be equivalent to L-dopa in early disease, but L-dopa was more effective for late stage disease.

When used with L-dopa in patients with motor fluctuations the new dopa-agonists significantly reduced awake 'off' time by approximately 2 hours a day, and a 30% mean reduction in L-dopa dosage was achieved. It remains to be seen whether the use of these dopa agonists as monotherapy in early disease will result in a delay or a reduction in the incidence of motor response fluctuations and dyskinesias by delaying L-dopa treatment. The known adverse effects of these new drugs include nausea, insomnia, hallucinations and dyskinesias. The dose should be built up slowly, and domperidone may be useful as an antiemetic in the initial few weeks of treatment.

The short plasma half-life of L-dopa, and hence the brief rise in brain dopamine, is a result of its rapid absorption and metabolism. L-dopa is metabolized by two enzyme pathways: it is decarboxylated by aromatic aminoacid decarboxylases (AAAD) and undergoes O-methylation by catechol-O-methyl transferases (COMT). Inhibitors of AAAD (carbidopa and benserazide) have been used routinely for many years to increase the bioavailability of L-dopa. These drugs do not, however, substantially prolong L-dopa's plasma half-life. O-methylation of L-dopa prevents its conversion to dopamine in the brain, whereas O-methylation of dopamine itself is one step in the metabolic inactivation of L-dopa.

Entacapone and tolcapone are newly developed catechol-O-methyl transferase (COMT) inhibitors. Tolcapone was withdrawn in Europe in November 1998 following reports of hepatic failure. COMT inhibition slows the elimination of L-dopa from the plasma, increasing its plasma half-life but without altering the time to plasma peak or its maximum concentration. The introduction of a COMT inhibitor allows a reduction in the daily dose of L-dopa, either by reducing each dose or by increasing the dosing interval. Entacapone has been shown to increase the duration of action of L-dopa by 57% and reduce the dose by up to 30%. It increased awake 'on' time by approximately 2 hours a day. The adverse effects of entacapone are mostly those due to increased dopaminergic stimulation.

Drugs with new forms of action, such as dopamine reuptake inhibitors and adenosine antagonists, are being investigated in animal and early human trials. In addition, with an increasing understanding of the genetics and pathophysiology of the neurodegenerative process, treatments aimed at neuroprotection and neurorescue are being investigated which may in the future enable us to halt or reverse the underlying disease process.

References

MCA/CSM 1999 Withdrawal of tolcapone. Current Problems in Pharmacovigilance. 25 (Feb): 2

Nutt JG 1998 Catechol-O-methyltransferase inhibitors for the treatment of Parkinson's disease. Lancet 351: 1221–1222

Schapira AHV 1999 Science, medicine and the future: Parkinson's disease. British Medical Journal 318: 311–314

42. Neurosurgical treatments for Parkinson's disease

A.F   B.T   C.F   D.T   E.T

Acquired brain lesions, e.g. stroke, have long been known to modify the symptoms of Parkinson's disease (PD). Stereotactic neurosurgical procedures aimed at countering the imbalances in basal ganglia circuitry thought to result in the motor symptoms of Parkinson's disease and essential tremor were popular in the 1950s and 1960s. Unilateral thalamotomy (a neurosurgically produced lesion in the thalamus) was found to provide good relief from contralateral tremor and rigidity but had no effect on the akinesia of PD. Akinesia is the core disabling feature of PD. In addition, bilateral lesions were found to be associated with a 25% risk of pseudobulbar speech and swallowing difficulties. Although the popularity of surgery for PD declined steeply following the introduction of L-dopa in 1967, there has been a resurgence of interest in the last decade.

Stimulating electrodes are used during surgery (with the patient awake) to locate the correct site for surgical lesions and avoid speech areas. During thalamotomy operations it was discovered that high-frequency stimulation at the intended site of the lesion could abolish tremor. This observation paved the way for the use of high-frequency deep brain stimulating electrodes as an alternative to destructive lesions in the treatment of tremor. Bilateral Vim thalamic stimulators, or a stimulator on one side and a lesion on the other, do not carry the same risks of side effects as bilateral lesions, but there is still no effect on the akinesia of PD.

Models of basal ganglia circuitry suggest that in PD there is overactivity in both the subthalamic nucleus and the internal pallidum, the net effect of which is to reduce thalamic excitatory output to cortex. Lesions in the posteroventral pallidum in Parkinson's disease result in improvements in akinesia, rigidity, freezing, and L-dopa induced dyskinesias. Unilateral pallidotomy does not result in a significant reduction in medication and does not result in any improvement in gait or postural instability (the axial symptoms of PD), and its effect on tremor remains controversial. Most studies report little or no effect of unilateral pallidotomy on neuropsychological tests. Bilateral pallidotomy has been complicated by cognitive impairment and pseudobulbar symptoms such as hypophonia and drooling. Pallidotomy carries a risk of death and stroke.

Spontaneous lesions in or near the subthalamic nucleus are known to result in hemiballismus, and consequently the subthalamic nucleus has not been a popular target. However, a number of centres have reported major benefits in parkinsonism without increased dyskinesia following ablative subthalamic lesions.

More recently deep brain stimulators have been implanted in the internal pallidum and subthalamic nucleus for the experimental treatment of Parkinson's disease. Pallidal stimulation has been reported to improve all the cardinal motor symptoms of PD, as well as drug-induced dyskinesias and motor fluctuations. However, the internal pallidum is a relatively large structure and the effect of stimulation appears to be focal, with the site for the optimal relief of one symptom sometimes resulting in no improvement or the worsening of another.

Deep brain stimulators placed in the smaller subthalamic nucleus have been reported to be effective at relieving all of the motor symptoms of PD but appear to have little effect on L-dopa-induced dyskinesia. However, in contrast to the results from ablative lesions in the posteroventral pallidum, the antiparkinsonian effect is large enough to allow a reduction in L-dopa dosage, which in itself reduces dyskinesia.

Many of the complications of PD drug therapy may be attributable to dopamine being delivered to the wrong structures and the concentration of drug fluctuating in a non-physiological or erratic manner. Several hundred adult PD patients have received intrastriatal grafts of embryonic nigral and striatal neurons. In about two-thirds of these patients clinically useful reductions in motor fluctuations and improvements in parkinsonian symptoms have been reported. In the most successful cases patients have been able to stop all L-dopa treatment.

Surgical treatments for Parkinson's disease remain experimental, with the definitive techniques and sites not yet established. The long-term outcome of these treatments is not yet known, and comparisons between surgical techniques and optimal medical treatments have not been performed.

References

Golbe LI 1998 Pallidotomy for Parkinson's disease: hitting the target? Lancet 351: 998–999

Lindvall O 1999 Cerebral implantation in movement disorders: state of the art. Movement Disorders 14 (2): 201–205

Quinn N, Bhatia K 1998 Functional neurosurgery for Parkinson's disease. British Medical Journal 316: 1259–1260

43. Trinucleotide repeat disorders
A.T   B.T   C.T   D.T   E.F

Myotonic dystrophy is an autosomal dominant disorder. The genetic mutation consists of an unstable and expanded CTG repeat sequence at the 3′ end of the myotonin protein kinase gene on chromosome 19q. It has an incidence of 14 per 100 000 of the population. It is a slowly progressive disorder, presenting in young adults with myotonia, weakness and wasting of the distal limb muscles and the muscles of the face. There is ptosis and dysphagia. Frontal baldness, cataracts, cardiac conduction defects, impotence, a low intellect, impaired glucose tolerance, hypothyroidism and malignant hyperpyrexia are all recognized features of the disease.

Olivopontocerebellar atrophy is a slowly progressive neurodegenerative disorder presenting with features of parkinsonism, cerebellar and cortical tract signs and dementia.

Fragile X syndrome is an X-linked recessive disorder resulting from an expanded CGG repeat sequence in the FMR1-RNA binding protein. There is decreased head size, prominent forehead, large ears, macro-orchidism and mental retardation.

Kennedy's disease shows X-linked recessive inheritance and is caused by a CAG repeat expansion in the androgen receptor gene. It results in muscle wasting and weakness, often with bulbar signs.

Spinocerebellar ataxia (SCA) types 1, 2, 3, 6 and 7 are autosomal dominant diseases that cause ataxia. All result from expanded CAG repeat sequences in separate genes which encode abnormally long polyglutamine tracts in their respective proteins (ataxin 1, 2, 3 and 7 in SCA 1, 2, 3 and 7 and a subunit of a voltage-dependent calcium channel in SCA 6). Machado–Joseph disease (SCA type 3) is frequently associated with ophthalmoplegia but may also present with pyramidal signs, parkinsonism, dystonia and an axonal neuropathy.

Dentatorubropallidoluysian atrophy is an autosomal dominant disorder which results from a CAG expansion in the atrophin gene.

References

Hussain M, Brooks DJ 1999 Case report: ataxia and ophthalmoplegia. CPD Bulletin of Neurology 1: 25–27

Paulson HL, Fischbeck KH 1996 Trinucleotide repeats in neurodegenerative disorders. Annual Review of Neuroscience 19: 79–107

44. Diagnosis and management of migraine

A.F   B.T   C.T   D.F   E.T

Migraine is defined as an episodic disorder with complete relief from symptoms between attacks. There are two main types: migraine without aurae, which accounts for 75% of cases, and migraine with aurae. In migraine without aurae the headache is typically unilateral, severe, pulsating, and may be accompanied by photophobia, phonophobia and nausea. Symptoms last 4 hours to 3 days. In migraine with aurae the attacks are preceded by neurological symptoms such as visual disturbance, parasthesiae or dizziness. Aurae typically progress over minutes.

Migraine-type headaches are very occasionally associated with underlying pathology. Examples include arteriovenous malformations, internal carotid artery dissection, epilepsy, mitochondrial DNA disorders such as MELAS syndrome (mitochondrial encephalomyopathy, lactic acidosis and stroke-like episodes), and cerebral autosomal dominant arteriopathy with subcortical infarction and leukoencephalopathy (CADASIL). Migraine headaches are typically unilateral, pulsating in nature, moderate to severe in intensity, and aggravated by movement.

The management of migraine involves indentifying and avoiding triggers. A symptom diary may be helpful. Simple analgesics such as paracetamol or aspirin may be effective. Soluble preparations are absorbed more quickly, and an antiemetic which promotes gastric emptying, such as metoclopramide or domperidone, also helps to circumvent the problems of nausea and delayed gastric emptying. Analgesics containing codeine, dihydrocodeine and dextropropoxyphene should be avoided because of the danger of inducing rebound analgesic headaches. If simple analgesics are ineffective 5-hydroxytryptamine (5-HT)$_{1B/D}$ agonists can be tried. They are contraindicated in patients over 65 and those with ischaemic heart disease, uncontrolled hypertension or previous myocardial infarction. The oldest on the market is sumatriptan. It is available in oral, subcutaneous or intranasal formulations. The oral bioavailabity is 14%. Zolmitriptan and naratriptan are available as tablets only and have better oral bioavailability. Adverse effects include malaise, dizziness, nausea and sensations of pressure, especially on the throat and chest. The chest pressure symptoms are thought to be mainly non-cardiac and may relate to oesophageal spasm. Ergotamine is now rarely prescribed as a symptomatic treatment for migraine. Its adverse effects include nausea, abdominal cramps and arterial vasoconstriction. Rebound analgesic headache is also a problem.

If migraines are frequent, for example more than two per month, or are severe and prolonged, responding poorly to symptomatic treatments, a prophylactic treatment should be tried. β-Blockers without partial agonist activity should be tried first, unless contraindicated. Pizotifen, low-dose amitryptiline, NSAIDS and sodium valproate (not licensed for this use) have also been found to be effective at reducing the frequency of the attacks. Once started, the effectiveness and need for prophylactic treatment should be reviewed every 3 months.

References

Anon 1998 Managing migraine. Drug and Therapeutics Bulletin 36: 41–44

Headache Classification Committee of the International Headache Society 1988 Classification and diagnostic criteria for headache disorders, cranial neuralgias and facial pain. Cephalgia 8 (suppl 7): 1–96

Schoenen J 1997 Acute migraine therapy: the newer drugs. Current Opinion in Neurology. 10: 237–243

45. Pathophysiology of migraine
A.F   B.F   C.F   D.F   E.T

It is thought that genetic factors which determine ion channel function set individual thresholds for migraine. Internal and environmental triggers, such as hormonal fluctuations, tiredness, relaxation after stress, substance misuse, hunger or certain foods, may then alter this set point. In patients with migraine there is evidence for increased cortical hyperexcitability between attacks. The physiological basis for this may be defective mitochondrial oxidative phosphorylation, low intracellular magnesium, increased neurotoxic aminoacids or an inherited dysfunction of calcium channels.

The traditional explanation of the pathophysiology of migraine was that aurae were the result of vasoconstriction and headache of vasodilatation. Aurae are now thought to result from a cortical spreading depression (CSD), with a wave of depolarization propagating across the cortex at a speed of 2–3 mm per minute. This is associated with a transient depression of spontaneous and evoked neuronal activity. The depression wave lasts several minutes and is preceded by a front of brief neuronal excitation. In animal experiments CSD is associated with profound cortical blood flow changes similar to those seen in migraine with aurae. Oligaemia propagates across the cortex from occipital to frontal lobes at a rate of 2–3 mm/min and is preceded by a short phase of hyperaemia. Interestingly, visual aurae are characterized by positive scintillations followed by negative scotomata progressing at a similar rate. This suggests that vascular changes during aurae may be epiphenomena secondary to neurogenic mechanisms. CSD can be induced in animals by local electrical, mechanical and biochemical stimuli. CSD has yet to be unequivocally demonstrated in humans.

In migraine, headache is thought to be caused by activation of the trigeminovascular system. Afferent fibres from trigeminal (V1) and upper cervical spinal cord segments (C1–2) innervate large cerebral vessels, pial vessels, large venous sinuses and dura mater. These sensory fibres carry nociceptive information to trigeminal nucleus caudalis and upper cervical cord and relay on to thalamus and cortical pain centres.

Experimental depolarization of trigeminal ganglia gives rise to central transmission of nociceptive information and retrograde perivascular release of vasoactive neuropeptides. Experimental CSD can activate the trigeminovascular system, providing a theoretical link between the aurae and the headache.

Complex genetic factors are involved in migraine. Half of all cases of the rare familial hemiplegic migraine have been linked to missense mutations in a gene on chromosome 19p which encodes the α_1 subunit of a brain-specific voltage-dependent calcium channel. Interestingly, small expansions in a CAG repeat sequence at the 3′ end of the same gene can cause the autosomal dominant spinocerebellar ataxia type 6 or episodic ataxia type 2. Episodic ataxia type 2 is characterized by acetazolamide-responsive attacks of cerebellar ataxia, migraine-like symptoms, interictal nystagmus and slowly progressive cerebellar atrophy. This gene has also been implicated in non-hemiplegic migraine with and without aurae. Thus disruption of calcium channel function is implicated in the pathogenesis of migraine, hemiparesis, epilepsy, ataxia and cerebral atrophy.

References

Ferrari MD 1998 Migraine. Lancet 351: 1043–1051

Goadsby PJ 1997 Bench to bedside: what have we learnt recently about headache? Current Opinion in Neurology. 10: 215–220

Ophoff RA, Terwindt GM, Vergouwe MN et al. 1996 Familial hemiplegic migraine and episodic ataxia type-2 are caused by mutations in the calcium channel gene CACNL1N4. Cell 87: 543–552

---

46.   Management of headache
A.**T**   B.**F**   C.**T**   D.**T**   E.**F**

20–25% of patients seen in the neurology clinic have headache, and only 2% of the general population has never experienced headache. Many patients have more than one type of headache, and asking them how many types they suffer from and then about the character of each type separately helps to clarify the history and diagnoses. The majority of patients who have had their headaches for more than a year and in whom there are no physical signs will not have an underlying structural lesion.

The differential diagnosis of headache includes migraine, tension headache or cervical spondylosis, vascular causes such as temporal arteritis, subarachnoid haemorrhage, trigeminal neuralgia, atypical facial pain, infections such as meningitis, a space-occupying lesion, tumour or abscess causing raised intracranial pressure, arterial hypertension and hypercapnia.

A common and important cause of daily headache is analgesia-induced headache or rebound headache. Ergotamine, opioids, opioid combinations, 5-hydroxytryptamine (5-HT)1 agonists and caffeine have all been causally associated with daily headache. Typically the patient describes relief on taking the analgesic, but the period of relief becomes shorter and shorter and the frequency of taking the analgesic increases. Withdrawal of the analgesic usually results in relief from headache, albeit after an initial worsening of symptoms. Other drugs that cause headache include alcohol, vasodilators, nifedipine, indomethacin and sympathomimetic agents.

Tension headache, or musculoskeletal headache, typically has qualities opposite to those of migraine. It is usually bilateral, non-pulsating, mild to moderate, and not aggravated by movement. This type of headache commonly occurs 4–7 times per week. There may be tenderness over the scalp and stiffness and pain in the neck muscles. There is mild or no nausea, photophobia and phonophobia.

Cluster headaches are highly stereotyped recurrent attacks of pain around one eye in the territory of the first division of the trigeminal nerve and the second cervical root. They are always without aura. The attacks, which last about an hour, occur one or more times daily for several weeks and are then interspersed by months or years of freedom from attacks. Cluster headaches are six times more common in males than in females. The pain is extremely severe and is usually associated with autonomic features such as ipsilateral conjunctival injection, lacrimation, rhinorrhoea and nasal stuffiness. Cluster-like headaches can be a feature of posterior fossa lesions and patients should be investigated with magnetic resonance imaging. In chronic paroxysmal hemicrania there is a similar pain syndrome to that of cluster headache, but the headaches occur daily for months. Females are more commonly affected than males. This syndrome reponds well to indomethacin.

In trigeminal neuralgia there is agonizing stabbing facial pain which typically lasts a few seconds to a minute. The pains always occur on one side of the face and usually start from near the corner of the mouth. The ophthalmic division of the trigeminal nerve (V1) is rarely involved. There may be one or many attacks per day, and bouts of attacks last days or weeks. The attacks can be triggered by touching the affected area, eating, brushing the teeth or cold winds. Very occasionally an underlying pathology is found, such as multiple sclerosis, cerebellopontine angle tumours, fifth-nerve neurofibromas or basilar artery ectasia. Carbamazepine is usually a very effective symptomatic treatment.

References

Goadsby PJ 1997 Bench to bedside: what have we learnt recently about headache? Current Opinion in Neurology 10: 215–220

Headache Classification Commitee of the International Headache Society 1988 Classification and diagnostic criteria for headache disorders, cranial neuralgias and facial pain. Cephalgia 8 (Suppl 7): 1–96

Warlow C 1991 Handbook of neurology. Blackwell Scientific Publications, Oxford

RESPIRATORY MEDICINE

47. Brittle asthma

A.F   B.T   C.F   D.F   E.F

Brittle asthma is an increasingly recognized condition that is distinct from steroid-resistant asthma. Most cases demonstrate a response to high-dose steroids. These patients have peak flow rates that demonstrate a marked and chaotic variation. There is no accepted unifying definition; however, O'Driscoll (1988) described it as 'a diurnal peak flow variability of greater than 40% for more than 50% of the time despite maximal medical treatment'. However, this definition is limited as a subset of patients may actually have well preserved peak flow measurements but develop acute severe life-threatening attacks.

This has led to the recent classification of this condition into two distinct types. Type 1 patients have marked peak flow variability as previously described for at least 150 days per year. Type 2 patients have well preserved peak flows but develop severe acute asthma within 3 hours of onset of an attack, without any obvious precipitating factor. This latter group has a considerably increased mortality rate.

The aetiology of this disease is not known. It is more common in females than males, suggesting a possible hormonal link. This is supported by the fact that there is an association with the menstrual cycle, with a subgroup of patients showing marked premenstrual worsening of symptoms. However, it is clear that other factors play a role. Atopy is recognized to be present in over 90% of patients, as defined by a positive skin test, but serum IgE levels are not elevated. Furthermore, 60% of patients have evidence of food intolerance, suggesting an immunological cause. In addition, it is well recognized that psychosocial factors play a role, with an increased prevalence of personality disorder among sufferers. These patients also have an impaired perception of worsening airway function that may lead to delayed hospital presentation and possible death.

Patients with brittle asthma are treated along traditional guidelines although the response to treatment is often disappointing.

References

Ayres JG, Miles JF, Barnes PJ 1998 Brittle asthma. Thorax 53: 315–321

O'Driscoll BRC, Ruffles SP, Ayres JG, Cochrane GM 1988. Long term treatment of severe asthma with subcutaneous terbutaline. British Journal of Diseases of the Chest 82: 360–365

48. Bronchial asthma

A.F   B.T   C.F   D.F   E.T

The last few years have seen the development and introduction into clinical practice of drugs that modify responses to leukotrienes in asthma. Leukotrienes $C_4/D_4/E_4$ comprise what was known as the slow relaxing substance of anaphylaxis (SRS-A). SRS-A mediates the late phase of the asthmatic response. However, it is now increasingly recognized that leukotrienes play an important role in the initial asthmatic response. Leukotriene D_4 is at least 1000 times more potent than histamine at inducing smooth muscle cell contraction. It also has a longer duration of action than histamine.

The leukotrienes are produced from arachidonic acid via the activation of the enzyme 5-lipoxygenase (5-LO). 5-LO catalyses the conversion of arachidonic acid to leukotriene A_4, which is subsequently metabolized to LTB_4 or LTC_4. Further enzymatic action results in the production of LTD_4 and LTE_4.

In asthma and other inflammatory disorders leukotrienes are produced by eosinophils, basophils and mast cells. The cellular effects of leukotrienes are mediated by cell surface receptors, of which the most important is the LTD_4 receptor. Thus there are two possible ways of manipulating the effects of these cytokines: by blocking 5-lipoxygenase (zileuton) or by blocking the receptor (zafirlukast, montelukast).

To assess the clinical importance of modulating this system a number of clinical trials have been performed. These studies have demonstrated that antileukotriene drugs inhibit the bronchoconstrictor response to the inhalation of dry cold air, exercise and the ingestion of aspirin in susceptible patients. Furthermore, both the early and late phase of allergen-induced bronchoconstriction in asthmatics is reduced by these drugs. Repeated administration of antileukotrienes to asthmatics has demonstrated an increased morning and evening peak expiratory flow rate (PEFR) and FEV_1. Some studies show that long-term improvements are more marked than the acute bronchodilator response to these drugs. They have also shown that both daytime and night-time symptoms of asthma are reduced with reduced use of rescue bronchodilators. Their combined use with inhaled corticosteroids has resulted in significant improvement in lung function compared to inhaled steroids alone. These initial results show promise but further studies are necessary to demonstrate their proper place in chronic asthma management.

References

Drazen JM, Israel E, O'Byrne PM 1999 Treatment of asthma with drugs modifying the leukotriene pathway. New England Journal of Medicine 340: 197–206

O' Byrne PM 1997 Leukotrienes in the pathogenesis of asthma. Chest 111/2 (Supp): 27S–34S

Okudaira H 1997 Challenge studies of a leukotriene receptor antagonist. Chest 111/2 (Supp): 46S–51S

Roquet A, Dahlen B, Kumlin M et al. 1997 Combined antagonism of leukotrienes and histamine produces predominant inhibition of allergen-induced early and late airway obstruction in asthmatics. American Journal of Respiratory and Critical Care Medicine 155: 1856–1863

49. α_1 Antitrypsin (AAT)

A.F   B.T   C.T   D.F   E.F

α_1 Antitrypsin (AAT) deficiency is an autosomal recessive disorder that is currently the only genetic factor known to increase the risk of development of chronic obstructive pulmonary disease (COPD). It accounts for less than 1% of cases of COPD in the UK. AAT is one of a group of serpins (serum protease inhibitors) ,including α-macroglobulin and secretory leukoproteinase inhibitor (SLPI), that inactivates proteolytic enzymes released from inflammatory cells. The most important of these is elastase from neutrophils. Failure to inhibit the activity of this enzyme results in progressive destruction of alveolar walls and the development of emphysema.

The gene for AAT is located on chromosome 14. The serum proteinase phenotype (Pi type) is determined by the genotype of both alleles. Over 70 different alleles are currently recognized. The normal M allele, which occurs in over 95% of Europeans, results in the phenotype PiMM and is associated with normal functioning levels of AAT. Homozygotes for the Z allele (PiZZ) have levels of AAT less than 20% of normal and are at risk of emphysema. However, patients with the PiMZ phenotype are not at an increased risk of emphysema. Occasional individuals are born with normal levels of AAT but have a dysfunctional phenotype: they have normal protein levels but the protein is abnormal.

Patients with severe AAT deficiency develop premature (by the age of 60 years) emphysema, chronic bronchitis and occasionally bronchiectasis. If the patient is a smoker then the mean age of developing emphysema is 40 years. In addition to pulmonary complications, these patients are at increased risk of chronic hepatitis and cirrhosis.

As the genetic basis of this condition is known, attempts have been made to replace the deficient protein. Currently available products require intravenous administration and have a circulating half-life of less than 5 minutes. There is evidence to suggest that therapy with AAT may result in a reduced rate of loss of FEV_1. No trials have so far demonstrated a beneficial effect on survival.

References

Hutchison DC, Hughes MD 1997 Alpha-1-antitrypsin replacement therapy: will its efficacy ever be proved? European Respiratory Journal 10: 2191–2193

Seersholm N, Wencker M, Banik N et al. 1997 Does alpha1–antitrypsin augmentation therapy slow the annual decline in FEV1 in patients with severe hereditary alpha1–antitrypsin deficiency? European Respiratory Journal 10: 2260–2263

50. Pulmonary fibrosis
A.F   B.F   C.F   D.T   E.F

51. Pulmonary fibrosis
A.T   B.T   C.F   D.F   E.T

Pulmonary fibrosis is the name given to a heterogeneous group of disorders characterized by the excessive accumulation of extracellular matrix within the lung parenchyma. The excessive accumulation of collagen within the lung is pathognomonic of pulmonary fibrosis.

Recent evidence suggests that the prevalence of pulmonary fibrosis is increasing, with up to 7 per 100 000 population being affected. The disease is more common in men than women and appears to occur in the older age group, with a mean age of presentation of 67 years. Mortality from this condition is increasing in the UK, with approximately 1200–1400 deaths per annum. Recent evidence suggests that life expectancy for an incident case is only 2.9 years, with a reduction in life expectancy of approximately 7 years. This represents a worse prognosis than stage I non-small cell lung cancer.

Pulmonary fibrosis can follow a range of insults to the lung. If there is no recognisable aetiology the disease is termed cryptogenic fibrosing alveolitis (CFA) or idiopathic pulmonary fibrosis. Inhalation of organic dusts, including asbestos, silica and wood dust, has been implicated in the aetiology. Asbestos is a collective term applied to a number of naturally occurring fibrous materials comprising chrysolite, crocidolite and other fibres, exposure to which results in a slow progressive fibrosis. The degree of fibrosis depends on the quantity of inhaled fibres. In addition, longer fibres are more fibrinogenic than shorter ones. Fibrosis is also seen in association with a number of systemic diseases, including rheumatoid arthritis, systemic sclerosis and sarcoidosis. Recent evidence suggests that viral infections may also play a role. Many patients date the onset of their respiratory symptoms from the development of a viral upper respiratory chest infection. Viruses that have been implicated include hepatitis C (HCV) Epstein–Barr (EBV), cytomegalovirus (CMV) and, more recently, adenovirus.

There is considerable evidence that suggests hereditary factors may be important. There is a familial form of pulmonary fibrosis with an inheritance that is probably autosomal dominant with variable penetrance. Genetic linkage studies suggest an association with HLA B8 and HLA B12. Some strains of mice have different susceptibilities to intratracheal bleomycin (an animal model of pulmonary fibrosis). This suggests that there is probably a combination of genetic and environmental factors that lead to the development of fibrosis.

Despite the diverse range of potential aetiologies, following the injury there is an inflammatory response which results in a proteinaceous and cellular infiltration into the lung. Soluble mediators are then produced both from resident and activated inflammatory cells. These mediators activate effector cells, the most important of which is the fibroblast. Fibroblasts are the main producers of collagen and other extracellular matrix proteins.

A large number of mediators have been implicated in the pathogenesis of pulmonary fibrosis. The most potent of these thus far described is transforming growth factor (TGF)-β. Levels of this cytokine are elevated in humans and animal models of pulmonary fibrosis. TGF-β can influence collagen levels at a number of different points within the metabolic pathway. It increases procollagen gene transcription, promotes prolonged mRNA stability and also reduces intracellular degradation of procollagen. In addition, TGF-β can inhibit collagenase production, thus preventing degradation. These alterations of collagen metabolism by TGF-β all result in excessive deposition of the protein within the pulmonary parenchyma. Other cytokines can also alter the balance between synthesis and degradation of collagen, and have been implicated in pulmonary fibrosis. These include platelet-derived growth factor, endothelin-1 and interleukins.

The poor prognosis of cryptogenic fibrosing alveolitis (CFA) is related to the insidious onset of symptoms and the poor response to therapy classically seen in these patients. The usual presentation is with slow onset of progressive breathlessness, initially occurring on exercise but eventually at rest. In addition, patients may have a non-productive cough. Non-specific symptoms are also recognized, which include arthralgia, fever and malaise. These symptoms are almost always associated with fine velvety crackles on auscultation in the chest and there is clubbing of the fingers in up to 85% of patients. As the disease progresses and the patient deteriorates they may become oxygen dependent and develop central cyanosis on exertion.

Current therapies for pulmonary fibrosis are unfortunately very limited. The major treatments are corticosteroids and immunomodulatory drugs such as azathioprine and cyclophosphamide. The anti-inflammatory action of corticosteroids is mediated by a number of mechanisms. Steroids can inhibit the activation of macrophages, neutrophils and lymphocytes. Furthermore, they can block macrophage and neutrophil chemotaxis, both of which are involved in the pathogenesis of pulmonary fibrosis. Only about 20% of patients show a clinical improvement with steroids. Patients with a CT scan appearance suggesting acute inflammation usually have a better response to corticosteroids. Treatment is usually commenced with a high dose of prednisolone 60–80 mg that is continued for 4 weeks before dose reduction. The beneficial effect of corticosteroids is limited and they are associated with significant adverse effects. Furthermore, in a double-blind study assessing corticosteroids there was no survival benefit compared to placebo.

Immunomodulatory drugs such as cyclophosphamide or azathioprine alter the inflammatory response and have been used as alternative or additional therapies to corticosteroids. They block lymphocyte and macrophage function and downregulate inflammation. They can be used in combination with high-dose corticosteroids, or they can be used in isolation. An early response to treatment is associated with a better overall long-term prognosis, but the response rate is low.

Lung transplantation is only available to a limited number of patients as there remains a severe shortage of donor organs, and patients with pulmonary fibrosis tend to be elderly and often have comorbid disease. This treatment has been successful in a number of patients, and experience so far suggests that single lung transplantation is as effective as double. Obliterative bronchiolitis, a consequence of chronic rejection, remains a significant problem in these patients.

References

Egan JJ, Stewart JP, Hasleton PS, Arrand JR, Carroll KB, Woodcock AA 1995 Epstein–Barr virus replication within pulmonary epithelial cells in cryptogenic fibrosing alveolitis. Thorax 50: 1234–1239

Hubbard R, Johnston I, Britton J 1997 Survival in patients with cryptogenic fibrosing alveolitis Chest 113: 396–400

Mutsaers SE, Foster ML, Chambers RC, Laurent GJ, McAnulty RJ 1998 Increased endothelin-1 and Its localization during the development of bleomycin-induced pulmonary fibrosis in rats. American Journal of Respiratory Cell and Molecular Biology 18: 611–619

52. Nebulizer therapy

A.**F**   B.**T**   C.**T**   D.**T**   E.**F**

Nebulizer therapy is important in a number of respiratory diseases, in particular asthma and cystic fibrosis. Over the last few years nebulizers have undergone significant improvements to enhance drug delivery to the lung. This has led to an increase in the number of drugs that can be delivered by this route. Currently these include bronchodilators, corticosteroids, antibiotics and nitric oxide.

Nebulizers have a number of distinct advantages over standard metered dose inhalers (MDIs). MDIs can be difficult to use, particularly for the young, the elderly, the infirm, and those with significant physical and mental problems. MDIs, even when used optimally, result in the deposition of less than 15% of drug into the lungs. This can be marginally improved by the use of a spacer device. Oropharyngeal deposition is also more marked with an MDI than with a nebulizer.

Nebulizers have other distinct advantages over MDIs. They can deliver doses over a longer period of time and result in enhanced deposition of drug to the lungs. This deposition is dependent on the size of the respirable particles. Larger particles in excess of 10 μm are usually deposited in the oropharynx and those between 5 μm and 10 μm in the larger airways. Deposition in the larger airways is associated with an increased incidence of coughing. Smaller particles of 1 μm to 3 μm are usually cleared by phagocytosis in the smaller airways. Thus the optimal particle size is between 3 μm and 5 μm. Particles of this size are more likely to be produced by nebulizers than by MDIs.

Other factors do, however, affect the efficacy of a nebulizer. There is increasing nasal deposition with age, and up to 20% of a nebulizer dose can be exhaled and another 20% can be retained within the tubing of the apparatus. These difficulties are now being addressed. *HaloLite* is able to produce up to 80% of particles in the respirable range and results in greatly enhanced drug deposition.

The respiratory pattern also plays a role in the efficacy of a nebulizer. Patients with a short or low inspiratory flow have reduced capacity for nebulization. This problem can now be overcome by adaptive systems which nebulize in response to inspiration. As these improvements continue it is likely that nebulizer therapy will be even more widely used for drug delivery.

References

Bisgaard H, Dolovich M 1997 Nebulizer technology: the way forward. European Respiratory Review 7: 378–392

O'Callaghan C, Cant M, Robertson C 1994 Delivery of beclomethasone dipropionate from a spacer device: what dose is available for inhalation? Thorax 49: 961–964

53.   Primary pulmonary hypertension
A.T   B.T   C.F   D.F   E.F

Primary pulmonary hypertension (PPH) is a disease with a poor prognosis characterized by the presence of pulmonary vascular obstructive disease. It is a rare condition that affects about 1 person per million. It is usually of unknown aetiology (cryptogenic PPH). However, there are a few known associations.

In less than 10% of patients there is a genetic predisposition. It can be inherited as an autosomal dominant condition with variable penetrance. There are associations with autoimmune disease and infections, including HIV. Drugs such as fenfluramine and dexfenfluramine are associated with the disease. In addition, other amphetamine-like drugs including phentermine, a serotonin uptake inhibitor, have been implicated.

The pathogenesis of the condition is unknown. Serotonin has been implicated and high levels have been found in patients with PPH. Recent evidence has also suggested that there are abnormalities in voltage-gated potassium channels, with a resulting reduction in intracellular potassium. A causal relationship with these factors has not been established.

Therapies for this condition are limited. The current treatments are anticoagulants (warfarin) and vasodilators. Recent studies have shown that intravenous treatment with prostacyclin is associated with a reduced overall mortality. An improved prognosis as a result of therapy with this drug is seen in younger patients and in those who demonstrate at least a 20% reduction in mean pulmonary arterial pressure following acute administration. Other drugs under investigation for this condition include calcium channel antagonists and nitric oxide.

As the response to medical treatment is often limited and has not been shown to reverse the condition, surgery is often the only option. Atrial septectomy may improve survival in those with recurrent syncope. The only other treatment is pulmonary transplantation, which has a 10-year survival rate of about 35%. A better understanding of the pathogenesis is now directing the development of novel therapeutic agents. These include serotonin inhibitors and drugs that modulate potassium channel activity.

References

Haworth SG 1998 Primary pulmonary hypertension. Journal of the Royal College of Physicians London 32: 187–190

Herve P, Launay JM, Scrobohaci ML et al. 1995 Increased plasma serotonin in primary pulmonary hypertension. American Journal of Medicine 99: 249–254

McLaughlin VV, Genthner DE, Panella MM, Rich S 1998 Reduction in pulmonary vascular resistance with long term epoprostenol (prostacyclin) therapy in primary pulmonary hypertension. New England Journal of Medicine 338: 273–277

Rich S, Dantzker DR, Ayres SM 1987 Primary pulmonary hypertension; a national retrospective study. Annals of Internal Medicine 107: 216–223

54. Lung volume reduction surgery

A.F   B.T   C.T   D.T   E.T

A number of surgical techniques have been performed to attempt to improve symptoms in patients with end-stage emphysema. These have included phrenic nerve ligation, costochondrectomy, the instillation of peritoneal air and procedures to denervate the lung. Unfortunately all of these have been terrible failures, often resulting in increased morbidity and mortality. Two procedures have, however, shown more promise, namely giant bullectomy and lung volume reduction surgery (LVRS).

In giant bullectomy, bullae that occupy more than one-third of the hemithorax are excised. In selected patients this results in long-lasting symptom relief and a significant improvement in pulmonary function. Surgical mortality for this operation ranges from 0 to 23%. The greatest functional improvement occurs in those with bullae that occupy more than 50% of the hemithorax. The majority of patients with emphysema, however, only have small bullae, and as a consequence alternative procedures have been investigated.

This has led to the resurgence of lung volume reduction surgery. This operation was originally performed over 40 years ago but fell into disrepute, only to reappear again in the early 1990s. Since that time several studies have been performed to confirm the benefit. Essentially, the operator uses a midline sternotomy to remove 20–30% of each lung from the upper zones. The lung is then stapled using strips of bovine pericardium. The procedure can also be performed using video assisted therapy (VATS), either with stapled tissue resection or with laser ablation of bullae.

The inclusion criteria for this operation are a history of emphysema, non-smoker for > 4 months, FEV_1<45%, total lung capacity >110%, residual volume >150%, and a carbon monoxide diffusion capacity of <70%. Patients are excluded if there is obesity (BMI>31), unexplained weight loss, $PaCo_2$ >9 kPa, pulmonary hypertension, previous chest or pleural surgery, and a 6-minute walk distance of <140 m after pulmonary rehabilitation.

Results from this operation have shown some promise, with a short-term improvement in blood gases, an increase in 6-minute walking distance and improvements in lung function. However, the mechanism for this is unknown; in the short term the benefit appears to be related to an increase in lung elastic recoil. Later improvements may be as a consequence of better diaphragmatic function. The operation is also not without risk, having an operative mortality ranging from 0 to 18%. Complications include empyema, recurrent pulmonary infections and phrenic nerve palsies. Further studies are currently being perfomed both in the UK and in the USA to identify which patients will benefit most.

References

Benditt JO, Albert RK. 1997 Surgical options for patients with advanced emphysema.Clinics in Chest Medicine 18: 577–593

Brantigan OC, Mueller E. 1957 Surgical treatment of pulmonary emphysema. American Surgeon 23: 789

Cooper JD, Trulock EP, Triantafillou AN, et al. 1995 Bilateral pneumectomy (volume reduction) for chronic obstructive pulmonary diseases. Journal of Thoracic and Cardiovascular Surgery 109: 106

Keenan RJ, Landreneau FJ, Sciurba FC, et al. 1996 Unilateral thoracoscopic surgical approach for diffuse emphysema. Journal of Thoracic Cardiovascular Surgery 111: 308

55. Lung transplantation
A.T   B.F   C.F   D.F   E.F

Lung transplantation is being increasingly performed around the world. The most common indication for lung transplantation is emphysema, but it is performed for a variety of other conditions, including cystic fibrosis, primary pulmonary hypertension and interstitial lung disease. For patients to be considered for transplantation they must have end-stage respiratory disease with a life expectancy of less than 2 years. The principal contraindications to transplantation are acute respiratory failure, neoplastic disease, active smoking, drug abuse, patients with poor compliance with previous medical regimens, obesity, and an inability to walk 180 m after pulmonary rehabilitation. Unfortunately, the number of eligible people who are on the waiting list for transplantation far exceeds the number of available donor organs. Survival rates for those who actually receive transplants is slowly beginning to increase.

One of the major contributors to this increased survival has been the emergence of better immunosuppression. The current recommendation is the use of a three-drug regimen consisting of corticosteroids, azathioprine and either cyclosporin A or tacrolimus (FK-506). Indeed many centres advocate the additional use of antilymphocyte globulins to augment this regimen.

Despite these therapies, up to 40% of patients show evidence of acute rejection within the first month. This is usually manifest as fever, chills, cough and chest pain, and is best managed with the use of high-dose methylprednisolone or occasionally by the administration of intravenous murine monoclonal T-cell antibody (OKT3). Fortunately, the majority of patients respond well to this treatment.

Indeed, the major cause of early mortality is related to acute infection. Bacterial pneumonia, for example, occurs in up to 35% of patients. CMV pneumonitis is also recognized to be a major problem in these patients. Several prophylactic regimens to prevent this infection are currently employed, including intravenous high-titre anti-CMV immunoglobulins and ganciclovir. The benefits of these treatments are currently under evaluation. *Pneumocystis casinii* (PCP) prophylaxis with septrin has virtually eliminated this infection as a cause of postoperative early mortality.

For those that survive the initial period the next major problem is chronic rejection, a problem known as bronchiolitis obliterans, which eventually occurs in up to 70% of patients. The severity of this appears to be related to the severity of the acute rejection. A major acute rejection episode is associated with an earlier and more severe onset of bronchiolitis obliterans. This is usually manifested as progressive dypsnoea on exertion and a gradual decline in FEV_1. These patients are treated with increased immunosuppression including corticosteroids; however, these therapies are usually ineffective and death occurs within 2 years in the majority of cases.

Disease recurrence has been observed in patients transplanted for sarcoidosis and lymphangioleiomyomatosis. To date, disease recurrence has not been observed in those transplanted for primary pulmonary hypertension or pulmonary fibrosis.

References

Hosenpud JD, Bennett LE, Keck BM et al. 1998 Effect of diagnosis on survival benefit of lung transplantation for end-stage lung disease. Lancet 351: 24

Levine SM, Bryan CL 1995 Bronchiolitis obliterans in lung transplant recipients: The 'thorn in the side' of lung transplantation. Chest 107: 894

Trulock EP 1997 Lung transplantation. American Journal of Respiratory and Critical Care Medicine 155: 789

ENDOCRINOLOGY

56. Causes of hirsutism in women

A.T   B.T   C.F   D.F   E.F

Hirsutism is the term used to describe excess hair growth in women. It can be androgen dependent or androgen independent. The distinction between these two types can be made on physical examination, as androgen-dependent hair growth follows the distribution of new hair growth seen in boys at puberty.

Causes of androgen-independent hair growth include drugs such as cyclosporin, minoxidil and the anticonvulsants, phenytoin and phenobarbitone. There is also a familial form of androgen-independent hirsutism called familial hypertrichosis. Androgen-independent hirsutism is treated by withdrawal of the offending drug and by mechanical hair removal.

Most hirsutism is androgen dependent and is caused by androgen overproduction (hyperandrogenism) and/or increased skin sensitivity to androgens. A common cause, idiopathic hirsutism, results from a combination of these two. The skin's sensitivity to androgens is determined by the level of 5α-reductase activity. The activity of this enzyme varies widely between women.

The most common pathogenic cause of hirsuitism is the polycystic ovary syndrome (PCOS). This syndrome and idiopathic hirsutism together account for 95% of cases. Other causes of androgen-dependent hirsutism include congenital adrenal hyperplasia, Cushing's syndrome, androgen-secreting tumours of the adrenal gland and ovary, severe insulin resistance and exogenous androgen intake.

Hirsutism developing rapidly, particularly outside of puberty, should be investigated to exclude an androgen-secreting tumour. Serum testosterone should be measured and, if raised, imaging with ultrasound and CT is indicated.

Laboratory investigations for other underlying causes of hirsutism include the measurement of serum 17-hydroxyprogesterone to investigate 21-hydroxylase deficiency, and serum prolactin and follicle-stimulating hormone levels, particularly in patients with amenorrhoea. Blood glucose and lipid levels may be raised owing to insulin resistance in the PCOS.

The treatment of androgen-dependent hirsutism is a combination of mechanical hair removal and medical therapy. Medical approaches to hirsutism include ovarian suppression, adrenal suppression, antiandrogen therapy and inhibition of 5α-reductase.

Ovarian hyperandrogenism is best treated with ovarian suppression using a combination of oral contraceptives and an antiandrogen. An alternative is to use gonadotrophin-releasing hormone analogues, which suppress pituitary sex hormones leading to ovarian suppression. They can cause oestrogen deficiency, and so supplementation with oestrogens and progestagens is required.

Corticosteroids have been used to suppress adrenal androgen secretion in hirsute women with adrenal hyperandrogenism, e.g. congenital adrenal hyperplasia. They are more effective when combined with antiandrogens.

The two most widely used antiandrogens are spironolactone and cyproterone acetate. Spironolactone binds to the androgen receptor, in competition with dihydrotestosterone. It can be used alone to treat idiopathic hirsutism and is used in combination with the oral contraceptive pill to treat PCOS. Spironolactone should be avoided in patients with renal failure and used cautiously in combination with other potassium-retaining medicines. Cyproterone acetate is a moderately effective antiandrogen. In combination with an oral contraceptive it is the treatment of choice for women with PCOS and elevated serum testosterone levels. Cyclic administration is advised and side effects include amenorrhoea, weight gain and hepatitis.

5α-reductase inhibitors can be used in the treatment of hirsutism. Finasteride should be discontinued before pregnancy as its use in the first trimester is associated with the development of ambiguous genitalia in male fetuses.

Reference

Rittmaster RS 1997 Hirsutism. Lancet 349: 191–195

---

57. Polycystic ovary syndrome
A.F   B.F   C.F   D.T   E.T

Polycystic ovary syndrome (PCOS) is the collection of symptoms associated with anovulation (amenorrhoea or irregular menses) and hyperandrogenism (hirsutism, acne and alopecia) in women with polycystic ovaries. It is the most common cause of hirsutism even in patients with regular menses. The aetiology of PCOS is unknown, but it is thought to result from an interaction between a small number of susceptibility genes and environmental factors. Hyperinsulinaemia and peripheral insulin resistance are now recognized as central features of PCOS. Impaired glucose tolerance is present in 10–40 % of obese patients with the syndrome. The estimated risk of developing non-insulin dependent diabetes mellitus (NIDDM) in later life in women with PCOS is 6–7 times that of weight-matched controls. Patients may suffer from dyslipidaemia.

PCOS is a heterogeneous condition with a spectrum of biochemical and clinical features. It is the underlying cause in 30%

of cases of amenorrhoea. This figure increases to 90% if the oestrogen level is normal. Obesity occurs in 35–40% of patients with PCOS. Other causes of menstrual disturbance with hirsutism include Cushing's disease, acromegaly, hyperprolactinaemia and tumours of the adrenal gland or ovary. In these conditions there are usually other clues to the diagnosis, such as a short history of hirsutism or a significantly raised testosterone level (greater than 5 nmol/l). Late-onset congenital adrenal hyperplasia due to 21-hydroxylase deficiency can be diagnosed by the measurement of 17-α hydroxyprogesterone.

The diagnosis of PCOS is primarily clinical. The typical biochemical features are elevated testosterone and luteinizing hormone (LH) levels, with normal serum follicle-stimulating hormone (FSH) levels. There is considerable variability in the biochemical indices and 50% of patients with all other features of PCOS have normal serum LH. Pelvic ultrasound confirming polycystic ovaries aids the diagnosis, but false negative results are common. Measurement of serum prolactin and oestrogen production should be done in patients with amenorrhoea to exclude prolactinomas and hypothalamic oestrogen-deficient amenorrhoea. Yearly fasting glucose measurements and lipid profile studies should be undertaken in patients with PCOS and obesity.

Treatment is largely symptomatic. Patients with anovulation may require induction of ovulation to achieve fertility. An antioestrogen such as clomiphene is usually effective. Specialist monitoring is suggested as multiple pregnancy can occur. If conception is not desired, oral contraceptives or cyclical progestagens are used. Symptoms of hyperandrogenism can be managed with antiandrogens such as cyproterone acetate. Calorie restriction improves the chances of ovulation and reduces the risk of non-insulin resistant diabetes mellitus.

References

Dunaif A 1997 Insulin resistance and the polycystic ovary syndrome: mechanism and implications for pathogenesis. Endocrine Reviews 18: 774–800

Franks S 1995 Polycystic ovary syndrome. New England Journal of Medicine 333: 853–861

58.   Endocrine hypertension

A.**T**   B.**F**   C.**T**   D.**T**   E.**F**

Hypertension affects 10% of the population at any given time and is thought to be secondary to endocrine causes in 2% of cases. Recognizing a cause of hypertension can often result in cure, and the morbidity and mortality of the underlying condition can be prevented.

Primary hyperaldosteronism has a prevalence of 0.5–3% in patients with essential hypertension. Most cases of primary hyperaldosteronism are due to an aldosterone-producing adenoma (Conn's syndrome). One-third of cases are due to bilateral adrenal hyperplasia and adrenal carcinoma. A rare cause of primary hyperaldosteronism is glucocorticoid-suppressible hyperaldosteronism.

Most patients with primary hyperaldosteronism are asymptomatic and are diagnosed when hypokalaemia is found incidentally. However, studies suggest that up to 30% have normal serum potassium. Patients with primary hyperaldosteronism demonstrate suppression of supine and erect plasma renin activity, with aldosterone levels either elevated or in the upper end of the normal range. The response to adrenocorticotrophin (ACTH) administration will differentiate between adrenal adenoma, adrenal hyperplasia and glucocorticoid-suppressible hyperaldosteronism (GSH). ACTH has no effect on plasma aldosterone in adrenal hyperplasia, a small effect in adrenal adenoma and produces a marked rise in plasma aldosterone in patients with GSH. Imaging by CT or MRI is also helpful, but should be interpreted in conjunction with other investigations as adrenal adenomas are common as an incidental finding.

GSH is a rare autosomal dominant form of low-renin hypertension characterized by aldosterone excess under the control of ACTH. In GSH a 'fusion gene' results in a hybrid enzyme containing components of 11β-hydroxylase 1 and 11β-hydroxylase 2. This synthesizes aldosterone and is controlled by ACTH. The condition can be diagnosed using PCR to confirm the presence of the chimeric gene. The condition is treated with dexamethasone to suppress ACTH, or with amiloride or spironolactone.

Other rare causes of endocrine hypertension are low-renin, low-aldosterone hypertension secondary to congenital adrenal hyperplasia (11β-hydroxylase or 17α-hydroxylase deficiency), Liddle's syndrome, apparent mineralocorticoid excess and liquorice or carbenoxolone ingestion.

Apparent mineralocorticoid excess is secondary to 11β-hydroxysteroid dehydrogenase deficiency. This enzyme catalyzes the inactivation of cortisol to cortisone, thereby preventing overstimulation of mineralocorticoid receptors. Mutatations of the enzyme result in a rare autosomal recessive condition with features of severe hypertension, hypokalaemia and suppression of plasma renin and aldosterone levels. Liquorice also inhibits the activity of this enzyme and produces a similar clinical condition. Treatment is with dexamethasone to suppress cortisol production.

Other endocrine causes of hypertension include states of glucocorticoid excess such as Cushing's syndrome and steroid therapy, phaeochromocytoma, acromegaly and primary hyperparathyroidism. Hypertension is also associated with both hyper- and hypothyroidism.

References

Cleland SJ, Connell JMC 1998 Endocrine hypertension. Journal of the Royal College of Physicians of London 32: 104–108

Ganguly A 1998 Primary aldosteronism. New England Journal of Medicine 339: 1828–1834

59. Phaeochromocytoma

A.F B.F C.T D.F E.T

Phaeochromocytomas are tumours that arise from chromaffin tissue and release catecholamines; 90% arise in the adrenal medulla and 10% from the carotid bodies (chemodectomas), postganglionic sympathetic neurons (ganglioneuromas), in the thorax, abdomen or, very rarely, in the bladder. Noradrenaline and adrenaline are the main hormones released, although other substances, such as endogenous opioids, endothelin and parathyroid hormone-related peptide, are also secreted. Phaeochromocytomas are the underlying diagnosis in 0.1% of patients with hypertension. 10% of phaeochromocytomas are bilateral and 10% malignant. Familial tumours include those occurring in association with multiple endocrine neoplasia type 2, neurofibromatosis and Von Hippel–Lindau disease.

The most common symptoms reported are headache (80%), sweating (70%), palpitations (70%), pallor (40%) and nausea (40%). Tremor, weakness, anxiety, chest pain and dyspnoea are less commonly reported. Sustained hypertension is found in 60% of patients and the remaining 40% have paroxysmal hypertension. 50% of patients are prone to the classic symptoms of headache, sweating, palpitations, chest pain and a feeling of impending doom. Postural hypotension may occur. This is thought to be due to reduced plasma volume and impaired sympathetic reflexes.

Diagnosis is made by measuring (at least three) 24-hour urinary catecholamines or catecholamine metabolites (vanillylmandelic acid or normetadrenaline). The clonidine suppression test involves the administration of clonidine, which suppresses catecholamine production in normal subjects but has no effect in patients with phaeochromocytoma. Once the diagnosis has been made other familial tumours, such as medullary thyroid cancer in multiple endocrine neoplasia, should be excluded.

The management of phaeochromocytoma is initially medical, with α-blockers such as phenoxybenzamine. Only when α-blockade is adequate can β-blockade be commenced. β-blocker therapy alone can result in a dangerous increase in blood pressure. Patients can then be considered for surgery. Preoperative localization of the tumour can be performed using CT or MRI and, with radionucleotide scintiscans after the administration of metaiodobenzylguanidine (MIBG). Operative mortality is 2–3%. The overall prognosis is good, with a 5-year survival rate of 95%. Long-term follow-up is necessary as the recurrence rate is 10%. Yearly catecholamine measurements should be undertaken.

References

MacDougall IC, Isles CG, Stewart H, Inglis GC 1998 Overnight clonidine suppression tests in the diagnosis and exclusion of phaeochromocytoma. American Journal of Medicine 84: 993–1000

Ross EJ, Griffith DNW 1989 The clinical presentation of phaeochromocytoma. Quarterly Journal of Medicine 71: 485 - 496

60. Multiple endocrine neoplasia
A.F   B.F   C.F   D.T   E.T

Multiple endocrine neoplasia (MEN) is an uncommon disease. There are two major forms, both inherited as autosomal dominant disorders. Occasionally MEN syndrome may arise sporadically. Patients with MEN-1 (Werner's syndrome) normally present in adolescence, whereas those with MEN-2 (Sipple's syndrome) present after the age of 20. MEN-2 can be further subdivided into types 2a and 2b.

MEN-1 is characterized by tumours or hyperplasia of the parathyroid glands and tumours of pancreatic islet cells and anterior pituitary gland. Rarely carcinoid tumours, tumours of the adrenal cortex and lipomas also occur. Parathyroid tumours occur in up to 95% of MEN-1 patients and are the first manifestation in approximately 90% of patients. Gastrinomas and insulinomas are the most common form of islet cell tumours. Gastrinomas, leading to the Zollinger–Ellison syndrome, are the most important cause of morbidity and mortality in MEN-1 patients. Anterior pituitary tumours occur in up to 30% of patients and are commonly prolactin or growth hormone (GH) secreting.

The pathogenesis of neoplasia in MEN-1 is thought to be an example of two-hit oncogenesis. Current evidence suggests that a mutation in a tumour suppressor gene occurs sequentially in both gene copies of a tumour precursor cell. The MEN-1 gene has been recently isolated by positional cloning and is located on chromosome 11q13. The 610 amino acid protein product of this gene is called menin, but its function is unclear. Genetic markers can identify patients with the affected haplotype with high sensitivity.

Constant surveillance is required in patients with MEN-1. Biochemical screening of serum calcium and prolactin is necessary in all patients. Measurement of gastrointestinal hormones and further endocrinological tests are required in patients with symptoms suggestive of these tumours.

MEN-2 consists of tumours arising from the thyroid 'C' cell (medullary cell carcinoma), the parathyroid and the adrenal medulla. MEN-2a is the commonest variant. In this variant medullary thyroid cancer (MTC) occurs with phaeochromocytoma in 50% of patients and less commonly with parathyroid tumours (20% of patients). MEN-2b represents 5% of all MEN-2 cases and is characterized by the occurrence of MTC, phaeochromocytoma, marfanoid habitus, mucosal neuromas, medullatoid corneal fibres, and intestinal ganglion dysfunction leading to multiple diverticulae and megacolon.

The genetic abnormality in MEN-2 is located at a region encoding the C-*ret* proto-oncogene on chromosome 10. Specific mutations of C-*ret* have been identified in all MEN variants and mutational analysis of the C-*ret* gene is used in the management of patients and families with this disorder.

Clinical and biochemical screening should be performed every 3–6 months in patients known to have MEN-2. Biochemical screening involves measurement of serum calcitonin, urinary catecholamines and serum calcium and parathyroid hormone levels.

As with MEN-1, the management of MEN-2 is with a combination of medical and surgical therapies. In MEN-2 surgery is the best option for the management of the thyroid and adrenal tumours.

References

Eng C, Clayton D, Schuffenecker I et al. 1996 The relationship between specific RET proto-oncogene mutations and disease phenotype in multiple endocrine neoplasia type 2. Journal of the American Medical Association 276: 1575–1579

Thakker R V 1997 Multiple endocrine neoplasia. Medicine 25: 86–88

61. Type 2 diabetes mellitus
A.F   B.T`   C.T   D.F   E.F

The incidence of type 2 diabetes mellitus is increasing in the UK. 20% of patients with type 2 diabetes will develop macrovascular complications, e.g. myocardial infarction (MI), peripheral vascular disease and stroke, within 10 years of diagnosis. Such complications are a significant cause of mortality in these patients, accounting for 59% of deaths. Microvascular complications will occur in 9% of patients over the same time. Good diabetic control has already been shown to reduce the development and progression of microvascular complications in type 1 diabetes. Readers are referred to the Diabetes Control and Complications Trial (DCCT) for further details.

The United Kingdom Prospective Diabetes Study (UKPDS) was started in 1977. Its aim was to establish whether intensive blood glucose control was of benefit in reducing the microvascular and macrovascular complications of type 2 diabetes. It also studied the outcome with different treatments. Patients were recruited from teaching hospitals and district general hospitals throughout the UK. Criteria for inclusion were newly diagnosed type 2 diabetic patients who had a fasting plasma glucose level between 6.1 and 15 after 3 months of dietary treatment. These patients were randomly assigned to one of three treatment groups: continued diet alone, treatment with a sulphonylurea, or treatment with insulin. Exclusions were made on the basis of existing renal failure, hypertension, retinopathy requiring laser treatment, and recent MI or other major vascular event. Additional treatment was given if patients had marked hyperglycaemia (fasting plasma glucose >15 or symptoms).

Three endpoints were studied. First, any diabetes-related endpoint, e.g. MI, renal failure, sudden death, amputation, stroke, hypoglycaemia, marked hyperglycaemia and blindness; second, any diabetes-related death, e.g. sudden death, MI, stroke, renal failure, peripheral vascular disease etc; third, all-cause mortality. The median follow-up time for endpoint analyses was 10 years and the comparative therapy analyses was 11 years.

Overall diabetic control as assessed by measurements of HbA1c was significantly better in drug treatment groups than diet alone. There was a 25% risk reduction of developing microvascular complications in the drug-treated groups compared to diet alone. However, intensive blood glucose control did not significantly decrease the risk of macrovascular disease, myocardial infarction or diabetes-related mortality.

There was no difference in endpoints between the three intensive agents, chlorpropamide, glibenclamide or insulin. It was noted that chlorpropamide was associated with higher blood pressure than glibenclamide or insulin. All intensive treatments increased the risk of hypoglycaemia and weight gain.

Metformin lowers fasting plasma insulin and acts as a hypoglycaemic agent by enhancing insulin sensitivity and inducing greater peripheral uptake of glucose. Improved blood glucose control can therefore be achieved without weight gain. Metformin has a low risk of causing lactic acidosis and, provided its use is avoided in patients with renal failure, can be used safely in type 2 diabetes.

The UKPDS included metformin in its treatment regimens. Metformin was added to a sulphonylurea or insulin in overweight patients, or in normal-weight patients if glycaemic control was inadequate. However, the addition of metformin to patients already on treatment with sulphonylureas resulted in a significant increase in diabetes-related death and all-cause mortality. This analysis included obese and non-obese patients. Metformin alone may have a useful role in the treatment of obese patients. Hence further study of this combination therapy is required.

A study of metformin plus diet in overweight type 2 diabetic patients compared with diet alone was performed. This trial revealed a risk reduction in any diabetes-related endpoint, diabetes-related death, or mortality from any cause in the metformin-treated group. These results may be explained in part by the action of metformin in decreasing plasminogen-activator inhibitor type 1 (PAI-1) levels, which in turn increases thrombolysis.

Metformin treatment was compared to treatment with a sulphonylurea or insulin in obese patients. Metformin therapy was associated with less weight gain and fewer hypoglycaemic episodes than insulin or sulphonylurea therapy, and may be the first-line therapy of choice in obese patients.

A new class of drug, the thiazolidinediones, is being developed for the treatment of patients with type 2 diabetes. These reduce insulin resistance in type 2 diabetes without producing hypoglycaemia. They also decrease PAI-1 production and increase insulin sensitivity.

References

Diabetes Control and Complication Trial Research Group 1993 The effect of intensive treatment of diabetes on the development and progression of long-term complications in insulin-dependent diabetes mellitus. New England Journal of Medicine 329 (14): 977–986

Inzucchi SE, Maggs DG, Spollett GR et al. 1998 Efficacy and metabolic effects of metformin and troglitazone in type 2 diabetes mellitus. New England Journal of Medicine 338: 867–872

UK Prospective Diabetes Study Group 1998 Intensive blood glucose control with sulphonylureas or insulin compared with conventional treatment and risk of complications in patients with type 2 diabetes. Lancet 352: 837–853

UK Prospective Diabetes Study Group 1998 Effect of intensive blood glucose control with metformin on complications in overweight patients with type 2 diabetes. Lancet 352: 854–865

62. Type 2 diabetes mellitus

A.T   B.T   C.F   D.T   E.T

Recent studies have changed the approach to the diagnosis and management of patients with diabetes mellitus. In 1997 the American Diabetes Association established new criteria which simplified its diagnosis. The fasting plasma glucose criteria were lowered to values greater than 7.0 mmol/l and the use of the oral glucose tolerance test was no longer recommended. Impaired plasma glucose was defined as a fasting plasma glucose level between 6.1 and 7.0 mmol/l. Up to one-third of type 2 diabetic patients are undiagnosed, and these recommendations were intended to simplify diagnosis.

Type 2 diabetes and hypertension are common medical disorders and both are associated with increased risk of cardiovascular and renal disease. The prevalence of hypertension in the type 2 diabetic population is increased compared with the normal population, especially in younger patients. The UK Prospective Diabetes Study provided evidence that, in addition to controlling blood glucose, control of hypertension in type 2 diabetics led to a reduction in diabetes-related deaths and complications, including progression to retinopathy and deterioration in visual acuity.

In terms of blood pressure control, the trial was divided into two arms. One arm was tight control aiming for BP values of less than 150/85 mmHg. The second arm was of less tight control with a target BP of less than 180/105 mmHg. The median overall follow-up was 8.4 years, and investigators found acceptable levels of compliance with treatment, indicating that the results of the trial might be reproducible in normal clinical practice. Overall the tight blood pressure control group had a 24% risk reduction in all diabetes-related endpoints and a 32% risk reduction in deaths due to diabetes. The risk reduction in microvascular disease was clinically and statistically significant, particularly when considering retinopathy. Although there was a clear trend towards a reduction in risk for macrovascular disease, the reported risk reduction in myocardial infarction and peripheral vascular disease failed to achieve statistical significance. There was a significant reduction in risk of stroke with tight blood pressure control. The study emphasizes the need for good blood pressure control in the management of type 2 diabetes.

The treatments used were either an ACE inhibitor (captopril) or a β-blocker (atenolol). A second concurrent analysis showed similiar benefits to blood pressure control irrespective of whether ACEI or β-blocker therapy was used, suggesting that blood pressure reduction itself was more important than the treatment used.

Patients with diabetes who suffer a myocardial infarction have poorer short- and long-term prognoses than patients without diabetes. 620 patients were studied and randomly assigned to receive standard care or standard care plus intensive glycaemic control for the first 24 hours postinfarction, followed by subcutaneous insulin for at least 3 months. Results at 3.5 years showed an absolute reduction in mortality of 11% with intensive glycaemic control. The effect was most apparent in patients who had not previously received insulin and who were at low cardiovascular risk.

References

Expert Committee on the Diagnosis and Classification of Diabetes Mellitus 1998 Report. Diabetes Care. 21: S5–S19

Malmberg K 1997 Prospective randomised study of intensive insulin treatment on long-term survival after acute myocardial infarction in patients with diabetes mellitus DIGAMI Study Group. British Medical Journal 314: 1512–1515

UK Prospective Diabetes Study Group 1998 Tight blood pressure control and risk of macrovascular and microvascular complications in type 2 diabetes. British Medical Journal 317: 703–713

UK Prospective Diabetes Study Group 1998 Efficacy of atenolol and captopril in reducing risk of macrovascular and microvascular complications in type 2 diabetes. British Medical Journal. 317: 13–20

63. Hypothyroidism

A.F B.T C.F D.F E.T

Hypothyroidism occurs as a result of a deficiency of the thyroid hormones, thyroxine (T_4) and triiodothyronine (T_3). The prevalence of hypothyroidism is approximately 15 per 1000 in females and 1 per 1000 in males. In the west 90% of cases of primary hypothyroidism are due to autoimmune (Hashimoto's) thyroiditis, idiopathic atrophy or previous treatment of hyperthyroidism with radioiodine or surgery. Other causes include iodine deficiency (common worldwide), antithyroid drugs, subacute thyroiditis, dyshormonogenesis, infiltrative disease and hypothalamic and pituitary disease. There are rare associations of hypothyroidism with cystic fibrosis, primary biliary cirrhosis and POEMS syndrome (polyneuropathy, organomegaly, endocrinopathy, M-protein band from plasmacytoma and skin pigmentation).

The most common features of hypothyroidism are tiredness, weight gain, cold intolerance, goitre, hyperlipidaemia, bradycardia, dry skin and myalgia. However, the presenting symptoms and signs are diverse and reflect the widespread tissue actions of thyroid hormones. The onset of hypothyroidism is often insidious and in mild illness symptoms and signs may be absent. A reduction in free or total T_4 with a rise in TSH indicates primary hypothyroidism. Secondary hypothyroidism is indicated by a reduction in free and total T_4 and a serum TSH level within or below the normal range. This biochemical picture can also be seen in patients with non-thyroidal illness or on corticosteroid or anticonvulsant therapy. An elevated serum TSH in association with normal serum T_4 is termed subclinical hypothyroidism. Measurements of T_3 and antithyroid antibodies are unhelpful in making the diagnosis. Associated findings are raised cholesterol and triglycerides, a normochromic, macrocytic anaemia and hyponatraemia. Elevated creatine kinase (CK), aspartate transaminase (AST) and lactate dehydrogenase (LDH) are also seen.

Patients treated with amiodarone commonly have a rise in free T_4 and fall in free T_3 but the clinical state is variable. 2% of patients exhibit clinically significant changes, which are the best guide to treatment requirements.

Treatment of patients with hypothyroidism is with lifelong thyroxine therapy. Symptomatic improvement can be seen within 2–3 weeks.

Serum TSH levels return to normal in 6 weeks, which is therefore the interval that should be allowed after a change in dose. The objective of therapy is to restore T_4 and TSH to normal levels and once stable, annual measurement of TSH ensures adequacy of therapy and compliance. Patients with ischaemic heart disease and the elderly should be commenced on a low dose of T_4 with close monitoring as T_4 therapy may precipitate angina or myocardial infarction. Effective thyroxine therapy is particularly important in patients with ischaemic heart disease because it corrects the hypercholesterolaemia of hypothyroidism.

After radioiodine treatment for hyperthyroidism many patients have subclinical hypothyroidism with a biochemical profile consistent with hypothyroidism. Thyroxine replacement in these patients may improve atheroma and hypercholesterolaemia. It is recommended that thyroxine is given to those patients with positive thyroid antibodies, organ-specific autoimmunity, previously treated Graves' disease or previous treatment with radioiodine because these patients have a higher risk of developing thyroid failure. In patients not treated, thyroid status should be checked every 6 months.

Reference

Vanderpump PM, Ahlquist JAO, Franklyn JA, Clayton RN 1996 Consensus statement for good practice and audit measures in the management of hypothyroidism and hyperthyroidism. British Medical Journal 313: 539–544

64. Primary hypothyroidism

A.T   B.T   C.F   D.F   E.F

Hypothyroidism is the term used to describe deficiency of thyroid hormone secretion from the thyroid gland. It can be primary (thyroid gland), secondary (pituitary) or tertiary (hypothalamus) and can be congenital or acquired.

Thyroid hormone secretion is under the control of a negative feedback loop including the hypothalamus, the anterior pituitary and the thyroid gland. Thyrotropin-releasing hormone (TRH) from the hypothalamus stimulates the release of thyrotropin (TSH) from the anterior pituitary which stimulates the release of thyroxine (T_4) and triiodothyronine (T_3) from the follicular cells of the thyroid. T_3 and T_4 suppress the release of TRH and TSH. Only 20% of total T_3 is produced by the thyroid. The majority is produced peripherally by deiodination of T_4. It is T_4 that is the more reliable of the two thyroid hormones in diagnosing hypothyroidism.

Detection of a low T_4 and a raised TSH is diagnostic of primary hypothyroidism. Secondary hypothyroidism due to pituitary failure is rare. In this case the TSH is also reduced. In the diagnosis of hypothyroidism other laboratory features may be helpful, including a normochromic, macrocytic anaemia, hyperlipidaemia and autoantibody detection.

The commonest cause of congenital hypothyroidism is thyroid dysgenesis. Although hypothyroidism occurs in 1 in 4000 live births, it is difficult to detect clinically. Clinical signs include macroglossia, prolonged neonatal jaundice and hypotonia. Thyroid hormones are important in intellectual development, and screening programmes exist to diagnose the condition at birth.

The commonest cause of adult acquired primary hypothyroidism is autoimmune disease. Hashimoto's disease is autoimmune thyroiditis with goitre, and may initially present with a transient hyperthyroidism. Autoimmune disease is diagnosed by the detection of antithyroglobulin and antiperoxidase antibodies in the presence of biochemical or clinical hypothyroidism.

Drugs are an important cause of primary hypothyroidism. They include the antithyroid drugs carbimazole and propylthiouracil, α-interferon therapy, lithium and amiodarone. Oral or topical iodine can cause hypothyroidism in the presence of autoimmune disease, whereas iodine deficiency is an important environmental cause of hypothyroidism.

Transient hypothyroidism is seen following subacute thyroiditis (de Quervain's thyroiditis), postpartum thyroiditis and post radioiodine treatment of Grave's disease or subtotal thyroidectomy. Transient causes of hypothyroidism may not require treatment unless the patient is symptomatic, in which case treatment can usually be reduced or withdrawn after a period of time.

Grave's disease is the commonest cause of hyperthyroidism and thyrotoxicosis. Hypothyroidism is seen in association with this condition as a result of the iatrogenic effect of treatment, not as a result of the disease per se. Treatment for this condition includes radioiodine therapy, which is safe, inexpensive and easily administered. Hypothyroidism is usually transient following this treatment. The alternative, indicated by goitre, patient preference or failure of radioiodine therapy, is total thyroidectomy, in which case lifelong thyroxine treatment will be needed for the subsequent hypothyroidism.

Medullary and follicular cell carcinomas of the thyroid rarely present with hyper- or hypothyroidism. Patients are usually euthyroid and the commonest presentation is with a thyroid nodule. Diagnosis is by fine needle aspirate and cytology, in conjunction with ultrasonography. In their early stages these cancers have a good prognosis, being amenable to surgery and radioablation. Hypothyroidism may occur as a result of therapy.

References

Lazarus JH 1997 Hyperthyroidism. Lancet 349: 339–343

Lindsay RS, Toft AD 1997 Hypothyroidism. Lancet 349: 413–417

Schlumberger MJ 1998 Papillary and follicular thyroid carcinoma. New England Journal of Medicine 338: 297–306

65. Primary hyperparathyroidism
A.F   B.F   C.T   D.F   E.T

Primary hyperparathyroidism is a common disorder of excessive parathyroid hormone secretion leading to hypercalcaemia. It is often asymptomatic and most patients are detected during routine blood testing. It most commonly presents between 40–60 years of age and is uncommon in childhood. It is more common in women than in men. The most common cause is a single parathyroid adenoma. Multiple adenomata and carcinoma are rare. Diffuse parathyroid hyperplasia occurs in about 20% of cases. Many of these cases will have other associated disorders as part of a familial syndrome such as Werner's or Sipple's syndrome (MEN-1 and-2).

Symptoms related to primary hyperparathyroidism are due to disordered calcium metabolism, with lack of the normal negative feedback control to the parathyroid glands. The classic bone disease is osteitis fibrosa cystica. In this uncommon condition there is increased cellularity of cortical bone, with both osteoclasts and osteoblasts. Bone resorption dominates over bone formation, with resultant bony cysts. On X-ray discrete lytic lesions of varying size, cysts and brown tumours can be seen, along with subperiosteal resorption. Tiny punched-out lesions in the skull produce a salt-and-pepper appearance. Osteoporosis is commonly seen as an X-ray feature in primary hyperparathyroidism.

Primary hyperparathyroidism is not associated with renal failure, but there is hypercalciuria and nephrolithiasis is the most common complication. Primary hyperparathyroidism is the underlying cause of 5% of renal calculi. Nephrocalcinosis is less common and is detected on X-ray as a diffuse deposition of calcium and phosphate throughout the kidneys.

Other clinical features of primary hyperparathyroidism include psychiatric symptoms, lethargy, muscle weakness and gastrointestinal symptoms.

Secondary and tertiary hyperparathyroidism are associated with chronic renal failure. In chronic renal failure hypocalcaemia is a common finding. This is partly due to vitamin D deficiency secondary to impaired production of 1,25-dihydroxycalciferol. As a result there is resistance to the metabolic effects of parathyroid hormone, which further exacerbates hypocalcaemia. The hypocalcaemia induces parathyroid gland hyperplasia and secondary hyperparathyroidism. Eventually parathyroid secretion becomes autonomous and tertiary hyperparathyroidism results.

The diagnosis of primary hyperparathyroidism is made using the intact parathyroid hormone (PTH) assay when a raised PTH level is found. Lithium therapy needs to be excluded as a cause of raised PTH with hypercalcaemia. Very occasionally patients with familial hypocalciuric hypercalcaemia will have a raised PTH level. However, in contrast to primary hyperparathyroidism these patients have low urinary calcium excretion.

Not all patients with primary hyperparathyroidism need surgery, as many will not develop symptoms or complications of the disease. Parathyroidectomy is indicated for young patients, those who have had an episode of symptomatic hyperparathyroidism, patients with renal disease or complications, bone disease including significant osteoporosis, and for patients with a serum calcium persistently greater than 0.25 mmol/l above the normal range. Complications of surgery include a transient hypocalcaemia, recurrent laryngeal nerve injury and hypothyroidism. Conservative management includes monitoring of serum and urinary calcium and renal function. Bone density monitoring is performed in some centres. Calcium and vitamin D supplements should be avoided and thiazide diuretics discontinued. Patients should maintain good hydration. In patients unfit for surgery bisphosphonates can produce short-term control of hypercalcaemia, but their long-term use for this purpose is not established. Phosphate supplements can lower serum calcium and increase urinary calcium excretion. Hormone replacement therapy can be used to help prevent osteoporosis in postmenopausal women.

Mucocutaneous candidiasis occurs in association with hypoparathyroidism and adrenal insufficiency in type I autoimmune polyglandular syndrome. Type II autoimmune polyglandular syndrome consists of adrenal insufficiency, autoimmune thyroid disease and insulin-dependent diabetes mellitus.

Reference

Al Zahrani A, Levine MA 1997 Primary hyperparathyroidism. Lancet 349: 1233–1238

66. Adult growth hormone deficiency

A.**T** B.**F** C.**T** D.**T** E.**F**

The importance of diagnosing and treating adult growth hormone deficiency (GHD) is increasingly recognized. GHD may have important adverse metabolic effects in adults which could be reversed or attenuated with GH replacement therapy. The true prevalence of adult GHD is unknown, but estimates vary between 1 in 10 000 and 1 in 100 000. Adult-onset GHD is predominantly secondary to structural abnormality in the pituitary gland, where growth hormone is produced under the regulatory influence of growth hormone-releasing hormone (GHRH). Two-thirds of cases are secondary to pituitary macroadenomas. Other causes include craniopharyngioma, parasellar meningioma and cranial irradiation. Rare causes include suprasellar germ cell tumours, lymphocytic hypophysitis, Langhans' cell histiocytosis, sarcoidosis, haemochromatosis, trauma and postpartum pituitary necrosis.

It is important to differentiate adult-onset GHD from childhood onset, which is normally secondary to isolated deficiency of GHRH rather than structural causes. Childhood-onset GHD often does not persist into adult life. Repeat investigation when the active growth period has finished is necessary to determine the need for continuing treatment in these children.

The clinical features associated with adult GHD are increased central adiposity, decreased muscle mass and decreased energy. Subjective and objective measures of physical and psychological wellbeing are impaired. There is a reduction in the regulatory response to hypoglycaemia but a paradoxical reduction in insulin sensitivity and an increased incidence of impaired glucose tolerance. Studies have revealed that there is a twofold increase in mortality from cardiac and cerebrovascular disease. A contributory factor in this may be impaired lipid metabolism. Growth hormone-deficient adults have significantly raised serum triglyceride and high-density lipoprotein levels compared to control populations. There is a reduction in bone mineral density, which predisposes affected adults to an increased risk of osteoporotic fractures, and significant psychological effects of depressed mood, anxiety and social withdrawal.

The diagnosis of adult GHD is made using the insulin hypoglycaemia test. Peak GH concentrations below 3 ng/ml are diagnostic of deficiency. Single measurements of serum insulin-like growth factor 1 (IGF-1) are in the low or low to normal range in 30–50% of patients, and are insufficient as a single diagnostic test.

Criteria to select patients suitable for GH replacement therapy include clinical features, the insulin hypoglycaemia test and evidence of normal or remaining pituitary function. Recombinant GH (rGH) is given via daily subcutaneous injection and serum IGF-1 levels can be used to titrate therapy. Patients often demonstrate an improvement in central adiposity, with favourable changes in low-density lipoprotein and high-density lipoprotein cholesterol within 3 months of starting treatment. Insulin sensitivity returns to baseline by 12 months. GH replacement therapy has also been shown to increase bone mineral density and improve psychological wellbeing. Long-term administration of rGH can have adverse effects, which include carpal tunnel syndrome, oedema, hypertension and arthralgia. These effects are mostly dose related, as reflected by increased plasma IGF-1 levels. The incidence of side effects may be reduced by starting GH replacement at low doses.

References

Labram EK, Wilkin TJ 1995 Growth hormone deficiency in adults and its response to growth hormone replacement. Quarterly Journal of Medicine 88: 391–399

Monson J P 1998 Adult growth hormone deficiency. Journal of the Royal College of Physicians of London 32: 19–22

67. Carcinoid tumours

A.F   B.T   C.T   D.F   E.F

Carcinoid tumours are neuroendocrine tumours that arise from the foregut, midgut and hindgut and derive from enterochromaffin cells. The commonest site for carcinoid tumours is the appendix. They are also found in the ileum, small intestine, stomach, colon and rectum, and can arise in the bronchi. Bronchial carcinoid tumours may present with features of Cushing's syndrome owing to ectopic corticotrophin release. Carcinoid tumours usually present insidiously with local symptoms. The carcinoid syndrome is an unusual presentation.

Carcinoid tumours may be multiple. They are associated with adenocarcinomas, most commonly synchronous adenocarcinoma of the colon, and other tumours arising in patients with multiple endocrine neoplasia type 1. Patients with MEN-1 may have gastrinomas, producing the Zollinger–Ellison syndrome.

The diagnosis of carcinoid is confirmed histologically by the detection of 5-hydroxytryptamine, a breakdown product of dietary tryptophan, in tumour cells. Other detectable peptide products include kinins, substance P and gastrin.

The carcinoid syndrome is an uncommon presentation of carcinoid tumours. The commonest symptoms of this syndrome are flushing, diarrhoea and abdominal pain. Patients may develop wheezing, right-sided heart failure due to tricuspid and pulmonary valve fibrosis, and pellagra. Pellagra is a feature of nicotinic acid deficiency. The latter develops as a result of the abnormal tryptophan metabolism, which is normally used to synthesize nicotinic acid. Clinically the diagnosis is made by detecting high urinary excretion of a breakdown product of 5-hydroxytryptamine called 5-hydroxyindoleacetic acid.

Surgery is the only curative treatment and isolated primary carcinoids are ideally managed with local excision and draining of lymph nodes. Symptomatic treatment with octreotide inhibits 5-hydroxytryptamine release and is useful for patients with carcinoid syndrome who suffer from diarrhoea. For symptom control, hepatic metastases can be effectively treated by hepatic artery embolization. Current research is investigating the neuroendocrine peptide receptors on carcinoid cells as a possible target for treatment.

References

Caplin ME, Buscombe JR, Hilson AJ, Jones AL, Watkinson AF, Burroughs AK 1998 Carcinoid tumour. Lancet 352: 799–805

Halford S, Waxman J 1998 The management of carcinoid tumours. Quarterly Journal of Medicine 91: 795–798

CARDIOLOGY

68. Cardiac physiology
A.T   B.F   C.T   D.T   E.T

Diastole is the period from closure of the aortic valve to closure of the mitral valve. It consists of four phases:

1. Isovolumetric relaxation (aortic closure to mitral valve opening)
2. Early rapid filling due to transmitral pressure difference. This phase involves energy-dependent myocardial relaxation and contributes to 80% of left ventricular (LV) filling
3. Slow filling
4. Atrial contraction, which contributes 15% of LV filling.

Diastolic dysfunction may be considered as impaired left ventricular (LV) filling or impaired diastolic function. Impaired LV filling may be due to either pericardial disease (constriction or tamponade) or mitral stenosis. Impaired diastolic function is due to impaired ventricular relaxation (e.g. ischaemia), increased compliance (LV hypertrophy due to hypertension, hypertrophic obstructive cardiomyopathy or aortic stenosis) or restriction of the LV (infiltrative disease, e.g. amyloid or cardiomyopathy).

Diagnosis usually relies on echocardiography. Technetium-99 (^{99m}Tc) labelled red cells can be used during angiography to derive LV diastolic volume measurements. Doppler echo of transmitral flow enables non-invasive serial measurements of diastolic function. As it takes longer for the LV pressure to decrease below left atrial pressure, an altered transmitral flow wave pattern is seen with an increased isovolumetric relaxation time.

Decreased LV compliance results in reduced LV filling and reduced stroke volume. Initially, this manifests as low-output cardiac failure; however, as diastolic dysfunction worsens LV filling pressures are increased, resulting in pulmonary congestion. Symptoms of heart failure may occur in the presence of normal systolic function.

Treatment includes treating the underlying cause (e.g. revascularization for ischaemia) and angiotensin-converting enzyme (ACE) inhibitors for concomitent systolic impairment. There is a paucity of clinical trials of treatments for isolated diastolic dysfunction; however, β-blockers have been shown to improve LV filling by reducing heart rate and increasing the duration of diastole. This has the added advantage of reducing myocardial oxygen demand.

References

Mayet J, Foale R A 1998 Diastolic dysfunction. Cardiology News 1(3): 6–10

Wheeldon N, Clarkson P 1994 Diastolic heart failure. European Heart Journal 15: 1689–1697

---

69. Unstable angina and non-Q wave myocardial infarction

A.T   B.T   C.F   D.F   E.T

In the acute phase both unstable angina and non-Q wave MI carry a poor prognosis. Despite treatment with unfractionated heparin (UFH) and aspirin, approximately 10% of patients suffer a myocardial infarction (MI) or die in the 30 days following an episode of unstable angina or a non-Q wave MI.

Rupture or fissuring of an atherosclerotic plaque triggers platelet aggregation and activation. The resultant tissue factor (TF) release induces the coagulation cascade. TF and factor VIIa activate factor Xa, which catalyses the formation of thrombin. This in turn converts fibrinogen to fibrin, stabilizing the thrombus. Antiplatelet and antithrombin therapies are used in acute coronary syndromes. Thrombolysis has not been shown to be of any benefit in unstable angina.

Low molecular weight heparins (LMWH) act mainly via antithrombin III-mediated inhibition of factor Xa. LMWH has many advantages over UFH, including a more predictable anticoagulant effect, no requirement for monitoring, improved bioavailability and a reduced incidence of heparin-induced thrombocytopenia (HITS).

The FRISC trial (fragmin during instability in coronary artery disease) was a double-blind placebo-controlled trial which compared the LMWH deltaparin with placebo in patients with unstable angina or non-Q wave MI. At 6 days the rate of MI or death was 1.8% in the deltaparin group, versus 4.8% in the placebo group. Benefit was seen at 40 days but was no longer apparent at 150 days.

The ESSENCE (efficacy and safety of subcutaneous enoxaparin in non-Q wave coronary events) trial showed beneficial effects of LMWH over UFH in unstable angina in the presence of aspirin. At 14 days the risk of death, MI and recurrent angina was 16.6% in the LMWH group and 19.8% in the UFH group. This benefit was still apparent at 30 days and 1 year. A lower requirement for revascularization was seen at 1 year in the LMWH group compared to the UFH group.

References

Cohen M, Demers M, Gerfinkel M et al. 1997 ESSENCE study group. New England Journal of Medicine 337: 447–452

Fox K 1998 The role of the antithrombins in improving outcome in unstable angina. British Journal of Cardiology 5 (2): S2–S11

Toss H, Lindahl B, Wallentin L et al. 1996 FRISC Study Group. Lancet 347: 561–568

70. Ventricular fibrillation

A.**T**   B.**T**   C.**T**   D.**T**   E.**T**

Few clinical trials have been conducted to study drug therapy in cardiac arrest. Those that have been performed have used restoration of a spontaneous circulation, hospital admission (for cardiac arrest in the community) and hospital discharge (indicating longer-term survival) as endpoints.

During resuscitation adrenaline increases aortic diastolic blood pressure and coronary perfusion, improving cerebral and coronary flow, but at higher doses reduces blood flow to other vital organs and induces increased myocardial oxygen demand and myocardial injury. Adrenaline may also induce ventricular arrhythmia. The few trials performed in cardiac arrest suggest that using standard-dose adrenaline (1 mg) increases rates of restoration of spontaneous circulation and hospital admission. These endpoints were further increased using high-dose (5 mg) adrenaline. No increase in hospital discharge rate was seen.

Lignocaine has been recommended as an adjunctive treatment for VF resistant to DC shock, although the European resuscitation council guidelines now recommend its use only in the late stages of VF management after 12 DC shocks. There is evidence that lignocaine is associated with a significantly increased restoration of spontaneous circulation and hospital admission rates, but increased survival has not been demonstrated.

Amiodarone decreases the defibrillation threshold and consequently improves the response to defibrillation in resistant VF. In the ARREST trial a bolus of intravenous amiodarone or placebo was given after three unsuccessful DC shocks. Amiodarone had significant beneficial effects on defibrillation and increased admission to hospital. This trial supports the earlier administration of Class III agents as defibrillation adjuncts.

Bretylium tosylate has class III antiarrhythmic action. It also releases noradrenaline from nerve terminals, inducing hypotension. However, this does not increase the defibrillation threshold. It has a direct antifibrillatory effect, leading to spontaneous reversion to sinus rhythm as well as increased success with DC shocks.

Class I antiarrhythmic agents (e.g. flecainide and mexiletine) increase the defibrillation threshold and are thus unhelpful in resistant VF.

The use of sodium bicarbonate to overcome metabolic acidosis during cardiac arrest is controversial. It can increase intracellular acidosis, decrease cardiac output and cause a left shift in the oxygen dissociation curve, leading to reduced oxygen release to the tissues. Trials have not produced definitive evidence of benefit, and concentrating on producing adequate alveolar ventilation remains the mainstay of control of acid–base disturbance in arrest. Sodium bicarbonate may be indicated in severe acidosis (pH <7.1, base excess >10), after prolonged arrest (10–20 min) and in arrest associated with hyperkalaemia or tricyclic antidepressant overdose.

References

Adgey A 1998 Approaches to modern management of cardiac arrest. Heart 80: 397–414

European Resuscitation Council 1998 Guidelines for adult advanced life support. Resuscitation 37(2): 81–90

71. Chronic heart failure
A.T   B.F   C.T   D.F   E.T

Decreased cardiac pump function, e.g. after myocardial infarction (MI) or in dilated cardiomyopathy (DCM), results in neurohormonal activation with increases in noradrenaline, angiotensin II, aldosterone and antidiuretic hormone (ADH). This results in vasoconstriction, renal salt and water retention and ventricular remodelling (hypertrophy and dilatation). These substances downregulate β_1 adrenoceptors by 50% and therefore decrease intracellular cAMP and calcium uptake by the sarcoplasmic reticulum (SR), with subsequent systolic and diastolic dysfunction. In severe heart failure both the force of myocardial contraction and cardiac output (CO) decrease at high heart rates, resulting in a worsening of heart failure. This is the rationale for using β-blockers to slow heart rate. Prolongation of diastole allows the SR calcium ATPase to pump more calcium into the SR for release during systole, improving CO and coronary flow.

β-Blockers have a biphasic effect on myocardial function and clinical symptoms. As the heart is withdrawn from adrenergic support, the acute pharmacological effect is myocardial depression. After 1–3 months of treatment there is an improvement in intrinsic systolic function, together with a reduction in systolic and diastolic left ventricular (LV) volumes and improvement in LV ejection fraction (LVEF). After 4–12 months there is reversal of remodelling with a decrease in LV mass, improvement in LV shape and reduced mitral regurgitation.

β-Blockers have major benefits in the treatment of chronic congestive cardiac failure (CCF). Three recent trials are of particular importance. These trials used either bisoprolol, metoprolol or the third-generation vasodilating β-blocker carvedilol. The MDC (metoprolol in DCM) trial demonstrated a significant increase in LVEF and reduction in hospitalization for cardiac decompensation but no effect on mortality. CIBIS (cardiac insufficiency bisoprolol study) included both idiopathic DCM and ischaemic cardiomyopathy with LVEF <40%. This study showed a 20% reduction in mortality (which was non-significant) and fewer hospitalizations, with the greatest mortality reduction in the DCM group (53%). Combined analysis of the US Carvedilol Heart Failure Study Program has shown a dose-related improvement in LVEF, reduced hospitalizations in mild heart failure (New York Heart Association II) and improved symptomatic status in moderate to severe heart failure (New York Heart Association III/IV). The ANZ (Australia and New Zealand) study also showed clear long-term benefit in terms of mortality and morbidity among patients treated with carvedilol. β-Blockers are well tolerated in heart failure patients with similar withdrawal rates to placebo (5–15%).

Most recently, CIBIS II was stopped prematurely when a highly significant mortality trend favouring bisoprolol was seen. Among patients treated with bisoprolol rather than placebo there was a 32% relative reduction of annual all-cause mortality in CCF, a 45% reduction of sudden death and a 30% reduction in hospitalisations for worsening heart failure.

References

Heidreich P 1997 Effect of β-blockade on mortality in heart failure (a meta-analysis). Journal of the American College of Cardiologists 30: 27–34

Packer M, Bristow M 1996 The effect of carvedilol on morbidity and mortality in patients with chronic heart failure. New England Journal of Medicine 334: 1349–1355

Remme W 1998 β-Blockade in congestive heart failure: time for consideration. Heart 79 (Supp): 2

72. Chronic heart failure

A.F   B.F   C.F   D.F   E.T

Digoxin has been used for many years in the treatment of heart failure and has now become established for patients in sinus rhythm. It increases calcium influx via the sodium/calcium exchanger in the sarcolemmal membranes, resulting in increased myocardial contractility. It also improves baroreceptor function and inhibits renin secretion. The RADIANCE and PROVED trials were short-term randomized trials which indicated that withdrawing digoxin worsens functional status, exercise capacity and left ventricular ejection fraction in patients with heart failure. The DIG (Digitalis Investigation Group) study was a randomized double-blind placebo-controlled trial of digoxin in patients with heart failure and normal sinus rhythm. After 3–5 years there was no overall effect on mortality of adding digoxin in patients receiving diuretics and ACE inhibitors but the overall number of hospitalizations and the combined endpoints of death and hospitalization attributable to worsening heart failure were reduced.

It is well established that angiotensin-converting enzyme (ACE) inhibitors reduce morbidity and mortality in patients with congestive cardiac failure (CCF). This is attributed to blockade of angiotensin II production and a decrease in bradykinin breakdown. Bradykinin reduces nitric oxide and prostacyclin, which improves endothelial function. These actions are also responsible for adverse reactions such as cough, angio-oedema, and renal dysfunction. Surveys have shown that in the UK ACE inhibitors are used in <30% of patients with heart failure.

Angiotensin II (ATII) receptor antagonists directly inhibit the ATII receptor. Several studies showed the efficacy of losartan in CCF. ELITE evaluated the effects of losartan compared to captopril when added to digitalis and diuretics for one year in 722 elderly patients with CCF and an ejection fraction <40%. Losartan produced a 46% absolute reduction in all-cause mortality compared to captopril, mostly owing to a decrease in sudden death (64%). In addition, losartan was better tolerated. However, this was a safety study and was not designed with mortality as a primary endpoint. The results of ELITE II (a larger definitive trial of losartan on morbidity and mortality) were disappointing.

In terms of mortality it is possible that patients who are intolerant of ACE inhibitors may benefit from ATII antagonists. These drugs may be an important step in the management of heart failure, either alone or in combination with ACE inhibitors. The RESOLVD trial (a randomized evaluation of strategies for LV dysfunction) is addressing this issue.

References

Garg R, Gorhin R, Smith T, et al. 1997 DIG (effect of digoxin on mortality and morbidity in patients with heart failure). New England Journal of Medicine 336: 525–533

Packer M, Gheorghiade M, Young J, et al. 1993 RADIANCE (withdrawal of digoxin from patients with CHF treated with ACE inhibitors). New England Journal of Medicine 329: 1–7

Pitt B, Segal R, Martinez F et al. 1997 ELITE (randomised trial of losartan vs. captopril in patients over 65 with heart failure). Lancet 349: 747–752

Struthers A 1998 Angiotensin II receptor antagonists for heart failure. Heart 80: 5–6

Urtsky B, Young J, Shahidi F et al. 1993 PROVED (randomised study assessing effect of digoxin withdrawal in patients with mild–moderate CCF). Journal of the American College of Cardiology 22: 955–962

73.   Ischaemic heart disease
A.F   B.F   C.F   D.T   E.T

Triglycerides (TG) are recognized to be associated with atherogenesis via several mechanisms, including effects on endothelial function, macrophage loading and thrombogenesis. Evidence from the PROCAM study showed a significant and independent association between serum TG concentrations and the incidence of major coronary events. A meta-analysis of over 28 000 patients, controlling for HDL cholesterol, showed that for every 1 mmol increase in serum TG concentration the relative risk of ischaemic heart disease (IHD) increases by 14% in men and by 37% in women. Angiographic studies have also confirmed that progression of coronary atherosclerosis and coronary events is reduced by lowering serum TGs.

The CARE (Cholesterol and Recent Events) trial demonstrated that pravastatin reduced the risk of stroke by 31% in patients post myocardial infarction (MI) with average cholesterol levels (mean LDL 3.6 mmol/l). LIPID (Long Term Intervention with Pravastatin) showed a 19% reduction in the risk of stroke in this patient group. Both studies showed a reduction in cardiovascular events (death, MI and need for coronary artery bypass grafting) of 24–30%, with no increase in non-cardiovascular causes of death. Evidence is compelling that patients with high cholesterol and a moderate to high risk of IHD and cardiovascular events should be given intensive lipid-lowering therapy.

In the United States guidelines on lowering LDL cholesterol recognize the following cardiovascular risk factors: age (men >45 years, postmenopausal women), family history of premature IHD, smoking, hypertension, diabetes mellitus, insulin resistance, obesity, combined hyperlipidaemia and HDL cholesterol (<35 mg/dl). The guidelines suggest lowering LDL to 2.6 mmol/l in patients with IHD, to 3.4 in patients with no IHD but two risk factors, and to 4.2 in patients with fewer risk factors.

The early reduction in cardiovascular mortality seen in clinical trials of statin treatment cannot be attributed only to LDL reduction and its subsequent reduction in plaque volume, lipid content and atherosclerosis regression. MAAS (Multicentre Anti-Atheroma Study), a quantitative angiographic assessment of the impact of statins on atherosclerosis, showed morphological improvement after 4 years of statin treatment, with no change evident at 2 years. However, the Scandinavian Simvastatin Survival and the West of Scotland Coronary Prevention (WOSCOPS) studies showed significant benefit at less than 2 years. Experimental evidence shows that statins have additional effects on the pathophysiological determinants of acute coronary syndromes, which account for the early clinical benefit observed. These effects include altered macrophage metabolism (decreased cholesterol synthesis, increased LDL degradation and decreased foam cell formation), decreased macrophage activation, decreased smooth muscle cell proliferation and improved endothelial function. In addition, statins have some antithrombotic activity.

References

Assmann G 1996 Hypertrigliceridaemia and elevated lipoprotein(a) are risk factors for major coronary events. American Journal of Cardiology 77: 1179–1184

Assmann G, Cullen P, Schulte H et al. 1998 The Munster heart study. PROCAM. European Heart Journal 19 (Supp) A: A2–11

Packard C 1998 End of triglicerides in cardiovascular risk assessment? British Medical Journal 7158: 553–554

Pederson T, Kjekshus J, Berg K et al. Scandinavian Simvastatin Survival Study 1994 Randomised trial of cholesterol lowering in 4444 patients with coronary heart disease. Lancet 344: 1383–1389

Sacks F, Pfeffer M, Moye L et al. 1996 CARE (effect of pravastatin on coronary events after MI in patients with average cholesterol levels). New England Journal of Medicine 335: 1001–1009

Shepard J, Cobbe S M, Ford I et al. (for the West of Scotland Coronary Prevention Study). 1995. Prevention of coronary heart disease with pravastatin in men with hypercholesterolaemia. New England Journal of Medicine 333: 1301–1307

Vos J, de Feyter P, Kingma J et al. 1997 Evolution of coronary atherosclerosis in patients with mild coronary artery disease studied by serial quantitative coronary angiography at 2 and 4 year follow up. The multicenter anti-atheroma study MAAS. European Heart Journal 18(7): 1081–1089

74. Antiplatelet agents in coronary artery disease
A.T   B.F   C.T   D.T   E.F

Glycoprotein (GP) IIb/IIIa is a platelet-specific adhesion molecule which acts as a receptor for fibrinogen on the platelet surface. It becomes a high-affinity receptor during episodes of platelet activation, for example during plaque fissuring. Intracellular platelet signalling is mediated by a variety of activators, including collagen, Von Willebrand factor, adrenaline, platelet-activating factor and thrombin. ADP and thromboxane A_2 are released by platelet activation and act as positive feedback to activate further platelets.

Clopidrogel (a teiclopidine derivative) interferes with ATP-binding sites on the platelet, preventing ADP-dependent activation of glycoprotein IIb/IIIa receptors and preventing the positive feedback pathway which further activates platelets. In the CAPRIE trial comparing clopidrogel to aspirin clopidrogel resulted in a relative risk reduction of 8.7% in terms of the combined endpoints of stroke, myocardial infarction (MI) and vascular death. Clopidrogel may cause neutropenia. However, haemorrhagic and gastrointestinal side effects were less common than with aspirin. It may prove useful alone or in combination with aspirin for the prevention of coronary stent thrombosis in place of teiclopidine, which acts in the same way but is associated with more frequent blood dyscrasias.

Glycoprotein IIb/IIIa receptor antagonists are very potent inhibitors of platelet aggregation. They act by competitively inhibiting fibrinogen binding at the common pathway of platelet activation. Abciximab, a monoclonal antibody directed at the fibrinogen-binding site on glycoprotein IIb/IIIa, is indicated as an adjunct to heparin and aspirin to prevent ischaemic cardiac complications in high-risk patients undergoing percutaneous transarterial coronary angioplasty (PTCA). The EPISTENT trial showed a 54% reduction in death, MI or urgent revascularisation when abciximab was used rather than placebo in patients undergoing coronary stenting. Compared to placebo, the CAPTURE trial and EPIC study showed that abciximab improved clinical outcome (death, MI or urgent revascularization) by 30–50% when given prior to and up to 12 hours post PTCA. This effect extended to 3 years (with a 20% relative risk reduction). Initial concerns over increased bleeding risk have been addressed by reducing heparin doses.

The PRISM and PRISM-PLUS trials demonstrated that tirofiban, a non-peptide glycoprotein IIb/IIIa inhibitor, significantly improved clinical outcome at 7 days in severe unstable angina when therapy with aspirin, heparin and tirofiban was compared to aspirin and heparin alone. There was a 32% relative risk reduction in death, MI or revascularisation in the group treated with tirofiban. Benefit from tirofiban was maintained to six months. PURSUIT, a large multicentre trial involving over 10 000 patients, has further demonstrated the additional benefits of glycoprotein IIb/IIIa inhibitors in acute coronary syndromes.

References

Anon 1998 Management of unstable angina. Drug and Therapeutics Bulletin 36(5): 36–39

Gent M, Beaumont D, Blanchard J et al. 1996 CAPRIE randomised blinded trial of clopidrogel versus aspirin in patients at risk of ischaemic events. Lancet 348: 1229–1239.

Moran N 1998 Novel antiplatelet agents. British Journal of Cardiology 5(8): 413–421

Simoons M, Rutsch W, Vahanian A et al. 1997 CAPTURE randomised placebo controlled trial of abciximab before and during coronary intervention in refractory unstable angina. Lancet 349: 1429–1435

Theroux P, Pelletier G, Davies R, et al. 1998 PRISM PLUS inhibition of glycoprotein IIb/IIIa receptor with unstable angina and non-Q wave MI. New England Journal of Medicine 338: 1488–1497

Topol E, Califf R, Simoons M et al. 1998 PURSUIT inhibition of platelet glycoprotein IIb/IIIa with eptifibrate in patients with acute coronary syndrome. New England Journal of Medicine 339: 436–443

Topol E, Lincoff A, Califf R et al. 1998 EPISTENT randomised placebo control and balloon PTCA trial to assess safety of coronary stenting with GP IIb/IIIa blockade. Lancet 352: 87–92

75. Arrhythmogenic right ventricular dysplasia
A.**T**   B.**T**   C.**T**   D.**T**   E.**T**

Arrhythmogenic right ventricular dysplasia (ARVD) is a cardiomyopathy of unknown cause characterized by fibrofatty replacement of myocytes with scattered foci of inflammation in the right ventricle. Segmental right ventricular disease is usual, but evolution to more diffuse right ventricular involvement with left ventricular abnormalities and heart failure may occur. The incidence is unknown, but ARVD usually presents in adolescence or young adulthood. Clinical manifestations of the disease include structural and functional abnormalities of the right ventricle, electrocardiogram depolarization/repolarization changes, and presentation with sudden death or arrhythmias of right ventricular origin. In 30% of cases the disease is familial with autosomal dominant inheritance. It is unclear whether the inherited forms of ARVD predispose to a degenerative disease with right ventricular atrophy and fibrofatty replacement or whether the inflammatory cells indicate a viral myocarditis or autoimmune pathogenesis.

Diagnosis is based on various criteria including right ventricular dilatation and regional dysfunction with little left ventricular involvement, fibrofatty replacement on endomyocardial biopsy, T-wave inversion and prolonged QRS complexes on right precordial ECG leads, left bundle branch block (LBBB)-type ventricular tachycardia and a positive family history. Dilatation of the right ventricle is defined by echocardiography or angiography. Recently, MRI criteria for diagnosing ARVD have been established. These include right ventricular thinning, fatty replacement of the myocardium and reduced RV systolic thickening. Other investigations include ECG exercise testing to induce ventricular tachycardia (VT), holter monitoring (frequent ventricular ectopics and VT are seen), and electrophysiological studies with programmed stimulation of the right ventricle to induce VT and to evaluate the risk of sudden death.

It was traditionally considered that ARVD was an isolated disease of the right ventricle but recent pathological data show that left ventricular involvement occurs in 76% of patients. This is associated with more severe cardiomegaly, inflammatory infiltrates and heart failure. The fibrofatty change in the right ventricular free wall delays intraventricular electrical transmission and allows the development of re-entrant ventricular arrhythmias of left bundle branch block morphology. These arrhythmias may be exacerbated by activated neutrophils in the infiltrate.

Treatment is based on antiarrhythmic therapy with either a single agent or a combination. Amiodarone, β-blockers and flecainide may all be effective. With treatment with these drugs the incidence of sudden death is approximately 1% per year. In cases of drug-resistant VT invasive treatment may be indicated. Radiofrequency ablation may be used to remove an inducible focus of VT. Insertion of an implantable defibrillator or surgery to resect the right ventricular free wall at the site of inducible VT may be indicated.

References

Fontaine G 1998 Arrhythmogenic right ventricular cardiomyopathies. Circulation 97: 1532–1535

McKenna W 1994 Diagnosis of arrhythmogenic right ventricular dysplasia / cardiomyopathy. British Heart Journal 71: 215–219

Zipes D, Wyse D, Friedman P, et al. 1997 AVID The antiarrhythmics versus implantable defibrillators investigators. New England Journal of Medicine 337: 1576–1583

76.   Right ventricular infarction
A.T   B.F   C.T   D.T   E.F

Haemodynamically important right ventricular (RV) myocardial infarction (MI) is an infrequent consequence of inferior MI. The clinical triad of hypotension, clear lung fields and elevated JVP occurs in less than 10% of inferior MI, and is associated with RV distension and wall motion abnormalities on transthoracic echocardiogram. RV function usually improves dramatically after infarction, even in the absence of revascularization. Electrocardiogram evidence of RV infarction (ST elevation in the right-sided precordial leads) is associated with a poor prognosis.

During RV contraction both the septum and the RV free wall contribute to RV stroke output, with a significant contribution from the left ventricle (LV) by ventricular interdependence. Acute ischaemia of the RV results in decreased systolic performance, resulting in decreased stroke output and RV distension in the fixed pericardial space. This compromises LV filling by increasing intrapericardial pressures, resulting in flattening of the interventricular septum during diastole and causing a low-output state of both the right and left ventricles. Inotropic therapy with volume loading may improve RV stroke output and systemic arterial pressure but can also increase LV oxygen demand, resulting in ischaemia and arrhythmias.

The lower afterload and myocardial oxygen demand of the RV explains its relative resistance to irreversible ischaemic damage during right coronary artery occlusion. When it does occur, however, it has devastating effects on systemic arterial pressure, and traditional treatment for acute LV failure (diuretics, nitrates, afterload reduction, balloon pumping etc.) can be ineffective or even detrimental.

Therapy involves volume loading, inotropic therapy and atrio-ventricular pacing. Recent studies have demonstrated that complete reperfusion of the occluded right coronary artery with balloon angioplasty improves RV function and reduces mortality in patients with RV infarction.

References

Bowers T, O'Neill WW, Grines C, et al 1998 Effect of reperfusion on biventricular function and survival after right ventricular infarction. New England Journal of Medicine 338: 933–940

Dell'Italia L 1998 Reperfusion for right ventricular infarction. New England Journal of Medicine 338: 978–980

GASTROENTEROLOGY

77.   Primary biliary cirrhosis

A.T   B.F   C.F   D.F   E.F

Primary biliary cirrhosis (PBC) is a chronic progressive autoimmune liver disease. Current estimates of prevalence range from 20 to 240 cases per million in the UK. The northeast region has data estimating prevalence at 128/million. Women are affected 8 times as commonly as men. It has not been reported in children. Clusters of cases have been reported, leading investigators to search for environmental aetiologies. There is a strong familial predisposition to acquiring the disease and the association with other autoimmune diseases is strong, indicating a likely genetic predisposition. The HLA association, however, is weak.

Diagnosis of primary biliary cirrhosis is made by finding positive titres of antimitochondrial antibodies (AMA), together with cholestatic liver function tests (LFTs) and compatible histology on liver biopsy. PBC patients also have raised IgM and IgG levels. C3 levels are normal. Antimitochondrial antibodies are found in 96% of patients. There are several subtypes, the E2 subtype being specific to PBC. The antibody is autoreactive against a component of pyruvate dehydrogenase. A small number of patients do not have AMA. They are diagnosed as having autoimmune cholangitis, which is likely to be an AMA-negative variant of PBC. Epidemiological evidence suggests that the presence of positive antibody titres alone indicates subclinical disease.

Patients with positive AMAs alone have slowly progressive disease. This contrasts with patients who are asymptomatic but have AMAs, abnormal LFTs and histology, where over 60% will progress to symptomatic disease within 5 years.

It is questionable whether liver biopsy has a role either diagnostically or prognostically in this disease. Histology characteristically shows a non-suppurative granulomatous cholangitis. Granulomata surround necrotic bile ducts and bile duct destruction leads to portal tract fibrosis and florid cirrhosis (the onion-skin lesion is seen in primary sclerosing cholangitis).

Symptomatic patients most commonly present with pruritus. This affects half of symptomatic patients and is more common in men. Lethargy and right upper quadrant pain are also common presentations. Hepatosplenomegaly can occur at any stage and without cirrhosis, as can variceal bleeding. Twenty per cent of patients present with symptoms of end-stage liver disease, with decompensated cirrhosis. The life expectancy for these patients without liver transplantation is approximately 3 years. Xanthelasma and xanthoma can be seen at any stage. Cholesterol levels are raised in about half of patients. The hypercholesterolaemia is predominantly of the high-density lipoprotein type and patients are not at increased risk of coronary heart disease.

PBC may first present in pregnancy and be mistaken for pruritus of pregnancy. It may also present primarily with symptoms of other autoimmune conditions. The sicca syndrome is present in 80% of PBC patients. Thyroid disease, Raynaud's syndrome and fibrosing alveolitis are seen in 20% of cases. Addison's disease, vitiligo and myasthenia gravis are rare associations.

Symptomatic treatment includes the prevention and treatment of malabsorption, bone disease and pruritus. Fat-soluble vitamin supplements may be necessary. Vitamin D replacement treats osteomalacia, which is rare. Osteopenia, which is common, should be treated with calcium supplements, etidronate and hormone replacement therapy. The best treatment for pruritus is cholestyramine. Rifampicin, ursodeoxycholic acid and naloxone are alternative therapies. Troublesome variceal bleeding without cirrhosis may be an indication for transjugular intrahepatic portosystemic shunting (TIPSS).

Ursodeoxycholic acid (UDCA) is a naturally occurring bile acid. Randomized placebo-controlled trials consistently show an improvement in liver function tests with UDCA, in particular a decrease in bilirubin. The trials have not assessed the use of UDCA in advanced disease and they have not specifically looked at its use in asymptomatic disease. It is not clear, however, whether improvements in biochemical indices translate to delayed disease progression.

End-stage liver disease is managed with paracentesis for recurrent ascites, nutritional support and treatment of encephalopathy. Liver transplantation is indicated for patients with life expectancy of less than a year, jaundice with bilirubin >170 µmol/l, recurrent ascites, recurrent spontaneous bacterial peritonitis, early hepatocellular carcinoma encephalopathy and unacceptable quality of life. Prognosis after transplantation is good, although the disease may recur in the donated organ.

References

Angulo P, Batts KP, Therneau TM, Jorgensen RA, Dickson ER, Lindor KD 1999 Long-term ursodeoxycholic acid delays histological progression in primary biliary cirrhosis. Hepatology 29: 644–647

Anon 1999 Ursodeoxycholic acid for primary biliary cirrhosis . Drug and Therapeutics Bulletin 37: 30–32

Kaplan MM 1996 Primary biliary cirrhosis. New England Journal of Medicine 335: 1570–1580

Metcalf JV, Mitchison HC, Palmer JM, Jones DE, Bassendine MF, James OFW 1996 Natural history of primary biliary cirrhosis. Lancet 348: 1399–1402

Neuberger J 1997 Primary biliary cirrhosis. Lancet 350: 875–879

78. Acute Pancreatitis
A.T   B.T   C.T   D.F   E.T

Acute pancreatitis is a common illness. The acute inflammatory process is reversible, distinguishing this disorder from chronic pancreatitis, where the inflammation is ongoing. Acute pancreatitis is often mild and self-limiting, but 20% of patients will have a severe attack. Overall mortality from acute pancreatitis is 5–10% and in severe cases is as high as 30%. Acute pancreatitis may be recurrent.

The pathological event in acute pancreatitis is the activation of pancreatic enzymes such as trypsin, which then activate many other enzymes, leading to autodigestion of the pancreas and surrounding fat and tissues. If this continues, peripancreatic and pancreatic necrosis ensues with the development of multiorgan failure. In these circumstances sepsis is common. Other sequelae of severe inflammation or necrosis include local complications such as fistulae and pancreatic pseudocysts.

The commonest causes of acute pancreatitis accounting for 80% of cases, are alcohol and gallstones, including microlithiasis. Other causes include drugs, e.g. azathioprine, pentamidine, 6–mercaptopurine and asparaginase. Local causes include penetrating peptic ulcer, pancreatic tumours or congenital anatomical anomalies such as pancreas divisum. Metabolic abnormalities (hyperlipidaemia and hypercalcaemia) are associated with acute pancreatitis, as is organ transplantation and end-stage renal failure. Trauma, major surgery and cardiac bypass surgery are risk factors. Pregnancy is associated with an increased risk. Infectious causes include mycoplasma, parasites such as ascariasis, and viruses, e.g. mumps, Coxsackie and HIV. In countries other than the UK rare causes include venoms from scorpion bites and some spider bites. In 10% of cases no identifiable cause is found.

Patients present with a continuous severe epigastric pain, sometimes radiating to the back and often worse in the supine position. Nausea and vomiting are common. There is local epigastric tenderness. Grey–Turner's and Cullen's signs are rare and are due to retroperitoneal haemorrhage. Hypoventilation is common, especially in severe cases, and may be exacerbated by atelectasis and pleural effusions. Abdominal distension and small bowel ileus is common. Hypocalcaemia is common and serum amylase is usually high. Serum lipase is more specific but not as widely available. With gallstone pancreatitis the serum aminotransferases may be elevated.

Management depends on both the severity of illness and the cause. In mild cases analgesia, intravenous rehydration and bowel rest may be sufficient. The commonly used Ranson's criteria are used to assess the severity of an attack. These criteria are valid for 0–48 hours after presentation. On admission a severe attack is indicated by age greater than 55 years, a white cell count of more than 16 000/mm^2, glucose greater than 11 mmol/l, lactate dehydrogenase greater than 350 iu/l and an aspartate transaminase greater than 250 iu/l. In the first 48 hours other poor prognostic indicators include hypoxaemia, hypocalcaemia, rising urea, decreasing packed cell volume, a base deficit and fluid sequestration. These latter criteria assess the systemic effect of circulatory toxins.

Intravenous fluids and adequate analgesia are essential. Nasogastric aspiration is needed in severe cases with vomiting. Enteral nutrition through a nasojejunal tube or parenteral nutrition is needed to improve the outcome if ileus or inflammation persist beyond 5 days. Antibiotics are not currently recommended for mild cases. In the event of sepsis or infected pancreatic debris, antibiotics are essential. Most practitioners recommend prophylactic antibiotics for patients fulfilling the criteria of a severe attack. Causative drugs should be withdrawn and precipitating metabolic disorders treated on resolution.

Acute pancreatitis due to biliary obstruction with sepsis is an indication for urgent endoscopic retrograde cholangiopancreatography (ERCP). Ultrasound is helpful in diagnosing obstruction if a dilated common bile duct is seen. This may take some time to develop, so a high index of suspicion must be taken in patients who have raised liver enzymes with hyperbiliruninaemia or who present jaundiced. There appears to be no advantage to early ERCP in patients with gallstone pancreatitis who do not have obstruction. Elective cholecystectomy is recommended for these patients once the acute attack has settled.

Patients with severe acute pancreatitis are best managed on a high-dependency or intensive care unit. Shock can develop suddenly, as can respiratory distress. Patients with pancreatic necrosis, pseudocysts and fistulae require surgical management. In all cases of pancreatitis there should be close liaison with a surgical team. The mortality in patients with severe disease is very high.

After recovery patients should abstain from alcohol: 6 months' abstinence has been recommended. A low-fat diet is also recommended.

References

Folsch UR, Nitsche R, Ludtke R, Hilgers RA, Creutzfeld W 1997 Early ERCP and papillotomy compared with conservative treatment for acute biliary pancreatitis. New England Journal of Medicine 336: 237–242

Johnson CD 1998 Severe acute pancreatitis: a continuing challenge for the intensive care team. British Journal of Intensive Care 8: 130–136

Mergener K, Baillie J 1998 Acute pancreatitis. British Medical Journal 316: 44–48

79. Barrett's oesophagus
A.F   B.F   C.F   D.F   E.T

Barrett's oesophagus has been defined as the replacement of distal oesophageal squamous epithelial lining by 3 cm or more of circumferential columnar epithelium in continuity with the gastric mucosa. There are some problems with this formal definition, as segments of metaplasia may be shorter than 3 cm (recently the term short-segment Barrett's has been adopted), and tongues of metaplastic epithelium are commonly seen at endoscopy which are not circumferential but clearly differ endoscopically and histologically from normal.

There are three types of metaplasia seen in the oesophagus. The commonest is columnar specialized intestinal metaplasia. The others are gastric metaplasia and junctional metaplasia. It is thought that adenocarcinomas arise in Barrett's oesophagus as a result of a metaplasia–dysplasia–neoplasia sequence. The increased risk of adenocarcinoma of the oesophagus is associated with intestinal metaplasia and is 30–40 times that of the general population. Adenocarcinoma of the oesophagus has increased fivefold in incidence in the last 50 years, making it currently the fastest-increasing cancer. The 5-year survival for adenocarcinoma arising in Barrett's oesophagus is 7%. The risk of carcinoma is increased in long segments (>5 cm) of Barrett's, areas of ulceration, and in smokers.

The mechanism of metaplasia is poorly understood. There is a disruption of normal cell–cell contact, mediated by cell adhesion molecules called cadherins. Epithelial or E-cadherin expression becomes disorganized in Barrett's epithelium compared to normal tissue and expression is also reduced compared to normal. In contrast, placental or P-cadherin, normally only found at the basal cell layer, is absent in Barrett's epithelium and dysplastic epithelium. At least part of the mechanism of progression from Barrett's to neoplasia is therefore associated with alterations in cadherins.

Gastro-oesophageal reflux is thought to play a part in the aetiology of Barrett's oesophagus, and bile reflux may also be important. Barrett's is found in 10% of patients undergoing endoscopy for gastro-oesophageal reflux disease. Treatment is difficult. Preventing reflux may prevent further damage and progression to dysplasia. Proton pump inhibitors will treat reflux and will also lead to the re-establishment of squamous epithelium, but this is patchy, in the form of squamous islands. Surgical measures for the treatment of reflux disease include Nissen fundoplication.

The detection and treatment of dysplasia in Barrett's oesophagus is even more controversial. Retrospective case-note studies have shown that only a small proportion of patients with Barrett's will develop or die of cancer of the oesophagus, and this raises the question of which patients to select for screening and what treatment to offer when dysplasia or carcinoma-in-situ is detected. In addition, there is likely to be a high chance of sampling error even when strict biopsy protocols are enforced.

The dysplasia–neoplasia sequence has led to the assumption that prevention of progression will prevent cancers developing. Some advocate oesophagectomy for high-grade dysplasia, as carcinoma has been found in 45% of these patients. However, other less radical therapies are being studied. These include laser therapy to restore squamous epithelium macroscopically and histologically, and photodynamic therapy. In the latter technique administration of the oral precursor molecule 5-aminolaevulinic acid results in intracellular accumulation of protoporphyrin IX in dysplastic cells. This is a photosensitizer that can be activated by laser light photoirradiation and causes destruction of dysplastic cells. The danger with both these techniques is that the Barrett's glands may be hidden beneath the restored epithelium, thereby burying the problem, not curing it. For overt adenocarcinoma the treatment is surgical after satisfactory staging.

References

Bailey T, Biddlestone L, Shepherd NA, Barr H, Warner P, Jankowski J 1998 Altered cadherin and catenin complexes in the Barrett's esophagus dysplasia–adenocarcinoma sequence: correlation with disease progression and dedifferentiation. American Journal of Pathology 152: 135–144

Barham CP, Jones RL, Biddlestone LR, Hardwick RH, Shepherd NA, Barr H 1997 Photothermal laser ablation of Barrett's oesophagus: endoscopic and histological evidence of squamous reepithelialization. Gut 41: 281–284

Barr H, Shepherd NA, Dix A, Roberts DJ, Tan WC, Krasner N 1996 Eradication of high-grade dysplasia in columnar-lined (Barrett's) oesophagus by photodynamic therapy with endogenously generated protoporphyrin IX. Lancet 348: 561–562

Biddlestone LR, Barham CP, Wilkinson SP, Barr H, Shepherd NA 1998 The histopathology of treated Barrett's oesophagus: squamous reepithelialization after acid suppression and laser photodynamic therapy. American Journal of Surgical Pathology 22: 239–245

Gore S, Healey CJ, Sutton R et al. 1993 Regression of columnar lined (Barrett's) oesophagus with continuous omeprazole therapy. Alimentary Pharmacology and Therapeutics 7: 623–628

Holscher AH, Bollschweiler E, Schneider PM, Siewert JR 1997 Early adenocarcinoma in Barrett's oesophagus. British Journal of Surgery 84: 1470–1473

Nandurkar S, Talley NJ, Martin CJ, Ng TH, Adams S 1997 Short segment Barrett's oesophagus: prevalence, diagnosis and assosciations. Gut 40: 710–715

Spechler S, Goyal RK 1986 Barrett's oesophagus. New England Journal of Medicine 315: 362–371

van der Burgh A, Dees J, Hop WC, van Blankenstein M 1996
Oesophageal cancer is an uncommon cause of death in patients
with Barrett's oesophagus. Gut 39: 5–8

Wright TA 1997 High-grade dysplasia in Barrett's oesophagus. British
Journal of Surgery. 84: 760–766

80.   Management of obesity

A.**F**   B.**F**   C.**F**   D.**F**   E.**F**

Obesity is a major public health problem in the western world and
its incidence is increasing. The body mass index is defined as the
weight in kilograms divided by the square of the height in metres.
Obesity, defined as a body mass index greater than 28, is
associated with increased morbidity, especially from stroke,
ischaemic heart disease and diabetes. The highest morbidity is
associated with a central fat deposition rather than a more
peripheral distribution. Waist circumferences of more than 102 cm
in men and 88 cm in women increase the development of disorders
such as breathlessness, hypercholesterolaemia, hypertension and
non-insulin dependent diabetes.

Dietary composition and weight fluctuations have no major role in
the pathogenesis of obesity. Both protein and carbohydrate can be
converted into fat, and weight loss does not result from changing
the proportions of fat, protein or carbohydrate in the diet without
reducing the caloric intake. Diets with reduced fat have fewer
calories, and fat in the diet promotes the palatability of food and
encourages increased intake.

Obesity in humans is multifactorial. There may be a genetic
propensity. Twin studies and studies on adoptees and families
suggest that as much as 80% of variance in body mass index is
attributable to genetic factors. These include adipose tissue
distribution, physical activity, resting metabolic rate, changes in
energy expenditure related to overeating, aspects of eating
behaviour, food preferences, lipoprotein lipase activity and basal
rate of lipolysis. Some of these are difficult to isolate from
environmental factors and highlight the probable polygenic nature
of genetic influences in obesity. These contrast with the single-
gene abnormality syndromes that are associated with obesity such
as the Prader–Willi, Bardet–Biedl, Alstrom and Cohen syndromes.
These are usually accompanied by marked morphological
abnormalities.

A protein that has recently caused a lot of interest in the field of
obesity research is leptin. This is a 167 amino acid protein
encoded by a gene on chromosome 7. It is produced in white
adipose tissue. The ob/ob strain of obese mouse is leptin deficient
and, when leptin is administered, a marked decrease in body
weight results. A search for mutations in the leptin gene in obese
humans has been elusive, with only one pair of consanguinous

identical twins, both extremely obese, identified. Leptin levels in humans are also proportional to adipocyte volume and therefore high in obese individuals, leading to a theory of leptin resistance in obesity due to a leptin receptor abnormality. This has foundations in another animal model – the db/db mouse, which lacks a functional leptin receptor and is obese with a propensity to develop diabetes mellitus.

The treatment of obesity is difficult. For the extremely obese, weight-reducing diets are rarely successful in the long term, although short-term weight loss is often successful. Weight for weight, fat provides more than twice as many calories as carbohydrate, so the aim should be to achieve a diet in which no more than 30% of the calories are provided by fat. After initial weight loss, an ad lib low-fat high-carbohydrate diet may be more successful at maintaining reduced weight than continuing with a strict calorie restricted diet. One reason for failure of the latter could be non-compliance. Many obese patients who lose 5% of their initial body weight show improvement in morbidity risk factors. Lifestyle changes, such as increased physical activity in combination with diet, are more effective than diet alone. Behavioural therapy may provide additional benefit.

The use of drug therapy is controversial. Few drugs have been successful in causing sustained weight loss, or are safe to use over long periods of time. The serotonin reuptake inhibitors fenfluramine and dexfenfluramine were withdrawn for the treatment of obesity because of adverse reactions, which included pulmonary hypertension and heart valve lesions, particularly aortic regurgitation. Orlistat is a relatively new antiobesity drug which is a gastrointestinal lipase inhibitor, promoting weight loss by inhibition of gastrointestinal tract lipase, which lowers the absorption of dietary fat by about 30% on average. Over 1 year, weight loss achieved using this drug in combination with diet was 10%, compared to a placebo effect of 6%. A small proportion of patients will lose more than 20% of initial body weight. After 2 years of continuous treatment weight regain is smaller in patients taking orlistat than those on placebo. The weight reduction was also associated with a reduction in hypercholesterolaemia, fasting blood glucose and blood pressure. Orlistat causes GI side effects which may limit compliance in a non-trial population. There is a potential risk of vitamin E and D deficiency developing with long-term treatment, but supplementation is not routinely necessary.

Surgery is usually reserved for obese patients with BMI greater than 40, or greater than 35 with obesity-related morbidity. Jejunoileal bypass is one effective option, although patients need to be carefully monitored for complications. In addition to a weight-reducing diet, patients need a low-oxalate diet to reduce the incidence of oxalate renal stones. Cholecalciferol, magnesium and vitamin B_{12} supplements are often needed. These patients are subject to bacterial overgrowth from blind loop syndrome. Gastroplasty is also effective, although continuous limitation of calorie intake is needed to maintain weight loss. There is no bypass of the small intestine, so vitamin absorbtion is normal.

References

Anon 1998 Why and how should adults lose weight? Drug and Therapeutics Bulletin 36: 89–92

Auwerx J, Staels B 1998 Leptin. Lancet 351: 737–742

Connolly HM, Crary JL, McGoon MD et al. 1997 Valvular heart disease associated with fenfluramine–phentermine. New England Journal of Medicine 337: 581–588

Khan MA, Herzog CA, St Peter JV et al. 1998 The prevalence of cardiac valvular insufficiency assessed by transthoracic echocardiography in obese patients treated with appetite-suppressant drugs. New England Journal of Medicine 339: 713–718

Lean MEJ, Han TS, Siedel JC 1998 Impairment of health and quality of life in people with large waist circumference. Lancet 351: 853–856

Sjostrom L, Rissanen A, Andersen T et al. 1998 Randomised placebo-controlled trial of orlistat for weight loss and prevention of weight regain in obese patients. Lancet 352: 167–173

Taubro S, Astrup A 1997 Randomised comparison of diets for maintaining obese subjects' weight after major weight loss: ad lib, low fat, high carbohydrate diet v fixed energy intake. British Medical Journal 314: 29–34

81. Hepatitis A infection

A.F   B.T   C.F   D.F   E.F

Hepatitis A infection is the commonest cause of acute viral hepatitis. Other viruses causing acute hepatitis include hepatitis B, Epstein–Barr, cytomegalovirus, yellow fever virus and herpes simplex virus.

Hepatitis A virus (HAV) is a small single-stranded RNA virus of the picornavirus family. Transmission is by person-to-person contact through the feco-oral route. It often occurs in epidemics in susceptible communities. Sources of infection include contaminated food, e.g. bivalve shellfish, or water from contaminated sewage or poor sanitary systems. It is common in developing countries and poor socioeconomic communities. Drug users who inject are at increased risk of infection. This may be due to fecal contamination of shared needles in conditions of poor personal hygiene.

Hepatitis A is usually an illness of children and young adults. It has an incubation period of 15–50 days with a mean of 30 days. During this time both virus and IgM antibodies can be detected, and viral shedding in faeces occurs. Fecal shedding of virus continues for at least a week after resolution of symptoms. IgG antibodies may be detectable immediately, but increase during the course of the illness and persist after the IgM levels drop at about 3 months. IgG antibodies confer lifelong immunity.

Clinical presentation is usually with non-specific prodromal symptoms. Headache, nausea, malaise, anorexia, arthralgia and myalgia are common. Jaundice is uncommon in children but quite common in adults. It is usually mild, with serum bilirubin rarely exceeding 170 µmol/l. Two uncommon exceptions to this occur: acute fulminant liver failure accompanied by a severe coagulopathy, and cholestatic hepatitis where jaundice persists for several months after the acute illness with relatively normal alkaline phosphatase and, in contrast to the acute illness, relatively normal aminotransferases. Cutaneous necrotizing vasculitis and mononeuritis multiplex are rare complications of the acute hepatitis. Overall the prognosis is excellent with most patients showing complete recovery both clinically and biochemically within 3–6 months.

For travellers from the UK, USA, western Europe and the Mediterranean visiting high endemic areas, vaccination is recommended. Passive immunization with human immunoglobulin pooled from HAV IgG-positive individuals is available, but more recently active immunization using inactivated whole virus vaccines has become available. Vaccination is recommended at least 2 weeks before travel. Immunoglobulin is recommended for children under the age of 2 and for postexposure prophylaxis.

Reference

Koff RS 1998 Hepatitis A. Lancet 351: 1643–1649

---

82. Haemochromatosis

A.T   B.F   C.F   D.T   E.F

Hereditary haemochromatosis is an autosomal recessive disorder. A major histocompatibility complex (MHC) class 1-like gene for haemochromatosis has recently been described on chromosome 6, explaining the HLA linkage previously observed. The gene has been called HFE and is an important mutation found at position 282 of the protein product, where tyrosine is substituted in place of cysteine. The mutation has been designated C282Y. Most, but not all (>60%), cases are homozygous for C282Y. A second mutation, H63D, has been found in some heterozygotes. The two mutations have not been described together on the same chromosome. A minority of people with haemochromatosis carry neither mutation, raising the possibility of a third or more mutations yet to be found. Conversely, some family studies have documented homozygotes for C282Y who do not show evidence of iron overload. This may suggest some environmental influence on the disease or other unidentified genes.

Organ iron overload due to excessive iron absorption characterizes the condition. Total body iron is normally 3–4g. In symptomatic haemochromatosis the total body iron is 20–40g. The serum iron level is elevated in this condition, which is most accurately diagnosed by a persistently elevated transferrin saturation level. A raised ferritin level in the absence of other causes of iron overload or acute illness is suggestive, and the diagnosis of iron overload is confirmed by liver biopsy.

Haemochromatosis has a prevalence of about 1 in 300 in the general population. In the early stages of iron overload patients are often asymptomatic or suffer non-specific symptoms such as malaise. The prevalence is therefore much higher than is recognized clinically. Clinical symptoms occur more often in men than in women, despite equal prevalence of the gene abnormality. It has been suggested that women are partially protected from the effects of iron overload by menstruation and pregnancy. The earlier onset of symptoms in women who undergo early menopause would seem to support this. However haemochromatosis can cause menstrual irregularity. In addition, if menstruation were protective women should present at a later age than men, but, this is not the case. Dietary iron intake and alcohol consumption may affect the severity of disease.

Clinically haemochromatosis may present in several ways. It may be detected at an asymptomatic stage through screening following diagnosis of an affected family member. Arthralgia, fatigue, impotence, menstrual irregularity, a bronzed appearance and abdominal pain may all be presenting features. Iron deposition in the gonads may cause hypogonadism and subfertility. It may be diagnosed during investigation of abnormal liver function tests. Patients frequently present with cirrhosis and complications of end-stage liver disease. Primary liver cancer arises in 30% of patients with cirrhosis. Haemochromatosis also commonly affects the pancreas and diabetes mellitus may be the first presenting feature. Iron overload resulting in cardiomyopathy may present as heart failure or arrhythmias.

Left untreated, the prognosis from symptomatic haemochromatosis is progression to end-stage liver disease, with death resulting from liver failure, complications of cirrhosis, hepatocellular carcinoma or diabetes mellitus. With adequate treatment before the onset of complications, life expectancy can be normal.

The treatment of choice is venesection. This is monitored by haemoglobin and ferritin levels. Initially patients may require once- or twice-weekly phlebotomy to achieve a normal ferritin level and improvement of symptoms. After about 1 year venesection needs to be maintained at intervals to prevent iron reaccumulation. Rarely patients cannot tolerate this treatment. The alternatives are much less satisfactory, but include chelation therapy with desferrioxamine.

There is no clear consensus on screening the general population for haemochromatosis. However, there is a clear case for screening family members of sufferers to detect early and asymptomatic disease. Genetic testing is available and is relatively simple and inexpensive.

References

Adams PC, Deugnier Y, Moirand R, Brissot P 1997 The relationship between iron overload, clinical symptoms and age in 410 patients with hemochromatosis. Hepatology 25: 162–166

Bacon BR 1997 Diagnosis and management of hemochromatosis. Gastroenterology 113: 995–999

Burke W, Thomson E, Khoury MJ et al. 1998 Hereditary haemochromatosis. Gene discovery and its implications for population based screening. Journal of the American Medical Association 280:172–178

Feder JN, Gnirke A, Thomas W et al. 1996 A novel MHC class 1-like gene is mutated in patients with hereditary haemochromatosis. Nature Genetics 13: 399–408

Tweed MJ, Roland JM 1998 Haemochromatosis as an endocrine cause of subfertility. British Medical Journal 316: 915–916

83. Assessment of nutritional status

A.F   B.F   C.F   D.F   E.F

The nutritional status of patients can influence mortality, morbidity and length of hospital stay but is often overlooked. In one study 40% of patients admitted to a general hospital were undernourished and in about a quarter of these it was of such severity as to threaten life. Body weight was recorded in the notes of only 23% of the undernourished patients, and any information regarding nutritional status was recorded in less than half. Only 10 out of 55 patients originally assessed as undernourished had seen a dietitian by the time they were reassessed at discharge.

There are several ways to assess nutritional status. The body mass index (BMI) can be calculated (BMI = weight (kg)/ height squared (m^2)). An optimal BMI is between 20 and 25 kg/m^2. The BMI is useful in comparing a patient's nutritional status to the general population, but on its own gives no indication of weight loss. A BMI of less than 20 kg/m^2 suggests undernutrition, and mortality is higher especially in the elderly when below 18 kg/m^2. Probably one of the best indicators of nutritional status is the percentage reduction in weight from usual for that individual. A loss of 35% of usual body weight is usually life threatening.

Anthropomorphic measurements such as the triceps skinfold thickness (body fat) and midarm muscle circumference (protein) can be useful in assessing body energy stores.

Albumin has a plasma half-life of approximately 21 days, whereas prealbumin has a half-life of just 2 days. This makes prealbumin more suitable in the assessment of changes in nutritional status. Transferrin is also used and has a half-life of 7 days. Transferrin levels are dependent upon several other factors, such as iron status and infection. The lymphocyte count also correlates with nutritional status, but is again determined by many other factors. A lymphocyte count of <800 cells/mm^3 suggests severe malnutrition and 1200–2000 cells/mm^3 mild malnutrition.

References

Anon 1996 Malnourished inpatients: overlooked and undertreated. Drug and Therapeutics Bulletin 34: 57–59

Silk D 1995 Nutrition for gastroenterologists: when, how and for how long? European Journal of Gastroenterology and Hepatology 7: 491–500

Payne-James JJ 1995 Enteral nutrition. European Journal of Gastroenterology and Hepatology 7: 501–506

84. Nutritional supplementation

A.F   B.F   C.F   D.T   E.T

A variety of techniques can be used to supplement patients calorie intake. Simple enrichment with natural ingredients such as cream and butter has been shown to increase energy intake by 40% and increase weight by 3.4% in long-stay elderly patients.

There are several types of oral supplement. Modular supplements are designed to increase the intake of one specific element of the diet, such as protein or fat. They can be added to normal food. Blenderized formulae are combinations of normal table food with additional vitamins and minerals. Most commercial formulae are lactose free, moderately osmotic and contain 1–2 kcal/ml. Some are fortified with extra protein. Elemental formulae consist of free amino acids, dipeptides, tripeptides, simple carbohydrates (maltodextrins) and simple fats (MCT oil). Elemental formulae are highly osmotic because of the small particle size.

In a prospective randomized study 501 long-term elderly patients, received either a standard diet or one with additional oral supplements (800 kcal/day) for up to 6 months. The oral supplement group had a 10% lower mortality than the control group.

There are many physiological benefits from enteral rather than parenteral nutrition. The enteral administration of nutritional support is generally safer, less expensive and more physiological than parenteral nutrition. Over recent years there has been a move towards using enteral nutrition wherever possible. A meta-analysis using data from eight randomized trials studying high-risk surgical patients demonstrated that 18% of enteral nutrition patients developed postoperative septic complications compared to 35% of those receiving parenteral nutrition. The biggest risk reduction was in the incidence of nosocomial pneumonia in patients who had suffered blunt abdominal trauma.

It has long been standard surgical practice to withhold oral nutrition in surgical patients after laparotomy until after bowel sounds have returned. It has now been shown that not only is it safe to start feeding, certainly a liquid diet, within 12 hours, but it is also advantageous, with a more rapid return of bowel sounds and the resumption of a normal diet.

Short-term oral dietary liquid supplements taken ad lib by surgical patients have been shown to not only improve total calorie intake but also to enable the maintenance of body weight and muscle strength compared to those taking a normal ward diet. Interestingly, the supplement group actually voluntarily took more of the ward diet. The difference in mean calorie intake was highly significant: 1833 compared to 1108 kcal/g ($P<0.0001$). Serious infections such as pneumonia were also significantly more common in the control group.

Percutaneous endoscopic gastrostomy (PEG) has been shown to result in a significantly higher prescribed feed intake than the use of nasogastric feeding tubes (93% vs. 55%). Long-term PEG feeding is associated with low morbidity. Patient selection is clearly important, as the procedure can be hazardous in those with severe pulmonary or cardiovascular disease.

References

Anon 1996 Malnourished inpatients: overlooked and undertreated. Drug and Therapeutics Bulletin 34: 57–59

Silk D 1995 Nutrition for gastroenterologists: when, how and for how long? European Journal of Gastroenterology and Hepatology 7: 491–500

Payne-James JJ 1995 Enteral nutrition. European Journal of Gastroenterology and Hepatology 7: 501–506

85. General malaise as a result of short bowel syndrome

A.F   B.F   C.F   D. F   E.T.

The short bowel syndrome occurs when the functional length of bowel is inadequate to absorb sufficient nutrients, fluid and electrolytes from a normal diet to maintain health. In normal individuals the length of the small bowel from the duodenojejunal flexure to the ileocaecal valve is between 275 and 850 cm. It is the amount of functional bowel left post surgery that is important. Bowel length can be measured at surgery or using a barium follow-through examination. The syndrome is influenced by the underlying disease and whether or not the colon remains in situ. Short bowel syndrome can lead to several problems. Fluid and electrolyte imbalance is common. Magnesium deficiency can result in fatigue, depression, irritability, muscle weakness, tetany and convulsions. Potassium loss is less commonly seen, but can result from secondary hyperaldersteronism or as a result of magnesium depletion. Malabsorption of nutrients also occurs. Gallstones occur in over 30% of patients and renal stones occur in patients with intact colons.

The bowel has a critical role in maintaining fluid and electrolyte balance. In health the bowel normally absorbs over 6 l of fluid each day, largely made up of intestinal secretions. For normal water and electrolyte homoeostasis in the absence of a colon a jejunal length of approximately 200 cm is required. In the presence of a colon only about 50 cm is sufficient. Jejunostomy patients with over 100 cm of jejunum in situ are usually net absorbers of water and electrolytes and can often be managed with oral supplements. If the remaining jejunum is less than this then intravenous supplementation is usually required.

Patients presenting with symptoms resulting from fluid and electrolyte depletion can have a normal supine blood pressure and a normal creatinine. Lying and standing blood pressure measurement and urinary sodium measurement are more sensitive assessments of fluid and electrolyte status. The creatinine is often falsely low as a result of low muscle bulk secondary to protein malabsorption. Changes in body weight and stomal output and careful fluid balance assessments are all essential.

In the emergency setting with severe depletion immediate intravenous replacement should be instituted, followed by an attempt to maintain balance with oral administration. If the patient has a treatable underlying disease such as Crohn's disease appropriate therapy should be instituted. Patients should drink as little hypotonic fluid as possible, as this can lead to leakage of sodium into the lumen, exacerbating sodium depletion. Glucose saline drinks should be administered, as sodium is absorbed with glucose in the jejunum (an electrolyte solution containing 3.5 g sodium chloride, 2.5 g sodium bicarbonate and 20 g glucose is recommended). If these first two steps do not work, drugs should be administered to reduce stomal output. Codeine phosphate, loperamide, proton pump inhibitors, H_2 receptor antagonists and somatostatin analogues all reduce intestinal secretion. Oral magnesium supplements or 1α-hydroxycholecalciferol may be required. In patients with intact colons a reduced dietary fat intake can reduce stool output, as unabsorbed dietary fats reaching the colon can exacerbate diarrhoea as well as increase calcium and magnesium losses. Orally active somatostatin analogues or peptide YY agonists may be available in the near future. If all these measures fail then parenteral fluids will be required for long-term management.

Careful nutritional management is also essential. Patients often absorb 60% or less of their daily calorie intake. Depending upon the severity, increased oral intake, nutritional supplements, nasogastric feeding at night and long-term parenteral nutrition may be needed.

The reversal of a 10cm length of small bowel to increase transit time can be beneficial. Small bowel transplantation can also be considered in selected patients. The use of growth factors such as epidermal growth factor to improve small intestinal function shows promise for the future.

References

Farthing MJG 1996 The role of somatostatin analogues in the treatment of refractory diarrhoea. Digestive Diseases. 57 (Suppl 1): 107–113

Nightingale J 1995 The short bowel syndrome. European Journal of Gastroenterology and Hepatology 7: 514–520

86.   Gastro-oesophageal reflux disease
A.F   B.F   C.T   D.T   E.T

There are several steps in the management of gastro-oesophageal reflux disease (GORD, or GERD in the USA). The management is tailored to the severity of the disease and the response to therapy, and can be divided into lifestyle interventions, drug therapies and surgical treatment.

Lifestyle advice should be given to all patients, but most of these recommendations are based on theoretical advantages rather than the results of randomized intervention studies. Advice includes avoiding fatty, fried and spicy foods, stopping smoking, losing weight and reducing alcohol and caffeine consumption. Fatty and spicy foods have been shown to reduce gastric emptying and therefore avoiding them has at least a theoretical advantage. Avoiding eating for at least 3 hours prior to lying down may be beneficial, especially if nocturnal symptoms are a feature. Elevating the head of the bed has been shown to be beneficial.

The first-line drug therapies for mild disease are antacids, alginates or alginate–antacid preparations. Alginate–antacid combinations have been shown to be more effective than antacids alone, and in mild disease most patients can remain in good clinical remission taking these therapies alone. They can also be useful for breakthrough symptoms in those taking more powerful acid-suppressing therapy.

Prokinetic agents such as cisapride and domperidone have also been shown to be effective. Cisapride is a 5-hydroxytryptamine (5-HT)$_4$ receptor agonist which increases oesophageal peristalsis, gastro-oesophageal sphincter tone and gastric emptying. In studies it has been shown to be almost as effective as H$_2$ receptor antagonists in reducing symptoms and healing mucosal lesions, and has also been shown to prevent relapses.

H$_2$ receptor antagonists alone for GORD have been shown to be beneficial and are probably more effective than prokinetics. In severe oesophagitis, however, over 80% of lesions fail to heal even with higher doses. They are generally very well tolerated, have an excellent safety profile and can be an ideal therapy for relatively mild disease.

Proton pump inhibitors (PPIs) are the most effective monotherapy agents in moderate to severe disease. PPIs irreversibly block the H+/K+ ATPase in gastric parietal cells. A meta-analysis of 43 trials comparing PPIs with H$_2$ receptor antagonists has confirmed their greater efficacy in moderate to severe disease. The proportion of patients cured is doubled, with faster healing and symptom reduction. They are also more effective in mild disease.

Despite their effectiveness there are some issues regarding the long-term use of PPIs that need to be discussed further. First, some patients remain symptomatic, especially at night, despite high-dose PPI therapy. This phenomenon of nocturnal acid breakthrough has been well documented with 24-hour oesophageal pH studies. Recently it has been shown that the addition of nocturnal H$_2$ receptor antagonist therapy can be highly effective at overcoming this problem, and is more effective than further PPI dose escalation. Secondly, concerns have been raised about the risk of neoplasia with long-term PPI-induced hypergastrinaemia. In rats this had been shown to lead to enterochromaffin-like cell hyperplasia and carcinoid tumours, but this has not been confirmed in humans (with the exception of one case report). Hypergastrinaemia in patients with hypochlorhydria is thought to contribute to the observed increased risk of adenocarcinoma of the stomach. In one study, PPI therapy in the presence of *Helicobacter pylori* infection was shown to lead to an increased rate of progression to atrophic gastritis, which is thought to be a premalignant lesion. The results of this study have not yet been reproduced and no study has shown an increased risk of adenocarcinoma of the oesophagus with PPI usage. Thirdly, the cost-effectiveness of long-term PPI therapy compared to surgery remains controversial. No long-term study has been published to help answer this.

Open and laparoscopic procedures, usually employing Nissen fundoplication or fundic wrap, can be highly successful and safe in experienced hands. Success rates of over 90% in terms of mucosal healing and symptom relief are quoted in the literature. The laparoscopic approach has many advantages, with patients spending less time in hospital and returning to work more rapidly.

Reference

Galmiche JP, Letessier E, Scarpignato C 1998 Treatment of gastro-
oesophageal disease in adults. British Medical Journal
316: 1720–1723

87. Coeliac disease

A.F   B.F   C.F   D.F   E.T

Coeliac disease can be defined as a permanent gluten-sensitive enteropathy. Several recent studies, aided by serological screening tests, have suggested that the incidence of coeliac disease is much higher than previously suspected, and may be in the region of 1 in 300 or less among Europeans. A study in Northern Ireland employed population screening of adults and found an incidence of 1 in 152,and a study screening Italian schoolchildren revealed an incidence of 1 in 184. An international study suggested a prevalence of about 1 in 250.

The disease appears to require a genetic predisposition and environmental factors. First-degree relatives of coeliac cases have a 10% risk of being affected. It rarely if ever occurs in Chinese, Japanese or blacks but is well documented in Asians from the Indian subcontinent. It is relatively rare in the USA. There are two peaks of onset: before the age of 5 and in the 30–50-year age group. In the second group twice as many women as men are diagnosed as suffering from the condition, but prevalence studies suggest that there is an equal sex distribution. Certain HLA types are more common among those with coeliac disease, such as HLA DR3, DR7 and DQ2.

Environmental factors almost certainly interact with genetic predisposing factors to produce overt disease. Several environmental factors have been implicated in the pathogenesis. The timing of the introduction of wheat to the diet may be important, with prolonged breastfeeding offering protection. Adenovirus 12 may be stimulating an autoimmune response through molecular mimicry (an amino acid sequence from this virus cross-reacts immunologically with a sequence from α-gliadin). Tissue transglutaminase has also been implicated as the autoantigen in the pathogenesis of coeliac disease. The presentation of peptide sequences by class II MHC molecules may also be important.

References

Ferguson A 1999 The coeliac iceberg. CME Journal of Gastroenterology, Hepatology and Nutrition 2: 52–56

Hill MD, McIntyre AS 1998 Coeliac disease: modern clinical practice. CME Journal of Gastroenterology, Hepatology and Nutrition 1: 36–41

Maki M 1997 Tissue transglutaminase as the autoantigen of coeliac disease. Gut 41: 565–566

McMillan SA, Watson RP, McCrum EE et al. 1996 Factors associated with serum antibodies to reticulin, endomysium and gliadin in adult population. Gut 39: 43–47

88. Coeliac disease

A.F   B.F   C.T   D.T   E.F

The diagnosis of coeliac disease was based on finding the classic small bowel mucosal changes, with resolution on a gluten-free diet and recurrence on gluten challenge. Over recent years the methods used to make a diagnosis have changed in several ways.

Endoscopic biopsies from the second part of the duodenum have superseded capsule biopsies. Gluten challenge is no longer required in children over the age of 2 in the revised European Society for Paediatric Gastroenterology and Nutrition (ESPGAN) criteria. IgA autoantibodies against endomysium have enabled more accurate screening and better use of endoscopy. IgA antigliadin antibodies were limited by sensitivity (46–90%) and specificity (85–98%) problems, with IgG antigliadin antibodies showing perhaps a minor improvement in accuracy (sensitivity 62–76% and specificity 88–97%). Antireticulin antibodies also have sensitivity (30–95%) and specificity (59–100%) levels that limit their usefulness. IgA antiendomysial antibodies (substrates include muscularis mucosae from monkey oesophagus and human umbilical cord) have been shown to offer a sensitivity up to 100% and specificity up to 99% in adults. This high accuracy makes these antibodies very useful in screening and targeting endoscopic biopsy to more appropriate cases. It must be remembered that selective IgA deficiency occurs in up to 10% of coeliac disease cases and this reduces the sensitivity of all the IgA-based tests. Antigliadin antibodies may be the most useful in monitoring compliance, as they return to normal within 1–3 months on a gluten-free diet and rise quite rapidly on gluten challenge. The improved reliability of screening antibody tests has enabled studies, which have demonstrated a higher prevalence than previously known. It is also apparent that there is a wide spectrum of disease, in terms of both symptoms and histological features. Cases may be asymptomatic, have mild symptoms, or the classic picture of malabsorption with weight loss, multiple nutritional deficiencies, low BMI, steatorrhoea and diarrhoea. The histological features can vary from the classic flat villous architecture with crypt hyperplasia to an isolated increase in intraepithelial lymphocytes.

There are a number of conditions associated with coeliac disease, including diabetes (with type I 'brittle diabetes' there is an estimated 50-fold increased prevalence), dermatitis herpetiformis, selective IgA deficiency, autoimmune thyroid disease, inflammatory bowel disease and rheumatoid arthritis. A low threshold for screening in these conditions is recommended. The long-term complications of coeliac disease include intestinal lymphoma (enteropathy-associated T-cell lymphoma: EATCL), carcinomas of the gastrointestinal tract and osteoporosis. All of these complications are dependent upon compliance. One study demonstrated that the carcinoma risk in untreated coeliacs was 11 times that of the normal population, a reduced-gluten diet reduced the relative risk to 5 times, and a gluten-free diet to just 1.2 times that of the general population. In the same study none of those on a strict gluten-free diet developed lymphoma. The carcinomas with an increased risk in coeliacs include carcinoma of the oesophagus, pharynx/larynx, and especially the small bowel.

References

Ferguson A 1999 The coeliac iceberg. CME Journal of Gastroenterology, Hepatology and Nutrition 2: 52–56

Hill MD, McIntyre AS 1998 Coeliac disease: modern clinical practice. CME Journal of Gastroenterology, Hepatology and Nutrition 1: 36–41

Holmes GKT, Prior P, Lane MR et al. 1989 Malignancy in coeliac disease – effect of gluten free diet. Gut 30: 333–338

McMillan SA, Watson RP, McCrum EE et al. 1996 Factors associated with serum antibodies to reticulin, endomysium and gliadin in adult populations. Gut 39: 43–47

NEPHROLOGY

89.   The nephrotic syndrome
A.F   B.F   C.F   D.T   E.T

The nephrotic syndrome is defined as a 24-hour urinary protein loss exceeding 3.5 g/1.73 m² of body surface area, associated with hypoalbuminaemia and peripheral oedema. Diabetic nephropathy is the most common cause of nephrotic range proteinuria in adults. Several primary glomerulopathies account for the great majority of remaining cases, with membranous glomerulonephritis accounting for 40% of these. Although IgA nephropathy is the most common glomerular disease in adults, it only occasionally causes a nephrotic syndrome. HIV nephropathy typically causes nephrotic proteinuria and renal insufficiency, and may be the first clinical manifestation of the acquired immunodeficiency syndrome (AIDS).

Despite traditional theories that reduced plasma oncotic pressure causes hypovolaemia and sodium retention, adults with the nephrotic syndrome are often found to have normal or increased plasma volumes. High blood pressure and increased levels of atrial natriuretic peptide both suggest circulatory overfilling. Patients may, however, have episodes of hypovolaemia, particularly after treatment with diuretics. If severe, this can cause acute renal failure, particularly in the elderly.

During the initial phase of oedema formation sodium excretion may be as low as 10 mmol/day. This can be counteracted with a combination of a low-sodium diet and loop diuretics. Sodium excretion can be further enhanced by the addition of a thiazide diuretic such as metolazone.

Thromboembolic complications are a major hazard of the nephrotic syndrome. Renal vein thrombosis occurs in 20–30% of patients with membranous nephropathy, although it may only be clinically apparent in 10%. Procoagulatory factors such as factors V and VIII and fibrinogen are increased, but antithrombin III is decreased. Low levels of factor XII lead to a prolonged partial thromboplastin time but are not associated with a tendency to bleed. Sepsis is another important complication of the nephrotic syndrome and an important cause of death.

Reference

Orth SR, Ritz E 1998 The nephrotic syndrome. New England Journal of Medicine 338(17): 1202–1211

90.   Solid organ transplantation

A.F   B.F   C.F   D.T   E.T

Infection is the most common life-threatening complication of long-term immunosuppressive therapy, although its incidence has decreased over the past 30 years. The net state of immunosuppression (immunodepression) of a patient is the result of many factors. These include the immunosuppressive drug regimen (dose, duration and temporal relation of individual agents), the effects of surgery, infection with immunomodulating viruses (e.g. CMV, Epstein–Barr (EBV), hepatitis B (HBV), hepatitis C (HCV) and HIV), uraemia, and coexisting conditions such as diabetes mellitus.

The immunosuppressive regimens used in all forms of solid organ transplantation are similar, resulting in similar patterns of infection and a consistent timetable for when certain infections occur. Three types of infection occur in the first month after transplantation: (1) rarely bacterial or fungal infection is passed on to the recipient via the allograft; (2) active infection in the recipient at the time of transplantation increases perioperative morbidity and can lead to bacterial or fungal colonization of the vascular anastomosis causing aneurysm formation; (3) however, more than 90% of infections occurring in the first month are the nosocomial infections of the surgical wound, lungs, urinary tract or vascular access devices that occur in all surgical patients. For this reason unnecessary lines should not be left in situ, and if a ureteric stent has been placed during the transplant procedure it should be removed within a few weeks. Opportunistic infections are very rarely encountered in the first month unless the patient was immunocompromised preoperatively.

From the second to the sixth month post transplant the most important pathogens are CMV and other herpes viruses such as Epstein–Barr. These predispose the patient to infection by the opportunistic pathogens such as *Pneumocystis carinii*, *Listeria monocytogenes*, fungi (e.g. *Candida* and *Aspergillus* sp.) and *Mycobacterium tuberculosis*.

After the sixth month post transplantation 80% of patients will have good allograft function and require minimal maintenance immunosuppression. These patients suffer from the same infectious diseases as the rest of the population. In addition, approximately 10% will continue to have chronic infection with CMV, EBV, HBV or HCV. These infections may damage organs such as the liver (HBV, HCV) or the retina (CMV). In 5–10% of transplant recipients acute, recurrent and chronic allograft rejection will have exposed them to higher levels of immunosuppression and therefore make them more susceptible to opportunistic infections.

CMV is the most important of the viruses that infect transplant recipients. It may lie dormant for years in the healthy carrier, to be reactivated in the second to fourth months after transplantation. Alternatively, infection will occur in about 70–80% of seronegative patients who receive an organ from a seropositive donor. In most patients features are confined to fever, malaise, elevated liver enzymes and leukopenia. However, occasionally thrombocytopenia, pneumonitis, gastrointestinal bleeding and encephalitis may occur. There is a 2% overall mortality. The best method of diagnosis is to detect antigenaemia, as serological tests are of little value and cultures take weeks to grow. Mild infections are usually self-limiting, but severe infections are treated with intravenous ganciclovir for 2–3 weeks. Some centres add specific CMV immunoglobulin. *Pneumocystis carinii* is closely linked with CMV and so should always be considered in a patient infected with this virus. Hypoxia is an early feature and may precede radiological changes. Diagnosis is by bronchoalveolar lavage and the treatment of choice is with high-dose co-trimoxazole.

Central nervous system infection is rare but has a high mortality, at over 50%. The immunocompromised patient may have few physical signs and so fever, headache, impaired consciousness or seizures should be investigated early with CT and lumbar puncture. Meningitis may be due to the conventional bacteria or to opportunistic organisms such as *Listeria* or *Cryptococcus*. Focal brain abscesses may be due to *Aspergillus*, *Nocardia* or, rarely *Candida* species. Encephalitis may occur with *Aspergillus*, *Toxoplasma*, herpes simplex or varicella viruses.

Septicaemia in a transplant recipient is usually due to *Staphylococcus aureus* and Gram-negative bacilli such as *Escherichia coli*, *Klebsiella pneumoniae* and *Pseudomonas aeruginosa*. Venous lines are the most likely source of staphylococci, whereas the coliforms tend to originate from the urinary or biliary tracts. If empirical antibiotic therapy is required initially, flucloxacillin and cefotaxime are an appropriate combination.

An increased risk of developing certain neoplasias is a well recognized complication of long-term immunosuppression. For example, the risk of developing a skin squamous cell carcinoma is increased by 40 times following transplantation. The risk of developing non-Hodgkin's lymphoma is markedly increased in patients on cyclosporin. Non-Hodgkin's lymphoma is commonest in the first year after transplantation, with the incidence falling to 0.06–0.08% per year. This pattern suggests that the causative agent was present at the time of immunosuppression and is almost always Epstein–Barr virus. For other post transplant malignancies the incidence increases with duration of follow-up.

References

Fishman JA, Rubin RH 1998 Infection in organ-transplant recipients. New England Journal of Medicine 338: 1741–1751

Newstead CG 1998 Assessment of risk of cancer after renal transplantation. Lancet 351: 610–611

91.   Solid organ transplantation

A.F   B.T   C.F   D.T   E.F

Azathioprine and corticosteroids have been the mainstays of immunosuppression in solid organ transplantation for over 30 years. Azathioprine is metabolized in the liver to the purine analogue mercaptopurine. Mercaptopurine is cytotoxic, preventing T- and B-cell activation and thereby affecting both cellular and humoral immune pathways. It is inactivated by xanthine oxidase, therefore concordant treatment with allopurinol, a xanthine oxidase inhibitor, can rapidly lead to toxic levels. Leucopenia is the most common side effect of azathioprine and is dose related.

Mycophenylate mofetil (MMF), introduced in 1995, is an inhibitor of de novo purine synthesis during cell division and particularly affects T- and B-cell proliferation. In a multicentre trial in the US comparing MMF and azathioprine in renal transplantation, MMF was shown to significantly reduce the risk of biopsy-proven rejection episodes. Data suggest that MMF has less bone marrow toxicity but gastrointestinal side effects are common and dose related.

Cyclosporin was introduced in 1983 and resulted in decreased rejection rates and an improvement in patient and graft survival in all solid organ and bone marrow transplants. It indirectly prevents the secretion of interleukin 2 (IL-2), a cytokine necessary for T-cell activation and proliferation. It is absorbed from the upper small intestine with a bioavailability of between 4 and 26% which can increase to 57% after a period of weeks. Metabolism occurs via the cytochrome P450 system, which is influenced by many other drugs. The metabolites, many of which are active, are excreted via the biliary tract. All of these factors necessitate careful monitoring of blood levels to ensure maintenance within the narrow therapeutic window. Adverse effects of cyclosporin include nephrotoxicity, hyperkalaemia and acidosis, hyperuricaemia and gout, hypophosphataemia, hyperlipidaemia, infection, tremor, gingival hyperplasia, hirsutism, hypertension, diabetes mellitus and haemolytic uraemic syndrome or thrombotic thrombocytopenic purpura.

Tacrolimus (FK506) has a similar mechanism of action to cyclosporin. It was initially approved for use in liver transplantation, but is now more widely used. It is at least as nephrotoxic as cyclosporin but causes less hyperlipidaemia, hirsutism or gum disease. It leads to a significantly higher incidence of new-onset insulin-dependent diabetes mellitus (IDDM). FK506 may be particularly useful as rescue therapy for renal transplant patients with recurrent or resistant rejection who are taking cyclosporin. Good results have been found using tacrolimus following combined kidney and pancreas transplantation.

References

First MR 1998 Clinical applications of immunosuppressive agents in renal transplantation. Surgical Clinics of North America 78:1: 61–76

Vella JP, Sayegh MH 1997 Maintenance pharmacological strategies in renal transplantation. Postgraduate Medical Journal 73: 386–390

92. Atheromatous renovascular disease
A.T   B.F   C.T   D.F   E.F

As many as 15% of patients reaching end-stage renal failure have a component of renal ischaemia. In patients over 60 atheromatous renovascular disease (ARVD) is the single most common cause of chronic renal failure, ahead of both diabetes mellitus and glomerulonephritis.

It may present in several different ways: hypertension, flash pulmonary oedema, acute renal failure (e.g. precipitated by ACE inhibitors), chronic renal failure, atheroembolic disease, as an incidental finding at angiography or at postmortem. Bilateral renal artery stenosis is common in the elderly and is usually accompanied by arterial disease at other sites.

ARVD is usually associated with no more than mild proteinuria. An ultrasound scan may show asymmetrical or bilaterally small kidneys. If suspected, a renal isotope scan with a captopril challenge can help make the diagnosis; in a patient with renovascular disease the administration of an ACE inhibitor may result in a decline in glomerular filtration rate and a prolongation in the transit time of the isotope through the kidney. The results are more difficult to interpret and are therefore less helpful in the face of moderate or severe renal impairment. The gold standard investigation remains renal angiography.

Although ARVD is an important cause of end-stage renal failure its treatment remains a matter of debate. In elderly patients generalized atheromatous disease is often associated with other medical problems, such as ischaemic heart disease. Intervention with percutaneous angioplasty or surgery carries risks and is therefore reserved to improve renal function rather than control blood pressure, which can usually be achieved with medication. Patients with acute or progressive renal failure due to atheromatous renal artery occlusion may achieve improvements in renal function following revascularization, thereby avoiding the need for dialysis and its associated complications. The main criteria for a favourable outcome include kidney size (> 9–9.5 cm), a patent renal artery distal to the stenosis, perfusion of the kidney on IVP and a serum creatinine of less than 400 µmol/l.

References

National High Blood Pressure Education Working Group 1995 Update of the working group reports on chronic renal failure and renovascular hypertension. Archives of Internal Medicine 156: 1938–1947

Nicholls A. 1997. Renovascular disease: the fifth frontier. Journal of the Royal Society of Medicine 90: 315–318

93. During pregnancy
A.F B.F C.T D.T E.F

In healthy pregnant women the GFR increases by 50% from the end of the first trimester and does not return to baseline until the end of pregnancy. Accordingly, serum creatinine concentration decreases by about 10% in the first trimester, and 30% in the last two trimesters with mean values declining from a pre-pregnancy average of 73 to 65, 51 and 47 μmol/l, respectively, in successive trimesters.

During normal pregnancy plasma volume increases continuously throughout gestation. Pre-eclampsia, however, is associated with a reduction in plasma volume, along with vasoconstriction and decreased renal blood flow. This leads to an increase in serum urate and eventually, creatinine.

Risk factors for developing pre-eclampsia include nulliparity, age over 40, family history, obesity, diabetes mellitus, fetal hydrops, multiple gestation, hypertension, renal disease, antiphospholipid antibody syndrome and vascular disease. The relative risk of pre-eclampsia developing in women with chronic renal disease is 20:1 and in women with essential hypertension it is 10:1. In these cases it may affect multiparous as well as nulliparous women and can occur earlier than the usual 32 weeks' gestation. It may also present as late as 48 hours postpartum. Laboratory findings in pre-eclampsia include elevated serum urate and creatinine, proteinuria greater than 250 mg/24 h, fragmented red cells, increased lactate dehydrogenase and thrombocytopenia.

Moderate hypertension occurring during pregnancy in the absence of other indicators of pre-eclampsia can be treated in the first instance with methyldopa, which is tried and tested and known to be safe during pregnancy. Second-line agents such as labetalol or metoprolol may be added if necessary, but atenolol has been reported to retard fetal growth. Hydralazine and calcium channel blockers have been used in patients unresponsive to the above. Diuretics should not be used, to avoid volume depletion, and ACE inhibitors are contraindicated after the first two trimesters, to prevent oligohydramnios.

The definitive treatment for established pre-eclampsia is delivery. Some clinicians advocate a trial of conservative management if the gestation is less than 34 weeks. However, most agree the pregnancy should be terminated if pre-eclampsia develops before 18 weeks.

Severe hypertension should be treated urgently. Hydralazine and labetalol can be given intravenously with cardiac monitoring, and sodium nitroprusside can also be used but only if delivery is imminent (because of the risk of fetal cyanide toxicity). Magnesium sulphate is a weak antihypertensive agent and is more effective than phenytoin in preventing seizures in pre-eclamptic women. Hypermagnesaemia may result in respiratory paralysis and should be treated with intravenous calcium. The dose of magnesium should be reduced in women with renal impairment.

The HELLP syndrome (haemolysis, elevated liver enzymes, low platelets) represents one form of severe pre-eclampsia and occurs in up to 12% of cases.

References

Jungers P, Chauveau D 1997 Pregnancy in renal disease. Kidney International 52: 871–885

Paller M S 1998 Hypertension in pregnancy. Journal of the American Society of Nephrology 9: 314–321

94. Kidney stones
A.T   B.F   C.F   D.T   E.F

In western societies the incidence of kidney stones is increasing. About 80% of stones consist of calcium usually as an oxalate or, less commonly, phosphate salt. The remaining 20% of stones are caused by substances such as uric acid, struvite or cystine.

Idiopathic hypercalciuria is found in 50–60% of patients with calcium stones and can be broadly classified into three groups. Absorptive hypercalciuria types I and II may be caused by increased calcitriol levels or increased numbers of calcitriol receptors in the gut. Type I is characterized by hypercalciuria on a low-calcium diet but normal urinary calcium while fasting. Type II is associated with a normal urinary calcium on a low-calcium diet but hypercalciuria as the dietary intake increases. Renal hypercalciuria resulting from a defect in renal tubular calcium reabsorption leads to high fasting urinary calcium and secondary hyperparathyroidism (with normal serum calcium levels). Calcium stones may also be associated with other disorders, such as primary hyperparathyroidism, sarcoidosis, prolonged immobilization, Crohn's disease and medullary sponge kidney.

The next most common group of patients with kidney stones are those with hyperuricosuria followed by hypocitraturia and hyperoxaluria. Uric acid stones are most common in middle-aged men. They are associated with gout, myeloproliferative disorders and the use of uricosuric drugs. Inborn errors of metabolism, such as Lesch–Nyhan syndrome and glycogen storage diseases, can cause uric acid stones in children. Citrate is a natural urinary inhibitor of stone formation along with other substances such as nephrocalcin. Hypocitraturia occurs with acidosis or acid retention and is therefore associated with renal tubular acidosis, metabolic acidosis of chronic diarrhoea, physical exercise and a meat-rich diet. Hyperoxaluria can either be primary, due to an inborn error of metabolism, or secondary to enteric malabsorption. In the latter, calcium ions are sequestered by long-chain fatty acids in the intestine and are unable to bind to free oxalate ions. These free ions are then absorbed and excreted in the urine.

Struvite stones primarily affect patients with neuropathic bladders, and are caused by recurrent urinary tract infection with urease-producing organisms such as *Proteus* species. Urease converts urea into ammonia, raising the urine pH and damaging the lining of the renal pelvis. This leads to the formation of stones containing struvite and apatite crystals, inflammatory cells and bacteria. They may grow rapidly and form staghorn calculi.

Cystine stones are uncommon and are caused by cystinuria, an autosomal recessive inborn error of metabolism. The stones are radio-opaque, usually multiple and can occur in children and young adults.

Investigations of patients with kidney stones should include urinalysis, urea and electrolytes, calcium and phosphate, plain abdominal X-ray and intravenous pyelography or ultrasound (bearing in mind that urate stones are radiolucent). If possible the stone should be retained and sent for analysis. In patients with recurrent stones a 24-hour urine sample should be collected and sent for calcium, uric acid, oxalate and citrate testing.

The advent of shockwave lithotripsy has dramatically improved the surgical management of patients with kidney stones, but there is much scope for medical management in both prevention and treatment. All patients should be advised to have a high fluid intake of at least 2 l/day. Dietary sodium should be restricted to 3–4 g/day and protein to 60 g/day. Patients with hyperoxaluria should avoid high-oxalate foods such as tea, nuts, chocolate and excess vitamin C, and in those who do not respond adequately calcium citrate supplements can be added. Calcium restriction is advisable only in patients with type II absorptive hypercalciuria. Thiazide diuretics may be useful in patients with renal hypercalciuria. Persistent urinary acidity exacerbates uric acid crystallization, and so treatment includes alkalinizing the urine with potassium citrate with or without the addition of allopurinol. Struvite stones should be fragmented and all calculus material removed, followed by long-term treatment with antibiotics. Cystine stones are treated by alkalinizing the urine and with chelating agents such as D-penicillamine.

References

Pak CYC 1998. Kidney stones. Lancet. 351: 1797–1801

Saklayen MG 1997 Medical management of nephrolithiasis. Medical Clinics of North America 81: 785–799

95. Acute renal failure

A.F   B.F   C.T   D.T   E.T

Acute renal failure (ARF) in the hospital setting is associated with a high morbidity and mortality. In critically ill patients invasive haemodynamic monitoring is required to accurately assess fluid balance in order to achieve adequate fluid replacement. Hypotension should be treated with fluid plus or minus inotropes to improve renal perfusion, and hyperkalaemia should be treated urgently as it may be life threatening. Many causes of ARF are treatable and, if recognized early, dialysis may be avoided. An early ultrasound scan is mandatory as obstruction is (usually) easy to relieve. Urinalysis revealing large amounts of blood and protein suggests a diagnosis of acute glomerulonephritis.

In animal experiments dopamine has been shown to dilate renal arteries. However, in humans the major factor causing an increase in renal blood flow is increased cardiac output, rather than any specific renal effect of dopamine, even at 'renal' doses. Although this increase in cardiac output is theoretically beneficial in the treatment of ARF no randomized controlled trials have been performed. Some studies have shown that prophylactic use of dopamine or dopexamine reduces the risk of ARF in high-risk patients undergoing surgery or intravenous contrast administration. Other similar studies, however, have not reproduced these findings. Diuretics are frequently used in the treatment of ARF, although they also have not been proved to be of benefit. Loop diuretics such as frusemide have the theoretical advantage of reducing the oxygen demand of the ascending loop of Henle by blocking the sodium pump. However, they do increase the nephrotoxic effects of other drugs such as gentamicin, and also acidify the urine, which can be detrimental in some causes of ARF, such as myoglobinuria and tumour lysis syndrome.

Prostaglandins are produced locally in the kidney and cause vasodilation of the surrounding arterioles. In the healthy individual they do not play a major role in the regulation of blood flow. However, under conditions of hypovolaemia when potent vasoconstrictors such as angiotensin are released they maintain adequate renal perfusion. Non-steroidal anti-inflammatory drugs (NSAIDs) block prostaglandin synthesis by inhibiting cyclo-oxygenase activity, and so may cause ARF in patients with low renal blood flow. Ibuprofen is less nephrotoxic than the other frequently prescribed NSAIDs. NSAIDs can also cause ARF by an immune-mediated interstitial nephritis.

The most frequent cause of renal failure in myeloma patients is cast nephropathy caused by the coprecipitation of light chains and Tamm–Horsfall protein in the tubules. It can be exacerbated by hypercalcaemia, dehydration, NSAIDs, infection and nephrotoxic antibiotics. Forced alkaline diuresis can prevent the precipitation of the proteins in the tubules. Chemotherapy should be started early to reduce production of the light chains, and recent studies have suggested that plasmapheresis is of benefit in the treatment of severe ARF.

Poisoning leading to ARF is uncommon but often easily treatable. Ethylene glycol is present in antifreeze and is sometimes ingested by alcoholics. It is converted to oxalic acid by alcohol dehydrogenase, and then precipitates in the tubules. Treatment is by ethanol infusion. A 600 mg/kg loading dose is followed by a maintenance infusion of 70–140 mg/kg/h. This acts by competing with ethylene glycol dehydrogenase, thereby reducing oxalic acid production. In severe poisoning haemodialysis should be considered early.

Lithium is not nephrotoxic if levels are maintained within the therapeutic range. Elevated levels and toxicity occur with dehydration, declining renal function and concomitant diuretic therapy. Deliberate self-overdose is less common than iatrogenic toxicity. Forced diuresis will enhance lithium excretion, but in patients with levels over 2.5 mmol/l haemodialysis should be considered.

References

Klahr S, Miller SB 1998 Acute oliguria. New England Journal of Medicine 338: 671–675

New DI, Barton IK 1996 Prevention of acute renal failure. British Journal of Hospital Medicine 55: 162–166

Turney JH 1996 Acute renal failure [editorial]. Journal of the American Medical Association 15: 275:19

96.   End-stage renal failure
A.T   B.F   C.F   D.F   E.T

The purpose of haemodialysis is to clear metabolic waste products while replenishing body buffers, and to remove excess body water. During haemodialysis, blood and an iso-osmotic dialysate containing electrolytes, buffers and glucose pass through the compartments of a dialysis filter in opposite directions on either side of a semipermeable membrane. Small molecular weight molecules diffuse between blood and the dialysate down a concentration gradient. Larger constituents such as proteins and cells are retained in the blood. Ultrafiltration is the process by which excess fluid is removed. By increasing the hydrostatic pressure in the blood compartment of the filter to greater than that in the dialysate compartment water molecules are forced across the membrane from blood to dialysate. A blood urea reduction of 65–70% can be achieved in a 3–4-hour dialysis session, and up to 3 l of excess fluid can be removed.

Symptomatic hypotension is very common during haemodialysis and may be associated with nausea and vomiting, muscle cramps, and eventually collapse. Inappropriate volume removal by ultrafiltration is the commonest cause. Ultrafiltration removes plasma water, which is replenished by fluid from the interstitial compartment. If water is removed more quickly than it can be replaced the vascular compartment contracts and eventually hypotension occurs. This can be treated simply by fluid replacement with normal saline. It is also important to recognize other causes of dialysis-associated hypotension. These include cardiac ischaemia or arrhythmia, bleeding, sepsis, pericardial effusion with tamponade, and (rarely now) membrane bioincompatibility. Conventional cellulose dialysis membranes can cause inflammatory reactions. They are known to induce complement activation by the release of C3a and C5a and to cause monocytes to generate lymphokines, such as tumour necrosis factor-α and interleukin-6. This can cause an anaphylactoid reaction. Modified cellulose membranes or the new synthetic membranes have much lower rates of bioincompatibility.

Forty years ago end-stage renal failure was universally fatal. Although the situation has been much improved by dialysis and transplantation, the annual mortality rate for patients on dialysis is still quite poor, ranging from 7.3% in France to 23% in the United States. International registries show that cardiovascular causes account for 40–50% of all recorded deaths, with infections ranking second at 12–15%. Numerous retrospective and prospective studies have found that protein–energy malnutrition and increased mortality are closely linked. A low serum albumin has been consistently found to be the laboratory test most correlated with increased risk of death.

To achieve peritoneal dialysis a catheter is tunnelled subcutaneously and implanted in the peritoneal cavity. A dialysis solution containing physiological amounts of sodium, magnesium, calcium and lactate (or occasionally bicarbonate) as the buffer is drained via the catheter in to the peritoneum, where it remains for a number of hours. During this dwell time metabolic waste products diffuse across the peritoneal membrane down a concentration gradient into the dialysis fluid. An osmolar gradient is created by different concentrations of glucose in order to achieve ultrafiltration. The volume of dialysate used for each dwell is

1.5–2 l, and this is changed 4–5 times a day. An alternative to CAPD is automated peritoneal dialysis, in which a mechanized cycler infuses and drains dialysis fluid to and from the peritoneum overnight, leaving the day free of exchanges.

The most common serious complication of peritoneal dialysis is peritonitis. This presents with cloudy dialysis fluid with or without abdominal pain. Microscopy of the fluid should demonstrate more than 100 white cells per ml. Micro-organisms will be evident in only 10–40% of cases. The most common causative organisms are Gram-positive cocci, followed by Gram-negative rods. Empirical antibiotic regimens are generally used as soon as the diagnosis is made. These are modified if the identity of the organism becomes known. Most commonly vancomycin and either a third-generation cephalosporin or an aminoglycoside are prescribed to be administered intraperitoneally. Yeast peritonitis is much less common but can be extremely serious. Although occasionally patients will respond to antifungal therapy, prompt catheter removal is usually necessary. Recurrent peritonitis may lead to peritoneal fibrosis and failure to dialyse adequately.

Reference

Eggers PW 1990 Mortality rates amongst dialysis patients in Medicare's end-stage renal disease program. American Journal of Kidney Diseases 15: 414–421

Ifudu O 1998 Care of patients undergoing haemodialysis. New England Journal of Medicine 339: 1054–1062

Pastan S, Bailey J 1998 Dialysis therapy. New England Journal of Medicine 338: 1428–1437

97. Management of rhabdomyolysis
A.F   B.F   C.F   D.T   E.T

Acute renal failure associated with muscle injury was originally described in victims of the Blitz during the Second World War. Although the majority of descriptions involve victims of crush injuries, so-called non-traumatic rhabdomyolysis is becoming increasingly prevalent. More common presentations to the medical registrar include drug or alcohol overdose victims who have lain in one position for a number of hours, compromising the circulation to one or more muscle groups. Other causes of rhabdomyolysis include strenuous exercise, seizures, heatstroke, viral infections, inflammatory myopathies, drugs (amphetamines, alcohol, phencyclidine, statins) and neuroleptic malignant syndrome. In these patients there may be generalized muscle involvement rather than isolated individual muscle groups.

Skeletal muscle contains up to 5 mg/g wet weight of myoglobin. When damaged, muscles release this myoglobin into the circulation which is freely filtered by the glomeruli, passing into the tubules. Under acidic conditions this myoglobin can precipitate with Tamm–Horsfall protein and directly block tubules. It also dissociates into haem and globin leading to the production of ferrihaemate, a nephrotoxic compound.

In order to prevent the rapid onset of acute tubular necrosis, the prompt diagnosis and management of rhabdomyolysis is needed. Careful history and examination are required, along with early consideration of the diagnosis. Tea-coloured urine that is strongly positive for blood on dipstick but reveals no red blood cells on microscopy implies myoglobinuria (or haemoglobinuria in the presence of intravascular haemolysis). Serum creatinine kinase (CK) is a useful test as it can rise rapidly with muscle damage. However, the absolute level of CK is not a reliable guide to the risk of developing renal failure. It is always important to look for and exclude a compartment syndrome. This occurs when local muscular ischaemia leads to increased pressure within an osteofascial compartment. Skeletal muscle is able to tolerate ischaemia for up to 1.5 hours with full recovery. When the blood supply is interrupted for periods longer than this, worsening muscle damage occurs. When ischaemic muscle is reperfused capillary permeability is increased, leading to tissue oedema. When the compartment pressure exceeds capillary perfusion pressure microcirculatory blood flow stops. Normal compartment pressures range from 0 to 15 mmHg; pressures over 30–35 mmHg halt tissue perfusion completely. Therefore, peripheral pulses are often palpable in the presence of a significant compartment syndrome. If the diagnosis is in doubt the intracompartment pressure can be measured directly and, if confirmed, fasciotomies should be performed to relieve the pressure. True compartment syndrome, however, is rare and unnecessary surgery should be avoided because of the high risk of infection of an open wound.

Initial treatment for the patient with rhabdomyolysis entails rapid fluid resuscitation, as they are invariably volume depleted. Renal hypoperfusion is a major contributing factor to the onset of acute renal failure. Patients are frequently acidotic from the catabolic effects of muscle injury. Intravenous bicarbonate should be administered to alkalinize the urine and minimize precipitation of myoglobin in the tubules. A urine pH of 7 should be gradually achieved while keeping a careful eye on arterial blood gases. The addition of mannitol has also been demonstrated to be beneficial in creating a diuresis to wash the myoglobin through the tubules. Mannitol is used in preference to frusemide as it is a volume expander and does not acidify the urine.

The marked acidosis often seen initially is frequently accompanied by profound hyperkalaemia. This will improve with a good diuresis and treatment of the acidosis, but may require urgent dialysis if the patient is oliguric. Hypocalcaemia also occurs owing to deposition of calcium in damaged muscles. This should not be treated unless tetani develop, as this calcium is eventually released back into the circulation and may lead to hypercalcaemia. Renal-dose dopamine may be helpful in producing a diuresis but has not been demonstrated to improve prognosis. Plasmapheresis is able to lower serum levels of myoglobin rapidly, but this does not effect the risk of developing acute renal failure.

References

Bywaters EG, Beall D 1998 Crushing injuries with impairment of renal function 1941 [classic article]. Journal of the American Society of Nephrology 9(2): 322–332

Slater MS, Mullins RJ 1998 Rhabdomyolysis and myoglobinuric renal failure in trauma and surgical patients: a review. Journal of the American College of Surgeons 186: 693–716

Szewczyk D, Ovadia P, Abdullah F, Rabinovici R 1998 Pressure-induced rhabdomyolysis and acute renal failure. Journal of Trauma 44: 384–388

98.   IgA nephropathy
A.**T**   B.**F**   C.**T**   D.**F**   E.**F**

IgA nephropathy was first described by Berger in the late 1960s and therefore often carries his name. It is the most common cause of glomerulonephritis in adults worldwide and has a male to female ratio of about 2:1. It usually presents in the second or third decade. People diagnosed under the age of 25 tend to be male and present with episodes of macroscopic haematuria associated with upper respiratory tract or gastrointestinal infections. Those diagnosed over the age of 25 are often asymptomatic, the sex ratio is 1:1 and are picked up by finding persistent microscopic haematuria on routine examination. A few patients (about 10%) present with either acute glomerulonephritis, nephrotic syndrome or end-stage renal failure. Patients have varying degrees of proteinuria, with heavy proteinuria being a bad prognostic sign. Other risk factors for progression to end-stage renal disease include older age at presentation, male sex, hypertension, persistent proteinuria, impaired renal function at the time of diagnosis, and the presence of glomerulosclerosis or interstitial fibrosis on renal biopsy. About 20% of patients with IgA nephropathy will eventually progress to end-stage renal failure.

IgA nephropathy is diagnosed on renal biopsy. It is characterized by glomerular mesangial deposition of IgA, as demonstrated by immunofluorescent microscopy. This is associated with varying degrees of mesangial cell proliferation and an increase in mesangial matrix. The histological changes can range from very mild to very severe, and are classified from grades I to V. The renal histology of Henoch–Schönlein purpura is indistinguishable from that of IgA nephropathy and in the acute phase of both conditions circulating levels of IgA and IgA immune complexes are elevated. Although there are differences between the two conditions the similarities are such that they are considered to be different manifestations of the same disease process. IgA nephropathy is occasionally associated with other systemic diseases, including hepatic cirrhosis, dermatitis herpetiformis and coeliac disease.

Although there is no curative therapy for IgA nephropathy, many treatment strategies have been tried in an attempt to delay progression. Trials of corticosteroids with or without adjunctive cytotoxic agents such as chlorambucil or cyclophosphamide have been undertaken, with mixed results. A meta-analysis of randomized controlled trials concluded that they reduce proteinuria, but was unclear as to whether they affect renal function in the long term. A recent prospective study has shown that a prolonged course of corticosteroids (6 months) may reduce proteinuria and delay the progression of renal failure in patients with mild renal impairment. Aggressive therapy tends to be reserved for patients with heavy proteinuria and severe lesions on renal biopsy. Fish oils have also been studied and have been shown to be of some benefit on short-term follow-up. A multicentre randomized placebo-controlled trial has demonstrated that angiotensin-converting enzyme inhibitors are more effective than other antihypertensives in reducing proteinuria and delaying progression to end-stage renal failure in patients with IgA nephropathy.

References

Ambrus JL, Sridhar NR 1997 Immunological aspects of renal disease. Journal of the American Medical Association 278: 1938–1945

Harper L, Savage COS 1999 Treatment of IgA nephropathy. Lancet 353: 860–862

Hricik DE, Chung-Park M, Sedor J R 1998 Glomerulonephritis. New England Journal of Medicine 339: 888–899

INFECTIOUS DISEASES

99. Leprosy

A.**T** B.**F** C.**F** D.**F** E.**T**

Despite an eradication campaign leprosy transmission remains common in most developing countries. There is a spectrum of disease, ranging from lepromatous leprosy with diffuse involvement of skin and nerves and high numbers of bacteria, to tuberculoid with a few skin patches or nerves involved and very few bacteria. The host's immune response rather than the bacillus determines the pattern of disease. A strong immune response tends towards the tuberculoid (paucibacillary) end of the spectrum, and a weak immune response to the lepromatous (multibacillary) pattern. Patients can move in both directions along this spectrum during a single illness ('upgrading' and 'downgrading').

The incubation period for leprosy is very long – up to 10 years or more – and multibacillary cases have often been excreting bacilli from the nose for many years before diagnosis. Despite these features transmission rates are very low. Patients become non-infectious within a couple of days of starting treatment, and isolation is therefore unnecessary. Multibacillary cases require treatment for 2 years, paucibacillary cases for 6 months, with a combination of rifampicin, dapsone and clofazimine. The WHO has recently accepted a 1-day treatment for those with a single skin lesion. In compliant patients the cure rate is close to 100%, though some can be left with severe lifelong disability owing to residual nerve damage. The nerve damage can follow either glove-and-stocking or mononeuritis multiplex patterns. Leprosy is probably the most important cause of peripheral neuropathy worldwide.

Steroids and thalidomide are sometimes helpful in treating the adverse reactions to antilepromatous therapy, which are common. In 1998 the US Food and Drug Administration (FDA) licensed thalidomide for this single indication. Although leprosy is a mycobacterium, HIV seems to make no difference to its transmission. BCG vaccination has, however, been shown to be highly protective against all forms of the disease.

References

Karonga Prevention Trial Group 1996 Randomised controlled trial of single BCG, repeated BCG, or combined BCG and killed *Mycobacterium leprae* vaccine for prevention of leprosy and tuberculosis in Malawi. Lancet 348: 17–24

Whitty CJM, Lockwood DNL 1999 Leprosy – new perspectives on an old disease. Journal of Infection 36: 38

100. Parasite presentation

A.F   B.T   C.T   D.F   E.T

It is extremely rare for the non-recurrent malarias (*Plasmodium falciparum* and *P. malariae)* to present more than a few months after return from the tropics. In contrast, *P. vivax and P. ovale* put down 'hypnozoites' (sleeping forms) in the liver at the time of infection, and these can reactivate months or sometimes years after return from a tropical area. Often the patient will not remember the initial attack. The hypnozoites are not killed by antimalarials used to treat malaria. Only primaquine is currently licensed to kill the liver forms ('radical cure'), and has to be used once the patient has recovered from the acute illness.

Strongyloides is the only worm that can complete its full lifecycle in humans, and can therefore persist for a lifetime. It may only become clinically apparent when the patient is old, or is immunosuppressed. Ex-Far East prisoners of war are still presenting for the first time more than 50 years after they returned to Britain. It is endemic in many warm climates, especially southeast Asia and the Caribbean. Diagnosis is by stool examination and serology.

Leishmania donovani, one of the causes of massive splenomegaly and pancytopenia, is another parasite which can survive at undetectable levels for a lifetime in the immunocompetent, only becoming apparent in the immunosuppressed, especially in patients with HIV. *Leishmania donovani* can be contracted around the Mediterranean and in various parts of Asia, Africa and South America.

Entamoeba histolytica can be carried asymptomatically in the gut for many years. Clinical disease follows tissue invasion, resulting in liver abscess, amoebic colitis or an amoeboma elsewhere. The trigger for this sudden switch to pathogenicity is unclear. Treatment of the invasive disease is with metronidazole or tinidazole, but this does not prevent cyst passage in the gut. This has to be treated with a subsequent luminal amoebicide to prevent invasive amoebic disease in the future. Diagnosis of the luminal amoeba is by stool microscopy, but *E. histolytica* is indistinguishable morphologically from the non-pathogenic (and more common) *E. dispar*. PCR can be used for successful differentiation. Diagnosis of invasive disease is usually by serology: often no cysts are identified in the stool at this stage.

References

Gonzalez-Ruiz A, Wright SG 1998 Disparate amoebae. Lancet 351: 1672–1673

Schneider JH, Rogers AI 1997 Strongyloides: the protean parasitic infection. Postgraduate Medicine 102: 177–192

101. Pathology mediated by exotoxins

A.T B.F C.T D.T E.F

Cholera is an archetypal exotoxin-mediated disease. The bacteria almost never invade, remaining in the gut lumen. The toxin binds to a receptor, resulting in changes to a GTP-binding protein, which in turn activates adenylate cyclase with an increase in cAMP and fluid secretion. In severe cases patients can secrete many times their body weight in diarrhoea.

Gram-negative septic shock is largely mediated by an endotoxin. The toxic element is part of the bacterial cell wall. During phagocytosis the engulfed bacteria can cause cell death, with the release of pyrogens and activation of the immune system. The term toxic shock syndrome is usually reserved for the exotoxin-mediated shock caused by release of exotoxin by strains of *Staphylococcus aureus*, which can build up in tampons. Gram-negative organisms can produce exotoxins. Important ones are the *Shigella* toxin, which can cause haemolytic uraemic syndrome, and the cholera-like toxins produced by the ETEC strains of *Escherichia coli*, the main cause of traveller's diarrhoea.

Clostridium tetani is usually localized to a very small wound where the point of entry is often not seen. It releases a highly potent exotoxin, tetanospasmin, which binds irreversibly with receptors in the presynaptic endplate. This prevents the release of inhibitory neuromediators, causing near-permanent depolarization and muscle spasm. The *Clostridium botulinum* exotoxin is an even more potent exotoxin, which binds to the presynaptic endplate and prevents acetylcholine release, causing a flaccid paralysis. *Clostridium diphtheriae* exotoxin causes both myocardial disease and peripheral neuropathy.

Entamoeba histolytica does not have an exotoxin. It is able to cause cell death by inserting an 'amoebapore'. This is a highly effective ion channel that causes an almost immediate change in the ionic balance of cells, resulting in cell death. How the amoeba holds such a universally cidal channel near the cell surface and manages to insert it without killing itself remains incompletely understood.

Reference

Sanchez JL, Taylor DN 1997 Cholera. Lancet 349: 1825–1830

102. Nematodes that migrate through the lung
A.T   B.F   C.F   D.T   E.F

The nematodes that affect humans include *Ascaris lumbricoides*, hookworms (*Ancylostoma duodenale* and *Necator americanus*) and *Strongyloides stercoralis*. They pass through the lung as part of their development. The larvae make their way to the lung and then penetrate the lung wall and climb to the larynx, where they are swallowed. They live the rest of their lives in the gut lumen. In intubated patients from the tropics it is not uncommon for *Ascaris* to appear up an endotracheal tube. Larvae of *Strongyloides* and hookworm penetrate the skin, usually from walking barefoot, and then migrate to the lungs and are swallowed.

The gut nematodes *Enterobius vermicularis* (threadworm), *Trichuris trichiura* (whipworm) and the muscle nematode *Trichinella spiralis* do not pass through the lung. The filarial worms *Loa loa*, *Wuchereria bancrofti* and *Brugia malayi* can cause lung problems, ranging from wheezing to tropical pulmonary eosinophilia. Microfilaria from these filarial worms live in the lung most of the time, but do not strictly migrate through it. Another important filarial worm is *Onchocerca volvulus*, the cause of river blindness, but microfilaria do not enter the lung.

Schistosomes are flukes (trematodes), not nematodes, that penetrate the skin from swimming in infected water, and migrate through the lungs. *Paragonimus westermani* is another fluke that lives in the lung. The other flukes of medical importance are the liver flukes, especially *Fasciola hepatica* and *Opisthorchis* (or *Clonorchis*) *sinensis*.

Tapeworms (cestodes), the other worm family of medical importance, do not usually enter the lung, although hydatid disease (from dog tapeworms) can cause lung cysts.

References

Burnham G 1998 Onchocerciasis. Lancet 351:1341–1346

Ong RK, Doyle RL 1998 Tropical pulmonary eosinophilia. Chest 113: 1673–1679

Sarinas PS, Chitkara RK 1997 Ascariasis and hookworm. Seminars in Respiratory Infections 12: 130–137

Wehner JH, Kirsch CM 1997 Pulmonary manifestations of strongyloides. Seminars in Respiratory Infection 12: 122–129

103. Diseases transmitted by specific vectors

A.F   B.T   C.F   D.T   E.F

Many diseases are transmitted by vectors but the following are perhaps the most important. Only the night-biting anopheles mosquito transmits all species of malaria. Anopheles mosquitoes occasionally transmit filarial disease. The culex mosquito family transmits a number of the filarial diseases. Aedes mosquitoes are vectors of several viral diseases that occur in epidemics, the most important being yellow fever and dengue fever. They also occasionally transmit filarial disease.

African trypanosomiasis (sleeping sickness) is caused by *Trypanosoma brucei* and is transmitted by tsetse flies. American trypanosomiasis (Chagas' disease), caused by *T. cruzei*, causes organomegaly and myocarditis and is transmitted by Reduviid (Triatome) bugs (assassin bugs) of various species which live in South America.

All species of leishmania are transmitted by sandflies of the *Phlebotomus* and *Lutzomyia* species. Mites, lice and ticks transmit different forms of rickettsial disease (especially typhus). *Onchocerca volvulus,* the cause of river blindness, is transmitted by the blackfly *Simulium damnosum*. Loa loa is transmitted by the chrysops fly.

Despite early fears that HIV might be transmissible by mosquitoes or other vectors there is now good epidemiological evidence that it is not.

Recent work suggests that genetically modifying vector species may lead to reduced disease transmission.

Reference

Conte JE 1997 A novel approach to preventing insect-borne diseases. New England Journal of Medicine 337: 785–786

---

104. Relative contraindications to the use of antimalarial drugs

A.T   B.T   C.F   D.T   E.F

Patients with the relatively common sex-linked enzyme defect glucose 6-phosphate dehydrogenase (G6PD) deficiency can have haemolytic crises caused by oxidizing drugs. Primaquine is probably the most important. Other antimalarials, including quinine and chloroquine, have occasionally been implicated, but this is not a major practical problem. Other important drugs to avoid in G6PD deficiency are dapsone, nitrofurantoin, naladixic acid and several of the sulphonamides. Primaquine needs to be prescribed to patients who have vivax or ovale forms of malaria to kill the liver hypnozoites ('radical cure'), but G6PD deficiency should be routinely excluded before administration.

Chloroquine can cause an exacerbation of psoriasis. Other adverse effects of chloroquine include slight increases in the risk of neuropsychiatric illness and epilepsy. Proguanil is well tolerated but can rarely cause alopecia. Mefloquine is contraindicated in epilepsy and psychotic illness and the risk of neuropsychiatric side effects is probably higher than with other antimalarials. Doxycycline can cause significant photosensitivity as well as oesophageal ulceration.

Quinine has a direct stimulatory effect on the pancreas and hypoglycaemia can occur during treatment of severe malaria, as the disease itself can also lower blood glucose levels. Pregnant women with malaria are at particular risk of hypoglycaemia.

Doxycycline and primaquine are contraindicated in pregnancy. Mefloquine should not be given in the first trimester. Quinine, chloroquine and proguanil are all safe in pregnancy.

References

White NJ 1996 The treatment of malaria. New England Journal of Medicine 335: 800–806

Whitty CJM 1997 Malaria prophylaxis for the 1990s and beyond. British Journal of Hospital Medicine 58: 545–546

105. Clinical diagnostic methods of choice
A.F   B.F   C.F   D.T   E.F

The number of diagnostic tools available for infectious diseases has increased enormously. Most of the new techniques have limited clinical indications but are useful in research.

The polymerase chain reaction (PCR) is a sensitive method of detecting tuberculous DNA in sputum but has a number of drawbacks that limit its clinical usefulness. It gives no indication of the viability of organisms, most people travelling in poorer countries will be exposed to tuberculosis (TB), and the presence of TB DNA does not necessarily mean active infection. It is important to know whether an individual has 'open' TB (and is therefore infectious). This depends on quantifying the amount of TB in sputum with microscopy. PCR is usually used as an all-or-none technique. Quantitative methods have been developed but have not yet been shown to be reliable diagnostically in pulmonary TB. In an era of drug-resistant TB it is also very important to be able to test sensitivity to antimicrobial agents, and this currently requires culture. In the future laboratories may be able to perform PCR to look for genes encoding resistance but such techniques currently remain research tools. Microscopy and culture of sputum or broncheolar lavage are the diagnostic methods of choice.

The Widal test in typhoid is of very limited usefulness. 'O' and 'H' antigens are detected. Unfortunately the test is not very sensitive early in the disease. In addition, anybody who has been vaccinated against typhoid will be 'H' positive, and both antigens cross-react with other *Salmonella* species. False positives and negatives are therefore common. Blood culture is diagnostic in most cases: although textbooks quote a sensitivity of less than 80%, modern culture methods are much more sensitive particularly in the first week of disease. Bone marrow culture has the highest sensitivity.

The leishmanin skin test is an antigen test similar to the tuberculin test. It is of no diagnostic use in visceral leishmaniasis, as almost all cases will be non-reactors. Individuals who are able to mount a strong immune reaction would not have the disease. The diagnostic method of choice is microscopy of splenic or bone-marrow aspirates looking for parasites. The leishmanin test has theoretical uses in cutaneous leishmaniasis, but in practice diagnosis of this condition also depends on light microscopy, with PCR for speciation.

Many new methods have been developed to aid the diagnosis of malaria. Antigen-detecting 'stix' tests are now available and are almost as sensitive as microscopy. These tests, however, are all-or-none (in malaria the parasite count is very important) and are species specific. At present only tests for *Plasmodium falciparum* are available routinely, but new ones are being developed. They are useful for screening and in situations where there is no technician competent to examine malaria films, but they do not provide as much information as microscopy. Fluorescent microscopy (QBC) of the buffy coat is much more labour-intensive than light microscopy and has no real advantages. PCR also takes longer and provides less information than light microscopy.

Diagnosis of the later stages of syphilis is serological. There is near 100% sensitivity for VDRL (venereal disease reference laboratory), TPHA (*Treponema pallidum* haemaglutination assay) and FTA (fluorescent treponemal antibody absorbed) tests in secondary syphilis. The TPHA remains elevated for life, and can therefore represent past infection. The VDRL fades with time and is more helpful in determining disease activity. The major drawback of the VDRL test is its lack of specificity. False positive reactions occur with systemic lupus erythematosus, TB, chronic infections, HIV and Lyme disease. The TPHA is the usual screening test for the later stages of syphilis. In primary syphilis the TPHA is less than 80% sensitive and the best serological test is the FTA. In very early primary syphilis this may also be negative, and occasionally dark-ground microscopy is needed.

References

Chiodini PL 1998 Non-microscopic methods for the diagnosis of malaria. Lancet 351: 80–81

Marshall BG, Shaw RJ 1996 New technology in the diagnosis of tuberculosis. British Journal of Hospital Medicine 55: 491–494

Nandwani R 1996 Modern diagnosis and management of acquired syphilis. British Journal of Hospital Medicine 55: 399–403

Zenilman JM 1997 Typhoid fever. Journal of the American Medical Association 278: 847–850

106. Infections
A.**F**   B.**T**   C.**T**   D.**T**   E.**F**

Immunity to malaria is difficult to acquire and easy to lose. The mechanisms behind it are incompletely understood. In vitro research seemed to suggest an important role for CD4 cells, but the advent of HIV has altered this view. HIV makes little impact on the course of malaria, except possibly in pregnancy. To date no vaccine has been developed that provides significant protection against malarial disease.

Septic shock is mediated by several elements of the immune system. Tumour necrosis factor (TNF), various interleukins, nitric oxide and platelet-activating factor have all been associated with its pathophysiology, and the overproduction of these mediators may be central to the observed high levels of morbidity and mortality. Clinical trials of antibodies to bind or block these elements have been tried in severe sepsis and malaria. So far none has demonstrated any significant clinical benefit. A trial of antiendotoxin, which did claim a benefit in septic shock, subsequently had to be retracted by the authors.

Salmonella typhi invade macrophages and are carried to areas of the reticuloendothelial system. Much of the pathology in typhoid disease is caused by interaction between the bacteria and the immune system. The inflammation and sloughing of Peyer's patches in the gut can lead to bowel perforation or haemorrhage, usually in the third week of the disease. In severe typhoid disease corticosteroids have been shown to have significant benefits in clinical trials. Corticosteroids should be used with great caution in bacterial and parasitic infections, but have a proven role in selected cases of bacterial and tuberculous meningitis, miliary and lymph-node TB and leprosy reactions. They have no role in most other causes of severe sepsis, or in malaria.

Eosinophils are central to the body's defences against worm invasion. An eosinophilia should always raise the possibility of a parasitic infection. Very high eosinophil counts are particularly common with *Strongyloides*, filarial worms and schistosomiasis. Other causes of eosinophilia include asthma and other atopic conditions and malignancies.

References

Bone RC 1996 Why sepsis trials fail. Journal of the American Medical Association 276: 565–566

Cobb JP, Danner RL 1996 Nitric oxide and septic shock. Journal of the American Medical Association 275: 1193–1196

Rothenberg ME 1998 Eosinophilia. New England Journal of Medicine 338: 1592–1600

107. Antimicrobials

A.T   B.T   C.T   D.T   E.T

The qinghaosu derivatives artesunate, artemether and arteether are drugs which have been recently developed from traditional Chinese medicine. They are highly active against malaria. Clinical trials show them to be as effective as quinine in severe falciparum disease and to be the drug of choice where quinine resistance is likely (such as in certain parts of southeast Asia).

The fluoroquinolones ciprofloxacin, ofloxacin and norfloxacin are currently the drugs of choice in typhoid. Chloramphenicol is the traditional drug, but resistance is now common. Third-generation cephalosporins also have some activity, but are probably less effective except in the currently rare cases where there is fluoroquinolone resistance.

Leishmaniasis continues to be treated with sodium stiboglutanate. The alternative drug of choice is amphotericin. Toxicity is common with amphotericin, but new liposomal forms have proved effective and have less toxicity.

Azithromycin is a relatively new antibiotic that can be used for almost any disease where erythromycin would be appropriate. It has an extremely long half-life.

Brucellosis is difficult to treat. Combination therapy is always necessary, and the standard combinations require some mixture of rifampicin, streptomycin and doxycycline for extended periods (weeks to months).

References

Russo R, Nigro LC, Minniti S et al. 1996 Visceral leishmaniasis in HIV infected patients: treatment with high dose liposomal amphotericin. British Journal of Infection 32: 133–137

Stout JE, Yu VL 1997 Current concepts –legionellosis. New England Journal of Medicine 337: 682–688

Tran TH, Day NP, Nguyen MD et al.1996 A controlled trial of artemether or quinine in Vietnamese adults with severe falciparum malaria. New England Journal of Medicine 335: 76–83

White NJ, Dung NM, Vinh H, Bethell D, Hien TT 1996 Fluoroquinolones in children with multidrug-resistant typhoid. Lancet 348: 547

HIV

108. Clinical features of acute HIV-1 infection
A.T   B.T   C.F   D.T   E.F

More than 30 million people worldwide are estimated to be infected with HIV-1, HIV-2 being confined mainly to West Africa. Globally there are estimated to be 16 000 new cases of HIV-1 infection daily. Between 40 and 90% of new HIV-1 infections are symptomatic. However, as the symptoms are frequently non-specific the diagnosis is often missed.

The signs and symptoms of acute infection typically occur days to weeks after initial exposure. Common signs and symptoms include fever, maculopapular rash, headache, aseptic meningitis, lymphadenopathy, pharyngitis, arthralgia, myalgia, nausea, vomiting, diarrhoea and mucosal ulceration. Routine blood tests may reveal leucopenia, thrombocytopenia or raised liver function tests (typically the transaminases, ALT and AST). The acute illness typically lasts less than 2 weeks but may last up to 10 weeks. Severe and prolonged symptoms are correlated with rapid disease progression. The diagnosis of acute HIV-1 infection should be considered in any patient with signs and symptoms consistent with infection and a history of possible exposure as well as any patient with a newly diagnosed sexually transmitted disease.

As standard serological tests (such as HIV-1 ELISA) do not become positive until 22–27 days after acute infection, laboratory diagnosis of acute HIV-1 infection depends on detection of viral p24 antigen or viral RNA in the plasma. Viral RNA is more sensitive and becomes detectable earlier in acute infection than p24 antigen. The detection of a high HIV-1 RNA viral load with a negative HIV-1 antibody test confirms the diagnosis. Viral load is typically greater than 50 000 copies/ml, and many patients will have more than 1 000 000 copies/ml. If low levels of HIV-1 RNA are found in the plasma in the context of a negative antibody test this may represent acute infection detected after the initial burst of viraemia or, more rarely, chronic infection without seroconversion. If both HIV-1 RNA and antibody are negative but the patient is symptomatic and at high risk, these should be repeated after 2–4 weeks.

In all patients with acute HIV-1 infection counselling should be given and, particularly as infectivity is very high at this time, this should include counselling about avoiding high-risk behaviours. In addition, other sexually transmitted diseases should be excluded and contact tracing initiated. The rationale for treatment of acute HIV-1 infection with antiretroviral drugs is based on the observation that early treatment restores virus-specific cellular immune responses; may limit viral dissemination, thereby restricting damage to immune and antigen-presenting cells; and may reduce the chance of disease progression. Clinical trial data to support antiretroviral therapy during acute infection are limited. Low-dose zidovudine continued for 6 months leads to a more marked increase in CD4 count than with placebo. Early therapy with two nucleoside analogues and a protease inhibitor resulted in undetectable viral load and an increased CD4 count. In addition, such therapy resulted in vigorous HIV-1 specific responses of CD4+ T-helper cells similar to those seen in non-progressive chronic infection. These data suggest that early therapy may help restore immune responses, which may result in slower disease progression. Despite this, the long-term benefit of such early treatment has not been demonstrated, and if patients are unable to adhere to a complex drug regimen viral resistance is likely to develop, which will severely limit future treatment options.

References

Kahn JO, Walker BD 1998 Acute human immunodeficiency virus infection. New England Journal of Medicine 339: 33–39

Quinn TC 1997 Grand round at the Johns Hopkins Hospital. Acute primary HIV infection. Journal of the American Medical Association 278: 58–62

109. Pathogenesis of acute HIV-1 infection
A.F   B.T   C.T   D.T   E.F

Animal models of intravaginal HIV-1 infection reveal that the first targets of the virus are Langerhans' cells (tissue dendritic cells) in the lamina propria beneath the epithelium. These cells then fuse with CD4+ lymphocytes, and within 2 days of infection virus can be detected in the iliac lymph nodes. In humans, the time from genital mucosal HIV-1 infection to viraemia varies from 4 to 11 days. Breaks in the mucosal barrier and inflammation which may be due to other sexually transmitted diseases increase the risk of acquiring HIV-1 infection. Infection can occur across the oral mucosa with the nasopharyngeal tonsil and adenoid tissues probably providing the initial target cells from which the virus is transmitted to CD4+ cells.

Transmitted HIV-1 is typically macrophage-tropic (not T-cell tropic). The HIV-1 viral envelope protein GP120 binds to the CD4 molecule. However, cell entry requires the presence of a coreceptor. The coreceptor for macrophage-tropic HIV-1 strains is CCR5, a surface chemokine receptor present on Langerhans' cells.

After infection there is a rapid rise in plasma viraemia with dissemination of the virus and seeding of lymphoid organs. High levels of virus are present in the genital tract at this stage, and so patients are likely to be highly infectious. After the initial peak of viraemia there is a marked reduction in viral load to a steady state of viral replication. This reduction is likely to be due to HIV-1–specific cytotoxic T lymphocytes. Neutralizing antibodies do not usually appear until weeks to months after the reduction in viral load. The level of viral load steady state or viral set-point is important, as individuals with the highest viral loads have the most rapid rates of progression to AIDS and death. The factors determining this set point include genetic differences in coreceptors, qualitative differences in the immune response and the virulence of the infecting strain.

References

Kahn JO, Walker BD 1998 Acute human immunodeficiency virus infection. New England Journal of Medicine 339: 33–39

Quinn TC 1997 Grand round at the Johns Hopkins Hospital. Acute primary HIV infection. Journal of the American Medical Association 278: 58–62

110. The effect of HIV infection on the immune system

A.T   B.T   C.F   D.T   E.T

Progressive depletion of circulating CD4+ cells, impaired function of remaining cells and inappropriate immune activation are hallmarks of the immune dysregulation associated with HIV infection.

The CD4+ cell compartment consists of two functional subsets; naive and memory cells. Naive cells express the cell surface markers CD45RA and CD62L. Memory cells express the cell surface marker CD45RO and lack expression of CD45RA. Naive cells can generate immune responses to newly encountered antigens but are not particularly adept at cytokine expression, nor at effector cell activity. Following exposure to antigenic peptides expressed on MHC class I molecules (for CD8+ cells) and MHC class II molecules (for CD4+ cells), naive cells evolve into memory cells. Memory cells are capable of cytokine expression and cytolytic activity. After antigenic exposure some cells die and others revert to a less activated memory state, where they are capable of rapid responses to previously encountered antigens. In healthy adults about half of circulating cells are naive and half memory. In HIV infection there is a selective loss of naive CD4+ cells early in the disease. However, functional studies show losses in antigen-specific responses that are mediated by memory cells.

Early HIV infection is characterized by a decrease in circulating CD4+ cells and an expansion in numbers of circulating CD8+ cells. In contrast, in advanced HIV infection all circulating lymphoid populations, including CD8+ cells, B lymphocytes and natural killer cells, decrease. CD8+ cells are major effectors of cell-mediated cytotoxicity. Their receptors can recognize foreign peptides expressed on the cell surface in association with MHC class I molecules. Recognition and binding trigger cytolytic mechanisms which can result in the destruction of cells serving as the factory for production of intracellular pathogens such as viruses. CD8+ cells are also important sources of β-chemokines and other soluble factors which prevent HIV propagation through inhibition of virus binding to cellular coreceptors. The development of a CD8+ cytolytic response is associated with downregulation of HIV propagation in early infection and is a critical mediator of host defence against HIV.

Maintenance of a strong cytolytic response against HIV also depends on the expression of 'helper' cytokines by CD4+ cells. CD4+ cell responses to HIV are profoundly altered in HIV disease. Preservation of interdependent CD4+ and CD8+ cell responses to HIV is associated with a better outcome in HIV infection.

HIV infection also induces a state of chronic immune activation in CD4+ cells, CD8+ cells and circulating monocytes. This is demonstrated by increased cell suface expression of markers of activation and increased levels of cytokines such as tumor necrosis factor α and interleukin 6. This may limit the ability of the host to provide defence against opportunistic pathogens and, as activated CD4+ cells are more permissive for HIV replication, enhance HIV propagation.

Reference

Powderly WG, Landay A, Lederman MM 1998 Recovery of the immune system with antiretroviral therapy. The end of opportunism? Journal of the American Medical Association 280: 72–77

111. Immune reconstitution in HIV-positive patients treated with HAART

A.T B.T C.F D.F E.T

The use of highly active antiretroviral therapy (HAART) has been associated with a dramatic decrease in the incidence of opportunistic infections and a reduction in hospitalizations for AIDS-related events. Opportunistic infections occur in HIV disease because of immunodeficiency caused principally by progressive loss of CD4+ T lymphocytes. HAART raises CD4+ cell counts by an average of 150 cells/ml over 12 months, and improves immunological competence. HAART can lead to resolution of infections previously thought impossible to treat, such as cryptosporidiosis, microsporidiosis, azole-resistant candida and progressive multifocal leukoencephalopathy. In addition, long-term remission can be achieved from CMV retinitis and disseminated Mycobacterium avium complex infection. This has allowed some patients to discontinue specific antimicrobial treatment. The reduced incidence of opportunistic infections following the initiation of HAART is due both to the prevention of further viral induced damage to the immune system and to partial reconstitution of the immune system.

Among patients with advanced HIV disease initiated on HAART, immune reconstitution has two main phases. The first takes about 3 months and is characterised by rapid increases in circulating naive and memory CD4+ and CD8+ cells, as well as increases in circulating B lymphocytes. Numbers of natural killer cells are unaffected. These rapid increases in circulating T and B cells are thought to be due to a decrease in cellular activation (which normally leads to apoptosis) and in adhesion. There is a redistribution of cells from lymphoid tissues, rather than generation of new cells. The second phase lasts for at least the first year of therapy. It is characterized by a slower increase in circulating naive CD4+ and CD8+ cells and a decrease in circulating memory CD8+ cells. The decrease in memory CD8+ cells may be due to a reduction of HIV-reactive CD8+ cell clones.

During the first phase of cellular restoration, perturbations in the T-cell receptor repertoire are not corrected. In contrast, evidence suggests that during the slower, second phase diversity of CD4+ cell repertoire improves. How much diversification is possible in adults is unclear, and full recovery of CD4+ cell numbers may take many years in patients with advanced disease. In HIV disease there is progressive loss of antigen reactivity and cell-mediated immune responses. This is demonstrated in vitro by failure of lymphocyte proliferative responses and in vivo by loss of delayed-type hypersensitivity responses to skin testing. Patients whose CD4+ cells show no proliferative response to CMV and tuberculin antigens in vitro have been demonstrated to regain these responses after starting HAART. This recovery is sustained and correlates with the amplitude of fall in HIV RNA viral load.

Responses to the application of skin test antigens progressively improve over the first year of HAART.

Chronic HIV infection is associated with immune activation. Following HAART, markers of activation fall, including plasma tumour necrosis factor-α levels and the cell surface markers CD38 and HLA-DR. In addition, cytokine expression and apoptosis rapidly decrease. These results suggest that it is HIV replication itself, rather than exposure to opportunistic pathogens, that drives the immune activation.

Control of viral replication is not achieved in all patients, and for those in whom even partial control is not possible immune deterioration and consequent opportunistic complications of AIDS will continue.

References

Cohen OJ, Fauci AS 1998 HIV/AIDS in 1998 – gaining the upper hand? Journal of the American Medical Association 280: 87–88

Li TS, Tubiana R, Karlama C, Calvez V, Ait Mohand H, Autran B 1998 Long-lasting recovery in CD4 T-cell function and viral-load reduction after highly active antiretroviral therapy in advanced HIV-1 disease. Lancet 351: 1682–1686

Powderly WG, Landay A, Lederman MM 1998 Recovery of the immune system with antiretroviral therapy. The end of opportunism? Journal of the American Medical Association 280: 72–77

---

112. BHIVA guidelines for treatment of HIV-1 infection

A.T   B.T   C.T   D.T   E.F

In April 1997 the British HIV Association (BHIVA) published guidelines for antiretroviral treatment of HIV-infected individuals. These were useful in ensuring that viral load testing and combination therapy are widely available in the UK. However, standards of treatment are rapidly changing as new evidence becomes available, and revised guidelines were published in July 1998. At the time of going to press a further update is being produced and readers are referred to http://www.aidsmap.com/nam/bhiva/bhivagd.htm.

The goals of antiretroviral therapy are to improve quality of life and prolong life. The virological goal is to achieve a viral load below detection limits of standard assays (usually 400–500 copies/ml) and ideally below detection limits of ultrasensitive assays (50 copies/ml). There is now evidence that the viral-load nadir on therapy is critical to the durability of the treatment response. Incomplete viral suppression with ongoing viral replication will eventually lead to the development of viral resistance, loss of treatment options and a poorer clinical outcome. To achieve an undetectable viral load, combination therapy should be selected which has highly active antiretroviral activity. For individuals with a viral load greater than 50 000 copies/ml a combination of two nucleoside analogues plus one or two protease inhibitors should be chosen, as data suggest that the inclusion of a protease inhibitor is required for these patients to reliably achieve an undetectable viral load. For individuals with a viral load less than 50 000 copies/ml triple therapy with two nucleoside analogues plus a non-nucleoside analogue reverse transcriptase inhibitor or a protease inhibitor is appropriate. Patients with very high viral loads and low CD4 counts at baseline, as well as those who have had extensive nucleoside–analogue therapy, are less likely to achieve an undetectable viral load on triple therapy, and therefore even more intensive antiretroviral combinations should be considered. An initial combination of two nucleoside analogues is no longer considered a reasonable standard of care and should only be considered in exceptional circumstances, such as patients with a viral load below 5 000 copies/ml at baseline.

Treatment should be initiated before irreversible damage has occurred to the immune system, such as at a CD4 count above 350 cells/ml, when the risk of opportunistic infections remains low. Those with high viral loads before treatment are significantly more likely to develop clinical illness over defined periods of follow-up than are CD4–matched individuals with low viral load. This suggests that individuals with very high viral loads should consider starting triple therapy even when their CD4 counts are relatively high. Management should be a balance between the potential benefit of therapy in delaying clinical events and the potential morbidities, both physical and psychological, associated with the commitment to lifelong multidrug therapy. Toxicity from therapy may be considerable and treatment adherence, which is crucial to virological suppression, is poorer in people with symptom-free disease.

Treatment failure after initiation of triple therapy may be primary owing to an inadequate treatment response (not achieving a viral load below assay detection within 24 weeks of initiating treatment), or secondary with virological rebound. Continuing treatment on a failing regimen and the presence of a higher viral load at the time of switch to another regimen are associated with an accumulation of greater numbers of mutations in the HIV genome and a greater chance of cross-resistance. If patients have virological failure on triple therapy, the subsequent choice of drugs will depend on the reason for treatment failure (toxicity, poor compliance or viral resistance). In general, adding one additional drug to a failing regimen is suboptimal and at least two drugs should be substituted, which should ideally include a drug from a new class.

References

BHIVA Guidelines Co-ordinating Committee 1997 British HIV
Association guidelines for antiretroviral treatment of HIV seropositive
individuals. Lancet 349: 1086–1092

Carpenter CCJ, Fischl MA, Hammer SM et al. 1998 Antiretroviral
therapy for HIV infection in 1998. Updated recommendations of the
International AIDS Society – USA Panel. Journal of the American
Medical Association 280: 78–86

Gazzard B, Moyle G on behalf of the BHIVA Guidelines Writing
Committee 1998 1998 revision to the British HIV Association
guidelines for antiretroviral treatment of HIV seropositive individuals.
Lancet 352: 314–316

113. Treatment of HIV infection with HAART

A.F   B.F   C.F   D.F   E.T

The number of drugs available for the treatment of HIV infection
has increased dramatically over the past few years, with new
classes of drug inhibiting different stages in the lifecycle of HIV.
The key target for HIV is the CD4–positive lymphocyte. The virus
attaches to the CD4 molecule and other cell membrane molecules
and then introduces its RNA into the cell. This RNA is used as a
template to generate DNA by the viral enzyme reverse
transcriptase. Two groups of drug have been developed which can
inhibit this enzyme: the nucleoside analogue reverse transcriptase
inhibitors (NRTIs: zidovudine, zalcitabine, didanosine, stavudine,
abacavir and lamivudine) and the non-nucleoside analogue
reverse transcriptase inhibitors (NNRTIs: nevirapine, efavirenz and
delavirdine). The DNA generated by reverse transcriptase is
incorporated into the host's genetic material, and is in turn
transcribed to produce new viral RNA. This RNA provides the
genetic material of new virus particles and is the template for the
production of viral precursor polyproteins. As the new viral particles
mature, the precursor polyproteins are cleaved by HIV protease
enzymes to form structural proteins and enzymes. The mature viral
particles then bud from the host cell and can infect other cells. HIV
protease inhibitors have been available in the UK since 1996, and
include saquinavir, indinavir, ritonavir and nelfinavir.

Numerous clinical trials have demonstrated that combinations of
antiretroviral drugs result in greater benefit than monotherapy.
Furthermore, three-drug combinations provide greater benefit than
dual therapy. Triple therapy including two NRTIs and a protease
inhibitor is a widely used initial combination and is often referred to
as highly active antiretroviral therapy (HAART). Triple-therapy
regimens can produce sustained increases in CD4 count,
reduction in viral load and reduced rates of progression to AIDS
and death, compared to mono or dual therapy.

Compliance with complex multidrug regimens is a major problem for HIV-positive individuals. Many of the drugs have to be taken at a certain interval from meals and most patients have to take 10 or more tablets a day. Patients who are unable to comply with triple therapy risk incomplete suppression of viral replication, with the development of resistance to their drugs and treatment failure. Drug toxicity is another frequent cause of treatment failure. Because of the difficulties in taking complex drug combinations, some studies have looked at the effectiveness of intensive initial therapy followed by less intensive maintenance therapy. The Amsterdam Duration of Antiretroviral Medication (ADAM) study enrolled 62 patients to an initial 26 weeks of stavudine, lamivudine, saquinavir and nelfinavir therapy. Patients were then randomized to continue on four drugs or be maintained on dual therapy (stavudine and nelfinavir or saquinavir and nelfinavir). Enrolment to the study was stopped when interim results showed that patients being randomized to dual therapy were showing increases in viral load.

Despite the difficult drug regimens the promising results from clinical trials have translated into normal clinical use, with a number of HIV cohort studies showing a marked reduction in progression to AIDS and death.

After an initial decrease in viral load following the initiation of HAART, treatment failure is often defined as a sustained increase in viral load. The choice of therapy following failure will depend on the reasons for failure, such as drug resistance and toxicity. Different combinations, for example including two protease inhibitors or four or five different drugs, are being studied as salvage therapy.

There is hope that the increase in treatment options for HIV-positive patients will mean that HIV infection can now be considered as a chronic disease. Many questions remain unanswered, however, such as the best time to start therapy, whether the immune system can be rebuilt and how to treat patients infected with virus resistant to the available drugs. Furthermore, with triple therapy costing about £7 000 per year the vast majority of the world's HIV infected population do not have access to therapy.

References

Flexner C 1998 HIV-protease Inhibitors. New England Journal of Medicine 338: 1281–1292.

Hammer SM, Squires KE, Hughes MD et al. for the AIDS Clinical Trials Group 320 Study Team 1997 A controlled trial of two nucleoside analogues plus indinavir in persons with human immunodeficiency virus infection and CD4 cell counts of 200 per cubic millimeter or less. New England Journal of Medicine 337: 725–733

Hogg RS, Heath KV, Yip B et al. for the EuroSIDA Study Group 1998 Changing patterns of mortality across Europe in patients infected with HIV-1. Lancet 352: 1725–1730

Montaner JSG 1998 Improved survival among HIV-infected individuals
    following initiation of antiretroviral therapy. Journal of the American
    Medical Association 279: 450–454

Reijers MHE, Weverling GJ, Jurriaans S et al. 1998 Maintenance
    therapy after quadruple induction therapy in HIV-1 infected
    individuals: Amsterdam Duration of Antiretroviral Medication (ADAM)
    study. Lancet 352: 185–190

Sepkoitz KA 1998 Editorial: Effects of HAART on natural history of
    AIDS-related opportunistic disorders. Lancet 351: 228–230

114. Reservoirs of HIV-1 in patients receiving HAART

A.F   B.T   C.T   D.F   E.F

Over the past few years there have been major advances in the
development of highly active antiretroviral therapy (HAART).
However, major obstacles remain to the eradication HIV-1 from
infected individuals. Inhibitors of HIV-1 reverse transcriptase and
protease enzymes can only inhibit actively replicating HIV-1. When
HAART was introduced it was observed that there are at least 2
phases of HIV-1 clearance from the blood. The first lasts about two
weeks and circulating HIV-1 declines by more than 99%. In this
phase, the estimated half-life of free virus is less than 6 hours and
the half-life of infected cells is about 1.6 days. In the second phase
of HIV-1 clearance the mean half-life of HIV-1 infected cells is
about 16 days. Based on these estimates of HIV-1 clearance
during HAART therapy, it was calculated that eradication of HIV-1
from an infected person might be possible in 2–3 years. However,
in practice the existence of reservoirs with slower rates of HIV-1
clearance and anatomical sites poorly penetrated by antiretroviral
drugs poses a major obstacle to eradication of HIV-1.

Reservoirs of HIV-1 can be divided into cellular and anatomical.
Cellular reservoirs may include latent CD4+ T cells containing
intergrated HIV-1 provirus, macrophages and follicular dendritic
cells (FDCs). Impediments to eliminating HIV-1 from cellular
reservoirs involve the existence of the virus in a physical state
capable of surviving for prolonged periods despite otherwise
therapeutic levels of antiretroviral drugs. The main anatomical
reservoir of HIV-1 is the central nervous system. With anatomical
reservoirs the difficulty is attaining adequate and consistent
antiretroviral concentrations in that anatomical space.

HIV-1 can infect activated or resting (memory) CD4+ T cells. In the
resting T cell the HIV-1 genome cannot integrate into the host
genome and is eliminated within hours. If the resting cell with the
HIV-1 genome in its cytoplasm is activated, the HIV-1 genome will
integrate into the host's DNA and production of new virus will
begin. Production of new virus is cytopathic to the T cell and most
of these cells will die. It has now been demonstrated that a small

proportion of activated T cells containing the HIV-1 genome will return to the resting state. Most of the integrated HIV-1 in resting T cells is defective. However, studies have demonstrated that a small proportion of the virus is capable of replication. These cells have a life-time of up to 3 years and, as HIV-1 is not replicating and HAART is therefore inactive against it, they are an important potential reservoir of HIV-1. Resting T cells containing replication-competent HIV-1 have been detected in patients after 30 months on HAART. There are two possible strategies to eliminate this reservoir. The first is for patients to continue HAART for long enough to outlive the T cells, calculated to be about 5 years. During this time the resting T cells will become activated and the HAART will kill any replicating virus, preventing the infection of new cells, and the activated T cell is likely to die. However, sustaining a patient on HAART which is completely suppressive of HIV-1 replication for such a prolonged period is unlikely to be achievable. The second strategy is to activate resting HIV-1 infected T cells, for example with antigens, mitogens or cytokines such as interleukin-2. At present it is not possible to selectively activate HIV-1 infected resting T cells, and activation of all resting T cells is likely to have serious adverse effects.

HIV-1 replication can occur in macrophages without cell death. In late-stage infection when CD4+ T cells are depleted, macrophages may be the main source of de novo HIV-1 replication. The lifetime of the macrophage is about 14 days, and these cells may represent the second slow phase of HIV-1 elimination from the blood. If some macrophages have a longer lifetime they may form an important reservoir of HIV-1 infection. P-glycoprotein is a membrane transporter that can pump protease inhibitors out of the macrophage. This may explain why very high levels of protease inhibitors are required to completely suppress HIV-1 replication in macrophages. Inhibition of P-glycoprotein, as an adjunct to protease inhibitor therapy, may allow this potential reservoir to be eradicated.

FDCs form networks in secondary lymphoid follicles and are implicated in maintaining B-cell memory. These cells hold antigen–antibody complexes on their surfaces by binding to Fc receptors. Large amounts of HIV-1–antibody complex are held on FDCs during HIV-1 infection. This HIV-1 reservoir is capable of infecting CD4+ T cells. The amount of HIV-1 held by these cells following initiation of HAART mirrors the amount of virus circulating in the blood. After a year of HAART this reservoir is essentially eradicated. However, even the transient low-level viraemia, which may occur after a brief interruption of HAART, leads to complete replenishment of this reservoir.

The central nervous system (CNS) is the most important anatomical reservoir for HIV-1. CNS involvement in HIV-1 infection is common and macrophages and macrophage-related microglial cells are the main sites of CNS infection. Most HIV-1 is macrophage-tropic in the CNS, even when the predominant HIV-1 strain in the blood is T-cell tropic. This, together with different viral load dynamics in the blood and CSF, suggests that the CNS forms an independent compartment of HIV-1 replication. If levels of antiretroviral drugs in the CSF are insufficient to completely suppress HIV-1 replication then resistant virus may emerge. Nucleoside analogue reverse transcriptase inhibitors penetrate the blood–brain barrier to a variable degree: zidovudine CSF levels reach 60% of those in the plasma, stavudine 40% and lamivudine 11%. Protease inhibitors are highly plasma protein bound and macrophages in the blood–brain barrier may pump them out of the CNS via P-glycoprotein. In addition, high levels of protease inhibitors are required to completely suppress HIV-1 replication in macrophages. Despite these factors, indinavir levels in the CSF are comparable to trough plasma levels, and the combination of saquinavir with ritonavir has been shown to effectively suppress CNS viral replication. The retina, protected by the blood–brain barrier, and the testes, protected by tight junctions between Sertoli cells, may also form anatomical reservoirs during HAART therapy.

These cellular and anatomical reservoirs pose obstacles to the eradication of HIV-1. Strategies to activate resting T cells and improvements in the penetration of antiretroviral drugs into anatomical reservoirs, together with improvements in antiretroviral therapy to allow long-term compliance, will be important if cure of HIV-1 infection is to become a reality.

References

Cohen OJ and Fauci AS 1998 HIV/AIDS in 1998 – gaining the upper hand? Journal of the American Medical Association 280: 87–88

Schrager LK, D'Souza PD 1998 Cellular and anatomical reservoirs of HIV-1 in patients receiving potent antiretroviral combination therapy. Journal of the American Medical Association 280: 67–71

115. Adverse effects of antiretroviral therapy

A.F   B.F   C.T   D.T   E.T

Combination antiretroviral therapy is being used in early HIV-1 infection and for many patients this therapy will continue for years. For maximum benefit patients must take complex regimens of drugs and compliance is crucial in maintaining suppression of viral replication and preventing the emergence of resistant viral strains. All the available antiretroviral agents have adverse effects, which may prevent patients achieving adequate suppression of HIV-1 replication and so deny them the immunological, clinical and survival benefits of therapy. In addition, as patients' lives are prolonged on therapy, adverse effects that reduce quality of life become more important.

Determining the adverse effect profile of antiretroviral drugs has been difficult for a number of reasons. Clinical trials of these agents often include only small numbers of patients and are designed to measure surrogate markers of disease, such as CD4 lymphocyte count and HIV RNA viral load. Antiretrovirals are usually used in combination, and often patients are also treated with antibacterial, antifungal, antiviral and antitumour drugs. Patients infected with HIV-1, particularly in the later stages of disease, may suffer frequent disease-related events such as infections, tumours and the direct effects of HIV on tissues such as the heart and brain. Drug toxicity may be difficult to distinguish from these disease-related events.

All nucleoside analogue reverse transcriptase inhibitors may cause liver toxicity, characterized by severe fatty infiltration of the liver (hepatic steatosis), often associated with lactic acidosis. Although uncommon, these reactions are often fatal. Zidovudine frequently causes nausea, fatigue and headache. Haematological toxicity with anaemia and leucopenia is also common and is the dose-limiting toxicity of this drug. Zidovudine may also cause myopathy, with ragged red fibres on light microscopy and abnormal mitochondria on electron microscopy. Didanosine causes pancreatitis, which may be fatal in up to 20% of patients. Pancreatic toxicity may also result in diabetes mellitus. Other important toxic effects of didanosine include peripheral neuropathy, diarrhoea, and possibly retinal toxicity in children. Peripheral neuropathy is the main dose-limiting toxicity with zalcitabine. This is usually sensory and may be painful and severe. Pancreatitis and stomatitis are also frequent. Stavudine causes peripheral neuropathy in up to 20% of patients, but pancreatitis in only about 1%. Other adverse reactions include anaemia and neutropenia. Lamivudine may cause headache, nausea, diarrhoea, insomnia, anaemia and, most frequently in children, pancreatitis and neuropathy. It has been proposed that some of the adverse effects of these nucleoside analogues, such as bone marrow suppression, liver failure, neuropathy, myopathy and lactic acidosis, may be due to their inhibition of mammalian DNA polymerases, including γ-polymerase. This enzyme is important to mitochondrial DNA replication and its inhibition may impair mitochondrial metabolism.

Non-nucleoside analogue reverse transcriptase inhibitors are the most recently introduced group of antiretroviral drugs. The main toxicity with this group of drugs is allergy, which may present as skin rashes, including Stevens–Johnson syndrome. Hepatitis may also occur.

The adverse effects of protease inhibitors have received considerable attention recently. All of the protease inhibitors (indinavir, ritonavir, saquinavir and nelfinavir) commonly cause GI symptoms, particularly nausea and diarrhoea, which may be severe. Protease inhibitors are also inhibitors of the liver isoenzyme cytochrome P450 3A, with ritonavir causing the most profound inhibition. This inhibition leads to important and potentially adverse interactions with a number of drugs commonly coprescribed in HIV-1 infected patients. There have been reports of an increased frequency of bleeding among haemophiliac patients treated with protease inhibitors. De novo diabetes mellitus, loss of control of existing diabetes mellitus and insulin resistance have been described following initiation of protease inhibitor therapy. Protease inhibitors have also been associated with dry lips, dermatitis, hair loss and nail dystrophy. Indinavir (but not the other protease inhibitors) causes crystalluria and renal stones (formed from indinavir crystals) in a high proportion of patients. This requires patients on indinavir to drink at least 2 l of fluid every day.

In late 1997 and 1998 reports were published of lipodystrophy occurring in patients treated with protease inhibitors. Lipodystrophy comprises loss of subcutaneous fat on the face, limbs and upper trunk, with an increase in intra-abdominal, breast and dorsocervical fat (buffalo humps). Overall, patients lose weight at a stage in their HIV infection when wasting would not be expected to occur. Hypercholesterolaemia and hypertriglyceridaemia also appear to be adverse effects of these drugs, and these reactions have frequently occurred in association with lipodystrophy. The long-term consequences of lipodystrophy, together with hyperlipidaemia and insulin resistance, are unknown. However, there is a theoretical risk of accelerated atherosclerosis which may limit the long-term survival benefits of HAART. It has been proposed that lipodystrophy, hyperlipidaemia and insulin resistance comprise a syndrome caused by protease inhibitors. However, other commentators have suggested that the body shape changes are a result of prolonged suppression of viral replication or recovery of the immune system.

References

Arlett P, Hooker M, Lee E, Darbyshire J, Breckenridge A 1997 Reporting adverse drug reactions in HIV infection. Genitourinary Medicine 73: 335

Carr A, Samaras K, Burton S et al. 1998 A syndrome of peripheral lipodystrophy, hyperlipidaemia and insulin resistance in patients receiving HIV protease inhibitors. AIDS. 12: F51– 58

Henry K, Melroe H, Huebsch J et al. 1998 Severe premature coronary artery disease with protease inhibitors. Lancet 351: 1328

Lo JC, Mulligan K, Tai VW, Algren H, Schambelan M 1998 'Buffalo hump' in men with HIV-1 infection. Lancet 351: 867–870

Miller KD, Jones E, Yanovski JA, Shankar R, Feuerstein I, Fallon J 1998 Visceral abdominal fat accumulation associated with the use of indinavir. Lancet 351: 871–875

Styrt BA, Piazza-Hepp TD, Chikami GK 1996. Clinical toxicity of antiretroviral nucleoside analogs. Antiviral Research 31: 121–135

116. Resistance to antiretroviral drugs
A.T   B.T   C.F   D.F   E.F

Resistance to antiretroviral drugs may represent the ultimate limit to the ability of current drug regimens to achieve long-term control of HIV infection. Drug-resistant HIV variants may pre-exist or be selected for during incompletely suppressive therapy. Patients with acute infection with HIV variants resistant to multiple reverse transcriptase and protease inhibitors have been described.

In untreated patients some 1×10^{10} new viral particles are produced per day. In view of the error-prone nature of HIV reverse transcriptase, this high level of viral turnover results in 1×10^4 to 1×10^5 mutations per day at each site in the HIV genome. However, the emergence of three or four mutations in the same genome at the same time is rare, and can be further minimized by the inhibition of viral replication. Because of this, the antiretroviral regimen should be selected to maximally suppress HIV replication, so minimizing the chances of resistant variants emerging.

Resistance has been described for all classes of antiretroviral drugs, and some level of cross-resistance exists between all members of the same class of antiretrovirals. Together with toxicity and poor compliance, resistance is an important and common cause of failure of viral suppression. It is likely that treatment failure on aggressive antiretroviral therapy will become increasingly common in clinical practice.

Reliable assays to measure viral sensitivity to different drugs may guide the choice of initial regimens and facilitate the design of salvage regimens. However, the currently available commercial assays are unable to detect minority viral populations (those comprising less than 20% of total plasma HIV RNA) and their place in clinical practice has not yet been established.

References

Hecht FM, Grant RM, Petropoulos CJ et al. 1998 Sexual transmission of an HIV-1 variant resistant to multiple reverse-transcriptase and protease inhibitors. New England Journal of Medicine 339: 307–311

Loveday C, Devereux H 1998 Clinical implications of antiretroviral drug resistance. Journal of HIV Therapy. 3: 48–54

Vella S. 1998. Prevention and detection of resistance: what does the future hold? Journal of HIV Therapy 3: 31–32

Wainberg MA, Friedland G 1998 Public health implications of antiretroviral therapy and HIV drug resistance. Journal of the American Medical Association 279: 1977–1991

ONCOLOGY

117. Radiotherapy

A.F   B.T   C.F   D.T   E.F

Radiotherapy uses ionizing radiation to deliver a precisely measured dose of irradiation to a defined tumour volume, causing as little damage as possible to surrounding normal tissue. Different types of ionizing radiation are used, each with its own characteristics. X-rays are the most common and are produced whenever an electron stream travelling at high speed is brought to rest in a solid target. Superficial tumours are treated with low-energy X-rays (50–150 kV) produced by relatively simple X-ray tubes. Megavoltage X-rays (4–25 MV) are used to treat deep tumours and are produced by linear accelerators, which accelerate electrons in a straight line using radiofrequency waves produced by a magnetron (a specially designed vacuum diode operating in a magnetic field) or klystron (a radiofrequency oscillator). γ-Rays are identical to X-rays except that they are emitted spontaneously from certain radioactive isotopes. These isotopes can be housed in substantial shielding to produce an X-ray beam for external beam radiotherapy, or made into needles or wires. These can be directly implanted into a tumour or arranged so that they irradiate the walls of a body cavity from the inside. This type of therapy is useful for easily accessible tumours, such as those of the oral cavity, anus, bronchus, oesophagus and cervix.

Ionizing radiation kills cells by damaging DNA, causing single- and double-strand DNA breaks; the latter are the more important as they are more difficult for the cell to repair. Cell death ensues when the cell attempts to divide, although cells may achieve several divisions before dying.

Normal tissues and tumours show a spectrum of radiosensitivity owing to the following factors: (1) the proportion of dividing cells in the tissue: those tumours and normal tissues with a high proportion of dividing cells undergo more cell kill with a given dose of radiation; (2) the intrinsic radiosensitivity of the cell; (3) the ability of the cells to repair radiation-induced damage; (4) tissue hypoxia: hypoxic tumours are known to be more radioresistant than well oxygenated ones.

It is often the radiosensitivity of the surrounding normal tissue that limits the dose of radiation that can be given to a tumour. Normal tissue responses to irradiation are divided into early or acute (within 3 months of radiotherapy) and late (after 6 months). Acute reactions are common, generally starting in the second and third weeks of conventionally fractionated radiotherapy (see next question) and occuring in those tissues that are rapidly dividing, such as skin and mucosa. This acute reaction will heal within 3 months of completing radiotherapy. For patients undergoing pelvic radiotherapy typical acute reactions are colitis and proctitis and radiation-induced cystitis. For patients undergoing head and neck radiotherapy acute reactions include skin erythema, which may progress to desquamation and mucositis, resulting in dysphagia and oral ulceration.

It is the late adverse effects that are of most concern to the radiotherapist, as these are irreversible and may occur years after completion of treatment. Late reactions are uncommon and thought to be the result of endarteritis obliterans, resulting in chronic vascular insufficiency in the tissue that has been irradiated. One of the most serious manifestations of this is myelitis following spinal cord irradiation. Other late adverse effects include bowel strictures following pelvic irradiation and osteoradionecrosis, cataract formation, and skin fibrosis following head and neck irradiation.

Acute reactions are dependent on total dose, dose per fraction, and time over which the radiation is given. Late reactions are dependent on total dose and dose per fraction, with little or no time factor. A second malignancy can be considered a late adverse effect but is not dose dependent. The dose of radiation that different normal tissues can tolerate before developing late adverse effects has been determined and is known as tissue tolerance. Radiotherapy often requires complex planning in order to deliver a tumoricidal radiation dose without exceeding the radiation tolerance of the surrounding normal tissue.

Reference

Anon 1997 Late complications of radiotherapy. Drug and Therapeutics Bulletin 35: 13–16

118. Radiotherapy

A.F   B.F   C.T   D.T   E.T

Radiotherapy is fractionated in order to reduce normal tissue damage. The Gray (Gy) is the unit of absorbed dose: 1 Gy is equivalent to 1 joule per kilogram. Conventional radical (curative) fractionation employs 2 Gy fractions given daily 5 times per week to a total dose of 50–70 Gy, depending on the radiosensitivity of the particular tumour being treated. Radiotherapy is a local therapy and may be used alone or together with surgery and/or chemotherapy, depending on the radiosensitivity of the tumour. It is the primary curative modality in about 30% of cancer patients. Examples of tumours that can be cured with radiotherapy alone are squamous cell carcinomas of the head and neck (such as laryngeal carcinoma), cervical carcinoma, prostate and bladder carcinoma, Hodgkin's disease and basal cell carcinomas.

Radiotherapy is also a very effective palliative modality for a variety of symptoms caused by advanced cancer. In patients with a very poor prognosis the concern regarding the development of late complications is lessened and the emphasis is on relief of symptoms with as little inconvenience to the patient as possible. It is not appropriate to put such patients through intensive radiotherapy, and 1–5 large fractions of radiation can produce good results in controlling bone pain, brain metastases and luminal obstruction.

One of the most important aspects of fractionated radiotherapy is the reproducibility of daily treatment set-up. Immobilization devices can be used to hold the patient in the treatment position when treating tumours close to late-responding normal tissues such as the spinal cord.

Before a patient undergoes a course of radical radiotherapy the treatment or target volume must be defined by the radiotherapist. This includes the tumour volume plus a margin for microscopic spread and daily treatment set-up variation. The target volume is defined using information from individual patient evaluation, diagnostic CT and MRI scans, details of any surgical findings and histology. The target volume and nearby late-responding normal structures are marked on CT scans taken in the treatment position. Radiation physicists then use multiple radiation beams to produce a plan giving coverage of the target volume with a dose variation ideally of around 5%, and minimizing the dose to nearby normal structures. This procedure is aided by the use of computer-based planning systems, which are becoming increasingly more sophisticated (see below).

A simulator is used to verify the beam positions. This is an isocentrically mounted diagnostic X-ray machine which can reproduce the treatment conditions in a linear accelerator and has the facility for screening using an image intensifier.

Recent advances in radiotherapy include conformal therapy, three-dimensional planning and fractionation studies.

Until recently, linear accelerators used simple beam collimation systems to produce square or rectangular beams. Clearly tumours are not rectangular in shape, and to conform the beam shape to that of the tumour (conformal therapy) customized lead blocks are made for each beam and each patient, which need to be manually positioned. This is very time-consuming and manual positioning can lead to inaccuracies in the daily treatment set-up. This can be avoided by the use of a multileaf collimator, which is a set of narrow tungsten leaves that can be individually positioned under computer control to create individually shaped beams.

Three-dimensional planning systems are rapidly being installed in radiotherapy departments. These have the ability to orientate beams in three dimensions and allow the development of complex plans involving multiple beams. They also allow the radiotherapist to view the target volume and normal structures in three dimensions, and therefore normal tissue within the target volume can be easily identified and shielded. It is hoped that 3D planning will enable higher doses of radiation to be given to the tumour without compromising the surrounding normal tissues.

Research-based trials are currently being performed to optimize fraction schedules for different tumours and minimize normal tissue damage. Options are: (1) Hyperfractionation: this is the use of smaller than standard fraction sizes without reducing total dose or increasing the treatment time. This can be achieved by treating six or seven times a week or treating with multiple fractions five times per week (these must be at least 6 hours apart to let late-responding tissues repair). The aim of this type of fractionation is to reduce late morbidity. (2) Accelerated fractionation: this is radiotherapy given in a shorter overall time to defeat tumour proliferation. However, this cannot be done by increasing the dose per fraction as this results in an increase in late tissue damage. This can be overcome by giving two conventional treatments per day 6 hours apart for the last 1–2 weeks of treatment.
(3) Accelerated hyperfractionation: a combination of the above.

Reference

Vijayakumar S, Hellman S 1997 Advances in radiation oncology. Lancet 349: (Suppl 2):1–3

---

119. Adjuvant chemotherapy

A.F   B.F   C.F   D.F   E.T

Colorectal carcinoma is the second most common cause of death from malignancy in the UK. Five-year survival according to Dukes' staging is as follows: Dukes' A – 80%, Dukes' B - 70%, Dukes' C (1–4 nodes positive) – 56%, Dukes' C (more than 4 nodes positive) – 26%.

Most of the large trials have been conducted in the USA – IMPACT, NCCTG, NSABP. All showed a survival advantage in Dukes' C carcinoma of 4–17% with adjuvant chemotherapy. The use of adjuvant chemotherapy in Dukes' B carcinoma is more controversial. The US studies suggested a decrease in relapse, but follow-up was too short to show an improvement in survival. The current recommendation is that those patients with B2 disease (through the muscle wall) should be entered in to a treatment trial. Debate continues over the optimal chemotherapy regimen but most regimens use 5-fluorouracil together with folinic acid as a bolus for 5 days every 4 weeks.

Every 5 years the Early Breast Cancer Triallists Collaborative Group (EBCTCG) has undertaken a systematic meta-analysis of an aspect of the treatment of early breast cancer (cancer restricted to the breast and local axillary lymph nodes). The data on adjuvant chemotherapy show that polychemotherapy reduced the rate of recurrence by 35% in patients under 50 years of age and by 20% in older patients. The decision to use chemotherapy should be based on the presence of poor prognostic factors, such as axillary lymph node involvement, tumour size and tumour grade. Most premenopausal patients with any of these factors would be offered chemotherapy. Owing to the results of the overview the use of chemotherapy is becoming increasingly common in postmenopausal women, particularly if the tumour has no oestrogen receptors, as these patients are unlikely to benefit from adjuvant tamoxifen.

Standard chemotherapy for breast cancer is most commonly CMF (cyclophosphamide, methotrexate, 5-fluorouracil), although the use of doxorubicin is increasing in patients with multiple poor prognostic factors. Alkylating agents can cause permanent gonadal failure, but this is dependent on age and dose. Many patients under 35 years will remain fertile following CMF chemotherapy.

Patients with spread to more than four axillary lymph nodes have the poorest prognosis. In this group more intensive chemotherapy can be given, either CMF plus doxorubicin or high-dose chemotherapy with peripheral stem cell rescue, within the setting of a clinical trial.

References

EBCTCG 1998 Polychemotherapy for early breast cancer: an overview of randomised trials. Lancet 352: 930–942

Hortobagyi GN 1998 Treatment of breast cancer. New England Journal of Medicine 339: 974–984

Kerr DJ, Gray R 1996 Adjuvant chemotherapy for colorectal cancer. British Journal of Hospital Medicine 55: 259–266

Rodenhuis S, Richel DJ, van der Wall E et al. 1998 Randomised trial of high dose chemotherapy and haemopoietic progenitor-cell support in operable breast cancer with extensive axillary lymph node involvement. Lancet 352: 515–521

Wils J 1998 The establishment of a large collaborative trial programme in the adjuvant treatment of colon cancer. British Journal of Cancer 77(S2): 23–28

120. Immunotherapy

A.T   B.T   C.T   D.T   E.F

Immunotherapy can be active or passive. Active immunotherapy is the immunization of the host with materials designed to elicit an immune reaction capable of eliminating or retarding tumour growth. It can be subdivided into non-specific and specific.

Early non-specific immunotherapy involved the use of adjuvants such as Bacille Calmette–Guérin (BCG) and was often unsuccessful. However, BCG still has a role in early bladder cancer, where intravesical installation results in delay of tumour recurrence in 50% of cases. The therapeutic use of cytokines such as the interferons and interleukin-2 has led to more sophisticated non-specific active immunotherapy. Recent trials have shown that both high-dose and low-dose adjuvant interferon-α improves relapse-free survival in high-risk localized melanoma.

Specific active immunotherapy involves the identification of tumour antigens and the development of cancer vaccines. Early attempts involved the use of autologous or allogenic tumor cells or cell fragments, alone or with immune adjuvants such as BCG. These were unsuccessful. However, the identification of specific tumour antigens and, more recently, the genes that encode them, means that recombinant viruses encoding the cancer antigens, alone or with genes of cytokines, are being investigated as a form of gene therapy. An alternative strategy involves the use of immunomodulatory peptides that increase binding to the major histocompatibility antigens. Much of this work has been carried out in melanoma. Techniques have been developed for the cloning of antigens that are targets of human cytotoxic lymphocytes. Antigens identified in this way in melanoma cells are MART-1, gp100 and tyrosinase. Current trials using these new antigens and recombinant viruses are ongoing.

Passive immunotherapy is based on the development of monoclonal antibodies with relatively unique antitumour specificity. Unmodified antibodies can induce cell tumour death via complement-dependent cytotoxicity or antibody-dependent cell toxicity. The advantage of this type of therapy is its selectivity for tumour tissue and relative lack of toxicity. However, except in lymphoma the ability of antibodies alone to destroy most tumours is minimal. Antibodies can be conjugated to radionucleotides, toxins and drugs to aid their effectiveness. Also, until recently these antibodies have been murine and induce human antibodies against mouse antibodies (HAMA). However, recombinant chimeric monoclonal antibodies reduce HAMA reactions. These approaches have been successful in relapsed or resistant follicular lymphoma, with response rates of 50% to unconjugated chimeric anti-CD20 antibody and even higher response rates when attached to [131]I. This antibody-targeted radiotherapy has been used to deliver both low- and high-dose radiation. In colorectal cancer (Dukes' C) adjuvant passive immunotherapy with antibody 17–1A resulted in improved disease-free and overall survival.

References

Grob JJ, Dreno B, de la Salmoniere P et al. 1998 Randomised trial of interferon-α-2a as adjuvant therapy in resected primary melanoma thicker than 1.5mm without clinically detectable node metastases. Lancet 351: 1905–1910

Kaminski MS, Fenner MC, Estes J et al. 1996 Phase 1/2 trial results of I-131 anti-B-1 (anti-CD20) non-myeloablative radioimmunotherapy for refractory B cell lymphoma. Proceedings of the American Society of Clinical Oncology 15: 1266

Kirkwood JM, Strawderman MH, Ernstoff MS et al. 1996 Interferon alfa-2b adjuvant therapy of high risk resected cutaneous melanoma: the eastern cooperative oncology group trial EST 1684. Journal of Clinical Oncology 14: 7–17

Press OW, Eary JF, Appelbaum FR et al.1995 Phase 2 trial of I-131 B1 (anti CD20) antibody therapy with autologous stem cell transplantation for relapsed B cell lymphomas. Lancet 346: 336–340

Reithmuller GS, Schlimck G 1994 Randomized trial of monoclonal antibody for adjuvant therapy of resected Dukes' C colorectal carcinoma. Lancet 343: 1177

Rosenberg SA 1997 Cancer vaccines based on the identification of genes encoding cancer regression antigens. Immunology Today 18: 175–182

121. Tamoxifen

A.F   B.T   C.F   D.F   E.T

Tamoxifen is an antioestrogen. It binds to oestrogen receptors, acting as a complete antagonist in some systems (the breast) and as an antagonist with partial agonist activity in other systems. The oestrogenic properties cause both its beneficial and its toxic effects. On the positive side tamoxifen reduces total cholesterol and coronary artery disease. It also preserves bone density in postmenopausal women. The most concerning adverse effect is the increase in endometrial cancer. Other troublesome adverse effects include hot flushes, vaginal discharge or dryness and increase in thromboembolic events, especially with concomitant chemotherapy. Retinal toxicity is a rare complication.

Tamoxifen is used in the treatment of breast cancer both as an adjuvant to radiotherapy and surgery and in metastatic disease. In patients with metastatic disease response rates are 30% overall and for oestrogen receptor-positive tumours 60%.

A recent overview of 55 randomized trials on the use of tamoxifen in early breast cancer (cancer restricted to the breast and local axillary lymph nodes) shows that only patients who have oestrogen receptor (ER)-positive tumours have a significant response to tamoxifen. In this group, 5 years of adjuvant tamoxifen resulted in a 47% proportional recurrence reduction after 10 years' follow-up. After only 2 years of adjuvant tamoxifen the reduction was less (29%). The mortality reductions were 26% and 17% respectively for 5 and 2 years of tamoxifen. As yet there are no data on a longer duration of therapy with tamoxifen, therefore 5 years of adjuvant tamoxifen is currently recommended in early breast cancer. Node-positive and node-negative patients benefited from tamoxifen, irrespective of age, menopausal status or dose of tamoxifen. Furthermore, the addition of tamoxifen to chemotherapy produced additional benefits in ER-positive tumours. There was a 47% reduction in contralateral breast cancer. However, the incidence of endometrial cancer was small but quadrupled compared to the control group. The absolute decrease in contralateral breast cancer was twice that of the increased incidence of endometrial cancer. There have been previous suggestions that tamoxifen might be associated with an increase in colorectal cancer, but there was no effect on the incidence of this cancer in this study.

The use of tamoxifen in the prevention of breast cancer is controversial. Three trials have been published recently. The first and largest is the NSABP breast cancer prevention trial from the USA, in which patients at increased risk of developing breast cancer were given either placebo or tamoxifen. 13 388 patients were entered and the trial was terminated early at an average of 4 years follow-up, as interim analysis revealed a 45% reduction in the risk of breast cancer. There was also noted to be a decrease in fractures of the hip, wrist and spine in the treated group. There was a threefold increase in endometrial cancer in the tamoxifen group. There was no difference in cardiovascular disease, but there was an increase in thromboembolic disease. The UK and Italian trials were smaller, with 2471 and 5408 patients, respectively, and showed no benefit with tamoxifen. The UK trial had the longest follow-up period (70 months) and recruited patients on the basis of family history. A proportion may have come from families carrying the BRCA1 gene, which tend to develop ER-negative tumours. The Italian trial had a similar follow-up period to the US trial but patients tended to be younger and compliance was lower. In the UK at present, routine use of tamoxifen for prevention of breast cancer in high-risk women is not recommended.

Raloxifene is a non-steroidal benzothiopene and has been classified as a selective oestrogen modulator. It has been shown to increase bone mineral density and lower serum concentrations of total and low-density lipoprotein cholesterol. It does not stimulate the endometrium in postmenopausal women and in animal models has been shown to inhibit oestrogen receptor-positive mammary tumours. At the American Society for Clinical Oncology in 1998 it was announced that this drug can also decrease the risk of breast cancer in some postmenopausal women. Trials will be taking place comparing raloxifene and tamoxifen in the prevention of breast cancer.

References

Delmas PD, Bjarnason NH, Mitlak BH et al. 1997 Effects of raloxifene on bone density, serum cholesterol concentrations, and uterine endometrium in postmenopausal women. New England Journal of Medicine 337: 1641–1686

EBCTCG 1998 Tamoxifen for early breast cancer: an overview of the randomised trials. Lancet 351: 1451–1467

Howell A and Dowsett M 1997 Recent advances in endocrine therapy of breast cancer. British Medical Journal 315: 863–866

Powles T, Eeles R, Ashley S et al. 1998 Interim analysis of the incidence of breast cancer in the Royal Marsden tamoxifen randomised chemoprevention trial. Lancet 352: 98–101

Veronesi U, Maisonneuve P, Costa A et al. 1998 Prevention of breast cancer with tamoxifen: preliminary findings from the Italian randomised trial among hysterectomised women. Lancet 352: 93–97

122. Screening
A.F   B.F   C.T   D.F   E.F

The decision to set up a screening programme for a disease depends on whether the following criteria are fulfilled: the disease must be an important public health problem; screening tests must be sensitive and specific and tolerable to the patient; treatment at an early stage of the disease must be more beneficial than intervention at a later stage; adequate facilities should exist for diagnosis and treatment; the programme must be cost-effective.

The debate regarding prostate cancer screening continues. Screening generally involves estimation of prostate-specific antigen (PSA), digital rectal examination (DRE), transrectal ultrasound or a combination of these techniques. PSA alone has a sensitivity of 57–79% and specificity of 59–68%. Screening detects more prostate cancers and at an earlier stage than in non-screened populations but until recently there has been no randomized control trial showing a decrease in cancer-related mortality using this approach. In May 1998 the results of a Canadian trial were presented to the American Society of Clinical Oncology. This trial involved 46 000 men aged 45–80 years who were randomly allocated to screening with PSA and DRE or no screening. There was a threefold reduction in prostate cancer deaths in the screened group. However, only 23% of patients offered screening accepted so the screened group was small (8137) compared to the control group (38 056).

Another problem in screening for prostate cancer is that once a cancer is detected the treatment is controversial. At present there are four possible options: radical prostatectomy, which results in a high incidence of impotence and incontinence; radiotherapy, with a lower incidence of impotence but the risk of long-term bowel damage; hormone manipulation (resulting in impotence and hot flushes); or watchful waiting. A Swedish study has shown that watchful waiting does not result in increased mortality over a 15–year period. The current recommendation in the UK is not to screen.

Randomized controlled trials have shown a 25% decrease in mortality from breast cancer by screening with mammography in women over 50. No significant benefit has been shown for screening in unselected women under 50. The current recommendations in the UK are 3-yearly mammograms in women between 50 and 64 years of age. The aim is to reduce the mortality from breast cancer by 30%. Mammography has a 15% false negative rate and a high false positive rate: only a third of those recalled turn out to have a malignancy. There is a higher than expected incidence of interval cancers, particularly in the third year after screening, and 2-yearly mammograms may be more effective.

There have been three trials which have shown a decrease in mortality from colorectal cancer using fecal occult blood testing. The problem with this method of screening is that it has low compliance among the public. It also has a low sensitivity: only 25–27% of cancers in the screened group were detected. The sensitivity can be improved by using rehydrated fecal occult blood testing but this is less specific. Despite this, these studies have shown a 15–18% decrease in mortality from colorectal cancer in the screened groups.

References

Charatan FB 1998 Prostate cancer screening reduces deaths. British Medical Journal 316: 1625

Hardcastle JD, Chamberlain JO, Robinson MHE et al. 1996 Randomised controlled trial of faecal-occult-blood screening for colorectal cancer. Lancet 348: 1472–1477

Johansson JE, Holmberg L, Johansson S et al. 1997 Fifteen year survival in prostate cancer, a prospective population-based study in Sweden. Journal of the American Medical Association 277: 467–471

Kronberg O, Fenger C, Olsen J et al. 1996 Randomised study of screening for colorectal cancer with faecal-occult-blood test. Lancet 348: 1467–1471

Sox HC 1998 Benefit and harm associated with screening for breast cancer. New England Journal of Medicine 338: 1145–1146

123. Non-small cell lung cancer
A.F B.T C.F D.F E.F

Only one-third of patients presenting with non-small cell lung cancer are suitable for curative surgery. The staging of lung cancer is important in defining these patients. The TNM system (T = size of primary tumour, N = regional nodal metastases, M = distant metastases) is an internationally agreed system of tumour staging and for non-small cell lung cancer is defined as follows:

T1: less than 3 cm
T2: greater than 3 cm or distant atelectasis
T3: extension to pleura, chest wall, diaphragm, pericardium or less than 2 cm from carina or total atelectasis
T4: invasion of mediastinal organs or malignant pleural effusion

N0: no nodal disease
N1: ipsilateral bronchopulmonary or hilar nodal disease
N2: ipsilateral or subcarinal mediastinal or ipsilateral supraclavicular nodal disease
N3: contralateral mediastinal, hilar or supraclavicular nodal disease

M0: no distant metastases
M1: distant metastases

Tumours can then be classified as follows:

Stage I   T1–2, N0, M0
Stage II   T1–2, N1, M0
Stage IIIa   T3, N0–1, M0
             T1–3, N2, M0
Stage IIIb   T4 or N3
Stage IV   M1

Early-stage (I, II, IIIa) non-small cell lung cancer should be treated with radical surgery. However, with stage IIIa disease those patients with N2 disease have a very poor survival following surgery: less than 10% at 5 years, compared to those with T3, N0–1 tumours who have a 40% 5-year survival following surgery. Radical (curative) radiotherapy is offered to those patients with early-stage disease who are medically unfit for surgery. In such cases radical radiotherapy can result in cure (up to 40% 5-year survival), but the results are not as good as would be expected for an equivalent surgical group.

Patients with localized inoperable disease can be considered for radical radiotherapy. However, this is not standard practice in the UK and there has never been a randomized controlled trial comparing radical and palliative radiotherapy in these patients. Palliative radiotherapy involves treatment with 1–10 fractions to try and alleviate symptoms, which it does successfully in 50% of cases. In contrast, radical radiotherapy gives higher doses of radiotherapy with increased toxicity and consists of 5 fractions per week for 6 weeks, aiming to improve survival in these patients. Two-year survival with radical radiotherapy is 15–20% in this group of patients. The CHART trial used a novel fractionation regimen of 54 Gy in 36 fractions over 12 days, treating three times per day including weekends. The rationale behind this is to overcome tumour repopulation by leaving no gaps in treatment and to try and prevent late toxicity by using small doses per fraction. This study showed a 9% improvement in absolute survival at 2 years in the experimental arm.

The role of postoperative radiotherapy following complete surgical resection was the subject of a recent meta-analysis and showed that the radiotherapy group had a significantly worse outcome than the group treated with surgery alone. One of the main reasons for this surprising result is likely to be the use of old treatment techniques and toxicity from undiagnosed radiation pneumonitis with radiation doses that may have been too high.

Non-small cell lung cancers are not chemosensitive. Palliative combination chemotherapy produces a 10% absolute increase in survival at 1 year in patients with metastatic disease.

Small cell lung cancer is much more chemosensitive and combination chemotherapy is the treatment of choice for patients with localiszed and metastatic disease, achieving 80% response rates. Despite this, most patients relapse within 2 years and less than 5% are cured. These patients are at high risk of developing brain metastases. Prophylactic cranial irradiation is now regarded as standard treatment for patients with limited disease small cell lung cancer who have achieved a complete response to chemotherapy. It has been shown to significantly reduce the risk of developing brain metastases and there is the suggestion of an improvement in survival.

References

Macbeth F 1996 Radiotherapy in the treatment of lung cancer. British Journal of Hospital Medicine 55: 639–642

Non-Small Cell Lung Cancer Collaborative Group 1995 Chemotherapy in non-small cell lung cancer: a meta-analysis using updated data on individual patients from 52 randomised clinical trials. British Medical Journal 311: 899–909

PORT Meta-analysis Trialists Group 1998 Postoperative radiotherapy in non-small cell lung cancer: systematic review and meta-analysis of individual patient data from nine randomised controlled trials. Lancet 352: 257–263

Saunders M, Dische S, Barrett A et al. 1997 Continuous hyperfractionated radiotherapy (CHART) versus conventional radiotherapy in non-small cell lung cancer: a multicentre randomised trial. Lancet 350: 161–165

124. High-grade B-cell non-Hodgkin's lymphoma
A.T B.F C.F D.F E.F

High-grade non-Hodgkin's lymphoma is a very chemosensitive tumour: 60% of patients are cured by conventional chemotherapy and radiotherapy. Standard treatment for all stages is CHOP (cyclophosphamide, doxorubicin, vincristine and prednisolone) chemotherapy. For localized disease three cycles of CHOP followed by radiotherapy have been shown to be superior to eight cycles of CHOP with no radiotherapy. For stage 3 and 4 disease 6–8 cycles of CHOP are recommended. Attainment of a complete response to primary treatment is the single most important indicator of prognosis. Patients who do not respond to primary therapy have a very poor outcome, which is not improved by high-dose chemotherapy. High-dose chemotherapy with stem cell transplantation can improve the cure rate in chemosensitive patients who relapse after first-line therapy.

Poor prognostic indicators at presentation are age over 60, raised lactate dehydrogenase, poor performance status, stage 3 or 4 disease and more than one extranodal site involved. These can be used to identify a group of patients with a poor outlook who may benefit from early high-dose chemotherapy. This treatment strategy is currently being investigated in randomized trials.

HTLV 1 is associated with adult T-cell lymphoma/leukaemia. This can be a highly aggressive disease with a raised white cell count, splenomegaly, hypercalcaemia, lytic bone lesions, or a more chronic picture with lymphadenopathy and extranodal disease. In both cases patients have a poor prognosis, relapsing rapidly after chemotherapy. There is some evidence that the nucleoside analogue zidovudine and interferon-α may be useful in the treatment of this type of lymphoma.

Gastric MALT (mucosa-associated lymphoid tissue) lymphomas belong to the group of indolent (low-grade) extranodal B-cell lymphomas that can involve the gastrointestinal system, salivary glands, breast, thyroid, orbit, conjunctiva or lung. Gastric MALT lymphomas are frequently associated with chronic gastritis and *Helicobacter pylori* infection, and can respond to antihelicobacter antibiotic therapy. There is currently a trial looking at this treatment in comparison to oral chlorambucil.

References

DeVita VT, Hellman S, Rosenberg SA 1997 Cancer, principles and practice of oncology. 5th edn. Lippincott-Raven

Gallo RC 1995 A surprising advance in the treatment of viral leukaemia. New England Journal of Medicine 332: 1783–1784

Miller TP, Dahlberg S, Cassady JR et al. 1998 Chemotherapy alone compared with chemotherapy plus radiotherapy for localized intermediate and high grade non-Hodgkin's lymphoma. New England Journal of Medicine 339: 21–26

Pettengell R 1996 High-dose therapy for aggressive non-Hodgkin's lymphoma. British Journal of Hospital Medicine 56: 5215–5228

125. Control of cancer pain

A.F   B.T   C.T   D.T   E.T

The first step in the management of cancer pain is to assess the cause, as patients may have more than one pain and each may have a different cause. In addition, radiotherapy, chemotherapy or surgery may control some symptoms that are not readily controlled by analgesics. However, 80% of cancer pain can be controlled with oral analgesics, the choice of which depends on the severity of the pain.

The World Health Organization (WHO) three-step analgesic ladder is a useful guide to management. Mild pain should be treated with non-opioids such as aspirin or paracetamol.

With moderate pain a weak opioid should be added, such as codeine or dextropropoxyphene. Some combination preparations of these opioids with aspirin or paracetamol do not contain therapeutic doses of the weak opioids and may not be effective.

With severe pain, the weak opioid should be replaced with a strong one. Morphine is the most commonly used strong oral opioid analgesic. It can be given as a 12- or 24-hour sustained-release preparation, but this should not be started until the required dose has been titrated using a quick-release formulation. Diamorphine is a semisynthetic derivative and a prodrug of morphine. It is not as effective as morphine when given orally. However, because of its greater solubility it is preferred to morphine for parenteral administration. The oral dose of morphine should be divided by three to obtain the equianalgesic dose of subcutaneous diamorphine. For patients who are unable to take oral medications, strong opioid analgesia can be administered transcutaneously using a fentanyl patch. This is changed every 72 hours and should only be used in patients whose pain is stable, as it takes 24–48 hours before peak plasma concentrations are achieved.

Common side effects of opioids are sedation, nausea and vomiting. These are common at the start of treatment but in most patients resolve within a few days. Constipation is very common and should be treated prophylactically. Dry mouth is another common complaint. Toxicity may present as agitation, hallucinations, confusion and myoclonic jerks. If the patient becomes sedated then dehydration can follow, with further accumulation of opioid metabolites and increasing toxicity.

At every step of the analgesic ladder adjuvant analgesic drugs may be added. These are drugs whose primary indication is not pain but which do have an analgesic effect in some painful conditions. These are particularly helpful in pain which is difficult to control with opioids such as neuropathic pain. Useful adjuvants for neuropathic pain include low doses of amitriptyline (mixed reuptake inhibitors are more effective than selective serotonin reuptake inhibitors), anticonvulsants such as sodium valproate and carbamazepine, and antiarrhythmic drugs, such as mexiletine, which are used when other options have failed. Corticosteroids can be very useful in reducing oedema and inflammation around nerves compressed by tumour.

Bisphosphonates are also adjuvant analgesics given for bone pain. In patients with metastatic breast cancer and bone metastases these pyrophosphate analogues significantly reduce the incidence of hypercalcaemia, bone pain and pathological fractures. They have also been shown to reduce the incidence of bone and visceral metastases in patients without overt clinical metastases but with tumour cells in the bone marrow.

References

Diel IJ, Solomayer EF, Costa S et al. 1998 Reduction in new metastases in breast cancer with adjuvant clodronate treatment. New England Journal of Medicine 339: 357–363

Hortobagyi GN, Theriault RL, Porter L et al. 1996 Efficacy of pamidronate in reducing skeletal complications in patients with breast cancer and lytic bone metastases. New England Journal of Medicine 335: 1785–1791

O'Neill B, Fallon M 1997 ABC of palliative care: principles of palliative care and pain control. British Medical Journal 315: 801–804

Sykes J, Johnson R, Hanks GW 1997 ABC of palliative care: difficult pain problems. British Medical Journal 315: 867–869

HAEMATOLOGY

126. Patients with multiple myeloma

A.T   B.T   C.T   D.F   E.T

The incidence of multiple myeloma (MM) is approximately 4 per 100 000 per year and in the USA in 1996 accounted for 14% of new haematological malignancies. The incidence is slightly higher in men than women and is twice as common in African Americans as in caucasians. The median age at diagnosis is approximately 65 years and less than 3% of patients are younger than 40. Putative causative factors include exposure to radiation, asbestos, agricultural and industrial toxins, including benzene. Genetic factors and viral agents have also been implicated.

Sequences from human herpesvirus 8 (HHV-8) have recently been detected by PCR in bone marrow stromal cells from >85% of MM patients and 25% of patients with monoclonal gammopathy. The HHV-8 genome shares homology with interleukin-6 (IL-6), a cytokine which plays an important role in MM. Cytogenetic abnormalities have been noted, but owing to low plasma cell proliferation the yield of evaluable metaphases is low. More sensitive techniques, such as fluorescent in situ hybridization (FISH) and Southern Blot assays, are now being used. Complex abnormalities are common (30–50%), with rearrangements of chromosome 14q32 (immunoglobulin heavy-chain switch region) and deletional mutations in chromosome 13 being well described.

The minimum diagnostic criteria for MM consist of more than 10% plasma cells in the bone marrow or a plasmacytoma with one of the following: serum M-protein (>3 g/dl), urine M-protein, or lytic bone lesions. High tumour mass is associated with increased serum β_2-microglobulin, calcium, paraprotein, C-reactive protein, lactate dehydrogenase, soluble IL-6 receptor, creatinine, circulating plasma cells, lytic lesions, bone marrow infiltration and anaemia. The bone marrow plasma cell-labelling index and β_2 microglobulin are the most important prognostic factors in previously untreated myeloma.

Without treatment MM follows a progressive course, resulting in death after a mean of 6 months. The current median duration of survival with chemotherapy is about 3 years. Approximately 25% of patients survive 5 years or more, but less than 5% live longer than 10 years. Treatment for patients under 65 includes the option of autologous stem cell transplantation as part of a prospective research trial. Stem cells are collected after the tumour has been 'eradicated' or maximally reduced, and so agents that damage haemopoietic stem cells (alkylating agents) should be avoided in initial therapy. For patients over 70, melphalan and prednisolone (M+P) or a combination of chemotherapeutic agents is suitable. In a meta-analysis of 18 published trials no difference in efficacy or survival was shown between M+P and combination chemotherapy when transplantation was not included in therapy.

In one study of 200 patients high-dose chemotherapy with or without radiotherapy followed by transplantation of either autologous bone marrow or peripheral blood stem cells showed an increased 5-year survival compared to chemotherapy alone (52% and 12%, respectively). However, it is unlikely that this treatment strategy will cure patients owing to contamination of the graft with tumour cells and the absence of graft-versus-myeloma effect. Methods for purging the graft and reducing relapse rates are being studied. These involve either the depletion of tumour cells or the positive selection of haemopoietic stem cells.

A treatment option which may result in cure is allogeneic bone marrow transplantation, but this is associated with a high transplant-related mortality (40–50%). A method proposed to reduce this mortality involves depleting the graft of T cells to reduce the complication of graft-versus-host disease. Experimental approaches to maintain the desired graft-versus-myeloma effect include infusing lymphocytes collected from the marrow donor (donor lymphocyte infusion) when relapse is detected.

The role of α-interferon (IFN-α) in the treatment of MM is controversial. α-IFN may produce a higher rate of complete remission and duration of response, but studies to date have demonstrated no survival advantage.

Osteolytic bone destruction is a major cause of morbidity and mortality in MM. Bisphosphonates are specific inhibitors of osteoclast activity and studies have demonstrated symptomatic benefit from their long-term use in MM. Reduction in the progression of lytic bone disease has been demonstrated with a reduction in new pathological fractures, bone pain, requirement for analgesic drugs and an improvement in quality of life.

References

Bataille R, Harousseau JL 1997 Multiple myeloma. New England Journal of Medicine 336: 1657–1664

Berenson JR, Lichtenstein A, Porter L et al. 1996 Efficacy of pamidronate in reducing the skeletal events in patients with advanced multiple myeloma. New England Journal of Medicine 334: 488–493

Rettig MB, Ma HJ, Vescio RA et al. 1997 Kaposi's sarcoma associated herpes virus infection of bone marrow dendritic cells from myeloma patients. Science 276: 1851–1854

Singer CRJ 1997 Multiple myeloma and related conditions. British Medical Journal 314: 960–996

127. Patients with sickle cell disease

A.F   B.F   C.T   D.T   E.T

Sickle cell disease occurs when both genes for the β-globin chain are abnormal due to an amino acid substitution. This produces the different electrical charge used in the detection of HbS by electropheresis. It also changes the behaviour of haemoglobin molecules, which tend to polymerize on deoxygenation. As a consequence red blood cells become less pliable, and some become deformed into the characteristic sickle shape. This results in their premature destruction (haemolysis) and blockage of blood flow (vaso-occlusion). The lifespan of a red blood cell is decreased from the normal 120 days to 10–12 days. At steady-state haemoglobin levels (6–9 g/dl), tissue oxygen delivery is maintained by the hyperdynamic circulation and the reduced oxygen affinity of HbS within the red cell.

Clinical consequences of haemolysis include jaundice and gallstone formation, megaloblastic erythropoiesis (due to increased folic acid demand) and risk of aplastic crises. The latter are caused by human parvovirus (B19) infection, which has a predeliction for erythrocyte precursors, causing anaemia and reticulocytopenia. The condition is self-limiting as bone marrow activity recommences after 7–10 days of aplasia, but transfusion may be necessary to maintain oxygen delivery in the interim.

Sequelae of vaso-occlusion include damage to the splenic vasculature. This may lead to acute enlargement of the spleen (splenic sequestration), chronic enlargement of the spleen (hypersplenism), overwhelming infection (especially pneumococcal septicaemia) and progressive splenic fibrosis and atrophy. The risk of pneumococcal septicaemia and acute splenic sequestration is greatest in the first 3 years of life and decreases after the age of 5. Prophylactic penicillin and pneumococcal vaccine administration reduces morbidity and mortality. Stroke is another devastating childhood complication, occurring at a median age of 6 years. It affects 8% of patients by 14 years but is infrequent after this age. There is a 50–70% chance of recurrence of stroke within 3 years of the first stroke if no active management is introduced, but chronic transfusion programmes have reduced this rate.

Risks of long-term transfusion programmes include red cell alloimmunization, transfusion reactions, transfusion-acquired infections, iron overload, and difficulties with venous access. Bone marrow transplantation (BMT) may be a viable option if there is an HLA-compatible sibling.

Painful bony crises result from avascular necrosis of active bone marrow and commonly affect the juxta-articular parts of the long bones. A potentially life-threatening complication is the acute chest syndrome. Infection, infarction, pulmonary sequestration and fat embolism are thought to be contributing factors. Genitourinary problems include enuresis, priapism and chronic renal failure. Other complications include chronic leg ulceration, retinopathy and impaired growth.

Indications for exchange transfusion include stroke, acute chest syndrome, fulminant priapism and the prevention of perioperative complications. However, a multicentre randomized study has demonstrated that prophylactic top-up transfusion to obtain a haemoglobin of greater than 10 g/dl is as effective as exchange transfusion in preventing perioperative complications. Compared to exchange transfusion top-up transfusion alone results in fewer transfusion-associated complications such as alloimmunization. Matching the patient for rhesus and Kell antigens also decreases alloimmunization.

A recent study of sickle cell disease (CSSCD) indicated that the median survival of patients with HbSS is 42 years for men and 48 years for women. Patients died from organ failure (18%), during an acute crisis (33%) or from a fatal stroke (22%). Deaths under the age of 20 are becoming less common and are usually due to pneumococcal sepsis. The CSSCD study showed that adults who had more symptoms of the disease were at increased risk of death and that the most reliable laboratory predictor of this risk was low levels of fetal haemoglobin.

Treatment with hydroxyurea (HU) reduces the frequency of vaso-occlusive events. A double-blinded randomized trial in the USA showed a significant reduction in painful crises, chest syndromes, hospitalization and transfusion requirement in patients with sickle cell disease suffering more than two crises per year assigned to HU treatment (15–35 mg/kg). HU blocks the synthesis of DNA by inhibiting ribonucleotide reductase. Proposed mechanisms of action include an increase in fetal haemoglobin (inhibiting intracellular sickle polymerization), decreased neutrophil count and reduced adhesion of red cells to endothelium. Adverse effects include nausea, rashes, alopecia, cytopenias and possibly teratogenicity. The possibility of long-term sequelae such as leukaemogenesis or carcinogenesis is not yet known. Other agents capable of augmenting fetal haemoglobin include erythropoietin and short-chain fatty acids such as arginine butyrate and valproic acid. Concerns about efficacy, biological half-life and route of administration have prevented their use clinically.

Allogeneic BMT is another experimental approach in the management of severe disease. More than 150 patients worldwide have been transplanted. Indications include neurological complications, severe chest crises and recurrent severe vaso-occlusive crises, and it has been restricted to children <16 years. The considerable cost, a short-term mortality of approximately 10%, the limited availability of HLA-compatible siblings and the long-term effects of the conditioning regimen on fertility and general health will limit the usefulness of this procedure.

Other new therapeutic approaches are based on the ability of magnesium and clotrimazole to decrease erythrocyte intracellular dehydration and the ability of nitric oxide to alter oxygen affinity. Interactions between red cells and endothelium are another potential target for future therapies.

References

Charache S, Terrin ML, Moore RD et al. 1995 Effect of hydroxyurea on the frequency of painful crises in sickle cell anaemia. New England Journal of Medicine 332: 1317–1332

Serjeant GR 1997 Sickle cell disease. Lancet 350: 725–730

Vichinsky EP, Charles MH et al. 1995 A comparison of conservative and aggressive transfusion regimens in the perioperative management of sickle cell disease. New England Journal of Medicine 333: 206–213

Walters MC et al. 1996 Bone marrow transplantation for sickle cell disease. New England Journal of Medicine 335: 369–376

128. Heparin-induced thrombocytopenia

A.F B.T C.F D.T E.F

Heparin-induced thrombocytopenia (HIT) is an important adverse immunological drug reaction that can be associated with catastrophic thromboembolic complications. Two types have been described: type I is a transient decline in platetet count (rarely <100 × 10^9/l) with no overt clinical consequences and type II is severe thrombocytopenia occurring approximately 5–15 days after starting heparin therapy. Cessation of heparin is followed by a return of the platelet count to normal levels within 5–12 days.

Type II HIT has been reported in patients receiving prophylactic as well as therapeutic doses of heparin. The incidence of type II HIT with porcine unfractionated heparin (UFH), the preparation used in the UK, is 1–5%, compared to 5–10% with the bovine heparin used in the USA. Type II HIT occurs less frequently (<1%) in patients receiving low molecular weight heparin (LMWH). Patients with HIT type II are at risk (>50%) of developing thromboembolic complications. Thrombotic arterial occlusion may have serious sequelae, such as limb gangrene requiring amputation, neurological deficit from stroke, or end-organ dysfunction. The mortality rate is about 30%, with a 20% risk of limb amputation.

Type II HIT is caused by a complex immunological mechanism. Affected patients develop antibodies (usually IgG) against a complex of heparin and platelet factor 4 (PF4). These immune complexes cause intravascular activation of platelets and vascular endothelial cells, with a marked increase in thrombin generation and thrombosis. Heparin chain length and negative charge are the major determinants of PF4 binding to heparin. LMWHs are made up of smaller oligosaccharides which bind less effectively to PF4, and these compounds are associated with a lower incidence of HIT type II.

Laboratory diagnosis of HIT type II can be difficult, so a high degree of clinical suspicion is necessary. Management of the condition can be initiated before the results of laboratory confirmatory tests are available. There are two types of assay: biological assays and enzyme 'immunoassays'. Biological assays include platelet aggregation tests, which observe the pattern of platelet activation (from selected donors) in the presence of patient serum and the heparin being used. This is labour intensive and neither sensitive nor specific. The gold standard is the serotonin-release assay, but this requires carefully selected control platelets and the use of radioactive markers, and is rarely performed. Assays based on the binding of patient immunoglobulin to a complex of heparin–PF4 complexes immobilized in wells using standard ELISA techniques are available but require further evaluation.

The first step in the management of a patient with HIT type II is cessation of heparin. Warfarin should not be started at this time as it can result in a precipitous fall in plasma concentrations of protein C, a natural anticoagulant. As a result, the thrombotic complications can paradoxically be aggravated. If there is a need to continue anticoagulation, other agents to consider include recombinant hirudin (a potent antithrombin derived from the leech), danaparoid (a heparinoid), ancrod (a defibrinogenating snake venom) or argatroban (a synthetic direct thrombin inhibitor). Unfortunately, although LMWHs are associated with a low incidence of HIT type II de novo, there is a high (40–100%) risk of in vitro and in vivo cross-reactivity of the HIT-IgG to LMWH. Thus LMWHs are not recommended as treatment for HIT.

Reference

Kelton JG, Warkentin TE 1998 Heparin-induced thrombocytopenia: an overview of the diagnosis, natural history and treatment options. Postgraduate Medicine 103: 169–171, 175–178

---

129. High homocysteine levels

A.T   B.F   C.F   D.T   E.T

Hyperhomocysteinaemia (sustained elevation of plasma homocysteine) is an independent risk factor for thrombosis and premature vascular disease. Whether homocysteine is pathogenetically related or incidental in this association, and whether lowering of homocysteine levels ameliorates the cardiovascular risk, remain to be determined.

The amino acid homocysteine is produced from the metabolism of dietary methionine and is normally present in the plasma at low concentrations (5–15 mmol/l). Its intracellular metabolism occurs through remethylation to methionine or transsulphuration, first to cystathionine and then to cysteine. These pathways are under tight metabolic control and involve several enzymes that require folate, cobalamin or pyridoxine as cofactors. Perturbation of homocysteine metabolism can result from either inherited or nutritional disorders.

The most frequent cause of severe (>100 μmol/l) hyperhomocysteinaemia is homozygous deficiency of cystathionine-B synthase, which has a frequency in the general population of approximately 1:200 000 – 1:335 000. Affected individuals have severe mental retardation, osteoporosis, ectopic lens, skeletal abnormalities, premature arterial vascular disease and venous thromboembolism.

Mild (15–25 μmol/l) or moderate (25–50 μmol/l) hyperhomocysteinaemia can be secondary to gene defects or acquired disorders. A common defect of the remethylation pathway is the presence of a thermolabile mutant of methylenetetrahydrofolate reductase, which has approximately

50% of the normal enzyme activity. The frequency of the homozygous state in the general population is 5%. The most common causes of acquired hyperhomocysteinaemia are nutritional deficiencies of cobalamin, folate or pyridoxine. Other factors include chronic renal insufficiency and compounds interfering with folate metabolism, such as anticonvulsants and methotrexate, or compounds interfering with metabolism of cobalamin, such as nitrous oxide. Raised plasma homocysteine levels have been reported in hypothyroidism.

Hyperhomocysteinaemia can be identified by simple measurement of plasma levels. To increase the sensitivity of detection, measurement of the peak plasma homocysteine level following administration of an oral methionine load is helpful.

Elevated homocysteine has been associated with an increased incidence of thromboembolism, myocardial disease and cerebrovascular and peripheral artery disease. Recent studies have demonstrated elevated homocysteine in 13–47% of patients with arterial occlusive disease. Numerous mechanisms have been proposed to explain the multiple vascular occlusive complications associated with hyperhomocysteinaemia. These involve disruption of normal endothelial cell function and/or blood coagulation pathways.

There is clear evidence that homocysteine levels can be lowered by administration of supplementary folate, with or without pyridoxine. However, it remains to be established whether lowering homocysteine levels with vitamin therapy will decrease the risk of arterial occlusive disease.

References

Malinow MR, Duell PB, Hess DL et al. 1998 Reduction of plasma homocysteine levels by breakfast cereal fortified with folic acid in patients with coronary heart disease. New England Journal of Medicine 338: 1009–1015

Nygard O, Nordrehaug JE, Refsum H et al. 1997 Plasma homocysteine levels and mortality in patients with coronary artery disease. New England Journal of Medicine 337: 230–236

130. Chronic myeloid leukaemia

A.F   B.T   C.F   D.F   E.T

Chronic myeloid leukaemia (CML) is a malignant myeloproliferative disease originating at the level of pluripotent haemopoietic stem cells. CML is characterized at the molecular level by the t(9;22) chromosomal translocation visible cytogenetically, or by fluorescence in situ hybridization (FISH) as the Philadelphia (Ph) chromosome. The resultant formation of the BCR-ABL fusion gene encodes a 210 kDa protein which functions as a protein, tyrosine kinase. These molecular changes are associated with expansion of the haemopoietic cell mass, predominantly of the myeloid series. Using FISH, a population of BCR-ABL-negative primitive progenitor cells have been identified in a substantial proportion of CML patients, both at diagnosis and during the course of their disease. Manipulation of this cell population is one approach to treatment and potential cure of CML.

There are various approaches to treating a newly diagnosed patient with CML. At diagnosis, leukapheresis can be used both to debulk disease (reducing symptoms and complications associated with hyperviscosity) and providing the opportunity for collecting and cryopreserving haemopoietic stem cells for later use as an autograft, if appropriate.

Allogeneic bone marrow transplantation, either from an HLA-identical sibling or an unrelated donor, offers the possibility of cure but is associated with a number of complications. The best outcome is achieved if patients are transplanted while still in the chronic phase, and preferably within 1 year of diagnosis. For patients transplanted with stem cells from HLA-matched donors, disease-free survival (DFS) at 5 years is 30–75%. In general, the results using unrelated donors are inferior to those using siblings. The increased incidence of acute and chronic graft-versus-host disease (GVHD), graft failure and life-threatening infections, with the resulting decrease in DFS and increased transplant-related mortality (TRM) is undeniably associated with the varying degrees of HLA disparity. Older age, advanced-phase disease, CMV positivity and prolonged interval from diagnosis to transplant all adversely affect DFS. With unrelated donors the use of molecular methods for HLA typing, especially in HLA-DRB1 matching, has improved results.

There are a number of treatment options for the patient who relapses after allogeneic transplantation. These include cessation of immunosuppressive therapy, the use of α-interferon (IFN-α) or a second transplant. Adoptive immunotherapy with the use of lymphocyte infusions obtained from the donor (DLI) has produced impressive results. The overall response rate is 30–90%, and is higher in those who receive DLI in molecular or cytogenetic relapse than in those whose leukaemia has progressed to haematogical relapse. Monitoring the level of BCR-ABL transcripts in the blood of post-transplant patients can identify candidates for early DLI. Acute and chronic GVHD and myelosuppression are the major side effects of this therapy.

For patients not eligible for any form of transplant procedure, initial treatment with IFN-α is becoming the standard approach. IFN-α induces haematological remission in 70–80% of previously untreated patients, and major or complete cytogenetic remissions in 5–27%. In one French study the addition of cytarabine to interferon has been shown to improve the results. Patients who achieve major or complete cytogenetic responses survive significantly longer than those who do not. The median survival of this group of patients is in excess of 6 years. However, in contrast to patients treated by bone marrow transplantation, almost all interferon-treated patients with a cytogenetic response have evidence of disease persistence at the molecular level (BCR-ABL transcripts). Intensification of chemotherapy with subsequent autologous stem cell support plus or minus IFN-α maintenance is under investigation.

IFN-α therapy is well tolerated but the majority of patients experience flu-like symptoms which last for 1–3 weeks after the start of treatment, or after an increase in dose. Other side effects described include anorexia, weight loss, depression, rashes, neurological disorders, vasculitis, autoimmune phenomena and thrombocytopenia. IFN-α appears not to impair fertility in either sex. Moreover, a small number of women who have conceived while receiving IFN-α have delivered normal children. However, further studies are necessary to exclude any teratogenic potential of IFN-α.

References

Guilhot F, Chastang C, Michallat M et al. 1997 Interferon alpha-2b combined with cytarabine versus interferon alone in chronic myelogenous leukaemia. New England Journal of Medicine 337: 223–229

Hansen JA, Gooley TA, Martin PJ et al. 1998 Bone marrow transplants from unrelated related donors for patients with chronic myeloid leukaemia. New England Journal of Medicine 338: 962–968

131. Essential thrombocythaemia

A.T   B.F   C.F   D.T   E.T

Essential thrombocythaemia (ET) is a myeloproliferative disorder characterized by clonal thrombocytosis. Diagnosis can be difficult because the disorder has no specific clinical or diagnostic features. Thrombocytosis can be found in other myeloproliferative disorders, in myelodysplasia, and as a reactive change in a variety of inflammatory and systemic diseases. Bone marrow morphology is often helpful in ET and reveals abnormal megakaryopoiesis. Abnormal platelet function is common, but this feature is not sufficiently specific to be applied diagnostically. Clonogenic cultures can be helpful as haemopoietic progenitor growth in vitro can be demonstrated to be growth factor independent in ET. Thrombopoietin concentrations are unhelpful as they tend to be normal or raised in both primary (ET) and reactive thrombocytosis. No specific cytogenetic abnormality has been described.

Life expectancy in ET approaches that of an age- and sex-matched control population. The risk of a life-threatening event in

ET, usually thrombosis, is related to the patient's age, history of previous thrombotic events or other coincident haemopoietic defects. Daily low-dose aspirin is widely recommended but may increase the risk of haemorrhage, particularly at very high platelet counts. Reduction of the platelet count by cytotoxic agents, such as hydroxyurea, reduces the incidence of vascular complications and appreciably improves survival in older patients (from about 3 years in untreated patients to 10 years or more in treated patients). The value of these agents in young patients is uncertain, and there is concern about the increased leukaemogenic risk that they may confer with long-term use. Therapeutic effects of interferon-α in ET include platelet reduction (80–100% response rate), resolution of splenomegaly and control of disease-associated symptoms. Interferon-α is not known to be leukaemogenic or teratogenic.

Anegrelide is an oral preparation of an active imidazoquinazolin derivative with species-specific thrombocytopenic activity in humans. In contrast, in animal studies potent antiaggregating activity occurs. Anegralide has been demonstrated to decrease the number of platelets by interfering with the maturation of megakaryocytes. Its efficacy in patients with ET has been described. Anegrelide treatment does not affect the neutrophil count or fertility, but cardiovascular side effects can limit its use in elderly people, who are at greatest risk of thrombosis.

References

Harrison CN, Linch DC, Machin SJ. 1998 Desirability and problems of early diagnosis of essential thrombocythaemia. Lancet 351: 846–847

Messinezy M, Pearson TC 1997 Polycythaemia, primary (essential) thrombocythaemia and myelofibrosis. British Medical Journal 314: 587–590

132. Severe haemophilia A
A.**T** B.**F** C.**F** D.**T** E.**T**

Haemophilia A is due to absent or decreased function of coagulation factor VIII (FVIII), resulting from mutations in the FVIII gene. The prevalence of haemophilia A is 1 in 10000 in the UK and it is an X-linked recessive disorder. In a third of cases there is no family history. The FVIII gene is among the largest known human genes, comprising 186 kb of DNA. The coding base consists of 26 exons. Over 80 different mutations have been characterized and these include deletions, insertions and point mutations. However, an inversion within the X chromosome at intron 22 has been found to underlie approximately 50% of cases of severe haemophilia (level of FVIII < 1%). Southern Blot analysis of a DNA sample for the common intron 22 inversion can be performed to aid prenatal diagnosis of severe haemophilia.

In the last decade HIV infection has overtaken fatal intracranial haemorrhage as the main cause of mortality in patients with severe haemophilia.

Infection with hepatitis C virus is almost universal for patients treated with clotting factors before 1985. Concern about viral transmission in concentrates has led to improvements in processing techniques designed to eliminate them. No cases of seroconversion from HIV, hepatitis B or C have been recorded in the UK since 1986 in this subgroup of blood product recipients. However, non-lipid coated viruses can escape inactivation procedures, with documented transmission of hepatitis A and parvovirus B19 in Europe. There is no evidence of transmission of Creutzfeld–Jakob disease from plasma-derived or recombinant products, although concern exists.

High-purity FVIII concentrates and recombinant FVIII concentrates are now in widespread use. The half-life of FVIII is 8 hours, and therefore 8–12-hourly dosing is advised. Treatment can be administered 'on-demand' or prophylactically. Development of inhibitors to FVIII can be problematic, and treatment strategies involving coagulation factors and immunomodulatory drugs have been employed.

Desmopressin is useful in patients with measurable FVIII (i.e. mild to moderate haemophilia). It is thought to work by releasing stores of FVIII from the endothelium. However, endothelial stores may be exhausted after several doses. Because of the associated side effects of fluid retention and hypertension, the use of desmopressin is not recommended for patients under 2 or over 60 years of age.

When patients with haemophilia A are treated with HIV protease inhibitors they may suffer an increased frequency or severity of bleeds, or an increased requirement for FVIII. The mechanism by which protease inhibitors produce this adverse affect is not known.

Gene therapy approaches to the treatment of haemophilia A are under development but to date there have been no major therapeutic successes in humans.

Reference

Cahill MR, Colvin BT 1997 Haemophilia. Postgraduate Medical Journal. 73: 201–206

133. Human T-cell leukaemia viruses

A.F   **B.**T   **C.**T   **D.**F   **E.**T

Human T-cell lymphotropic virus type I (HTLV-I) was first identified in 1980. It is a single-stranded RNA virus with reverse transcriptase activity that leads to DNA transcription of the virus and integration into the host genome. As with other retroviruses the genetic structure consists of a *gag* region, a *pol* region and an *env* region. HTLV-I also has a unique region at its 3′ end, referred to as the pX region, that encodes regulatory proteins such as *rex* and *tax,* thought to be crucial in the activation of host genes. Epidemiological studies have revealed regions of endemic HTLV-I in southern Japan, the Caribbean, Central and South America, and areas of Africa. HTLV-II, a virus with serological cross-reactivity to HTLV-I, has been found to be endemic in certain Native American populations and in intravenous drug users (IVDUs). These viruses are transmitted by sexual contact, blood transfusion, needle sharing among IVDUs, and from mother to child, primarily by breastfeeding.

HTLV-I has been implicated as the aetiological agent of adult T-cell leukaemia/lymphoma (ATL) and of a degenerative neurological disorder known as HTLV-I-associated myelopathy or tropical spastic paraparesis (HAM/TSP). The principal clinical features of ATL are lymphadenopathy, hepatosplenomegaly, skin lesions and hypercalcaemia. Opportunistic infections are common in late stages. The blood contains abnormal lymphocytes with characteristic lobulated nuclei ('flower cells'). These malignant cells are clonal and are activated CD4-positive T cells with increased expression of the α chain of the interleukin-2 receptor, which is the CD25 antigen. The lifetime risk among HTLV-I carriers for the development of ATL has been estimated at 1–4%. Combination chemotherapy, antiretroviral therapy, the interferons and monoclonal antibodies against the interleukin-2 receptor can all induce long-term disease-free survival in a minority of patients, but median survival is only 5 months.

HAM/TSP is a chronic progressive demyelinating disease that predominantly affects the spinal cord. It is reported to affect between 0.2 and 5% of infected individuals, and affects women more frequently than men. Onset is typically in the fourth decade, but it has been reported to occur within 6 months of transfusion of HTLV-I infected blood. Autoimmune or cytotoxic mechanisms may underlie the degenerative disease. The disease frequently progresses over a 5–10-year period and then stabilizes, with severe chronic disability. Corticosteroids and danazol have been used as treatment, but responses are unpredictable and transient.

References

Ferreira OC, Planelles V, Rosenblatt JD 1997 Human T-cell leukaemia viruses: epidemiology, biology, and pathogenesis. Blood Reviews 11: 91–104

Hollsberg P, Hafler DA 1993 Pathogenesis of diseases induced by human lymphotropic virus type I infection. New England Journal of Medicine 328: 1173–1182

134. Acute myeloid leukaemia

A.T   B.T   C.F   D.T   E.F

Acute myeloid leukaemia (AML) is a clonal malignant disorder. About 5% of cases are associated with inherited syndromes, which often involve genes encoding functions related to genomic stability and DNA repair. Other aetiological factors include exposure to ionizing radiation, organic solvents (benzene), alkylating agents (melphalan, chlorambucil), or transformation of a predisposing haematological disease (myeloproliferative disorder, myelodysplasia, or aplastic anaemia). Latencies for secondary AML associated with exposure to alkylating agents vary from 1 to 20 years. A period of myelodysplasia often precedes the presentation of therapy-induced leukaemia, and typically the chromosome abnormalities 5q- and monosomy 7 are seen.

There is also an association between exposure to the epipodophyllotoxin drugs (e.g. etoposide) and subsequent AML. Here latency is brief, usually between 1 and 3 years. A high proportion of these leukaemias are monocytic or myelomonocytic, with chromosome abnormalities at 11q23 involving rearrangements of the MLL gene. The epipodophyllotoxins are inhibitors of topoisomerase II which are enzymes that catalyse the breakage and resealing of DNA. Acute leukaemias arising de novo with 11q23/MLL gene rearrangements are a common finding in infant leukaemias. It has been proposed that in utero exposure to topoisomerase II inhibitors (benzene metabolites, flavonoids and quinolones) might be critical in the development of acute leukaemia in infancy. However, in most cases of AML the aetiology is not known.

The aim of chemotherapy for leukaemia is initially to induce a remission (<5% blasts in the bone marrow) and then to eradicate the residual leukaemic cell population by further courses of consolidation chemotherapy. In the UK, AML is currently treated with either intensive chemotherapy alone or intensive chemotherapy with allogeneic or autologous haemopoietic stem cell transplantation. The recently published MRC AML 10 trial investigated whether the addition of an autologous transplant to four courses of chemotherapy offered a survival benefit. It demonstrated a reduced relapse rate and a superior disease-free survival at 7 years with autologous transplant. The overall survival in patients aged <55 years at 7 years is 40–60%.

Good prognostic factors include the karyotype (cytogenetics) and less than 5% blasts after one course of induction chemotherapy. The cytogenetic abnormalities: t(15;17), t(8;21) and inv.(16) confer a good prognosis.

Acute promyelocytic leukaemia (APL) is characterized by the cytogenetic abnormality t(15;17) and accounts for 15% of all cases of AML. The addition of all-trans retinoic acid (ATRA) in remission induction regimens helps correct the coagulopathy that is commonly seen. ATRA induces terminal differentiation of blasts. Improved remission and long-term survival rates have been demonstrated in randomized trials of ATRA followed by standard remission chemotherapy.

Resistance of blasts to cytotoxic chemotherapy, at presentation or on relapse, has been a major hindrance to the success of leukaemia therapy. Mediators of drug resistance in leukaemias that have been identified include the multidrug resistance (MDR) P-glycoprotein and MDR-associated protein. P-glycoprotein is believed to act as a drug efflux pump. Expression of the MDR phenotype is an important determinant of outcome with chemotherapy. A number of agents are being studied which aim to restore drug sensitivity.

The use of growth factors (G-CSF and GM-CSF) has been studied in a number of trials. Although the period of post-chemotherapy neutropenia is shortened there appears to be no impact on incidence of infection or survival.

Other approaches under study include the role of immunomodulatory treatments and the use of novel drugs.

References

Burnett AK, Goldstone AH, Stevens RMF et al. 1998 Randomized comparison of addition of autologous bone-marrow transplantation to intensive chemotherapy for acute myeloid leukaemia in first remission: results of MRC AML 10 trial. Lancet 351: 700–708

Greaves MR 1997 Aetiology of acute leukaemia. Lancet 349: 344–349

Leisner RJ, Goldstone AH 1997 The acute leukaemias. British Medical Journal 314: 733–736

RHEUMATOLOGY

135. Antineutrophil cytoplasmic antibodies
A.F   B.T   C.F   D.F   E.T

Antineutrophil cytoplasmic antibodies (ANCA) are currently the only clinical serological test used in the diagnosis and management of vasculitis. They have also been identified in the sera of patients with other autoimmune rheumatic diseases, infections and inflammatory diseases.

Indirect immunofluorescence (IIF) techniques can be used to demonstrate typical cANCA (classic) and pANCA (perinuclear) staining patterns, but do not identify the specific antigen responsible for the immunofluorescence. In patients with vasculitis the target antigen of cANCA is usually serine proteinase 3 (90% cases) and of pANCA is myeloperoxidase (70% cases). These target antigens are found in neutrophil primary (or azurophilic) granules. Enzyme-linked immunoabsorbant assays (ELISA) can be used to confirm whether a cANCA staining pattern on IIF is due to serine proteinase 3 binding and a pANCA pattern due to myeloperoxidase binding. ANCA recognizing other target antigens should be interpreted with caution when being used to aid diagnosis of a primary vasculitis.

pANCA are commonly found in microscopic polyangiitis (75%) and Churg–Strauss syndrome (50%), but only rarely in polyarteritis nodosa (10%). cANCA has a high sensitivity (90%) and specificity (80%) for Wegener's granulomatosis. Antibody titres often correlate with disease activity and are a predictor of disease relapse, but high titres may sometimes persist despite apparent clinical remission.

cANCA specific for serine proteinase 3 are rarely seen in conditions other than vasculitis, exceptions being *Entamoeba histolytica* liver abscesses (75% of cases) and human immunodeficiency virus (HIV) infection. Many autoantibodies (including ANCA in 17–40% of cases) are found in HIV-positive patients, often in low titres. In this situation their presence typically does not correlate with clinical evidence of vasculitis or other rheumatic disease, and should be interpreted with caution.

References

Cambridge G 1998 Anti-neutrophil cytoplasmic antibodies. Arthritis and Rheumatism Council Topical Reviews series 3, no.13

Hoffman GS, Specks U 1998 Antineutrophil cytoplasmic antibodies. Arthritis and Rheumatism 41: 1521–1537

136. Scleroderma

A.F   B.T   C.T   D.T   E.F

Scleroderma is more common in females than males (4:1) with a prevalence of 15 per 100 000 population and a peak age of onset of 30–50 years of age. Althought its aetiology is unknown a large number of environmental factors have been associated with scleroderma (or similar conditions), such as chemicals (vinyl chloride, benzene) and drugs (bleomycin, pentazocine, contaminated L-tryptophan). Organ involvement in scleroderma is associated with extracellular matrix deposition (collagen, fibronectin, glycosaminoglycans) and microvascular injury. Inappropriate endothelial cell activation is believed to be a key feature in disease pathogenesis and elevated plasma levels of factor VIII–von Willebrands' factor provide evidence for this.

The degree of skin involvement is used to classify disease subtypes and provides important prognostic implications. Limited cutaneous (CREST) and diffuse cutaneous scleroderma are the two principal clinical syndromes. The limited disease group is associated with skin thickening on the limbs, restricted to sites distal to the knees and elbows, and on the face and neck but not the trunk. The diffuse disease is associated with skin thickening on the trunk and face, as well as the proximal and distal extremities. Other common clinical and laboratory features in the limited disease include Raynaud's phenomenon (99%), oesophageal dysmotility (90%), telangiectasia (90%), arthralgia (90%), calcinosis (40%) and anticentromere antibodies (50–90%). Isolated pulmonary hypertension occurs (25%) in limited disease but is usually asymptomatic for more than 5 years following diagnosis. The diffuse disease group has a much poorer prognosis with a 50% 10–year survival; pulmonary involvement is the major late cause of mortality. Other major organ involvement in diffuse disease includes oesophageal dysmotility (80%), interstitial lung disease (70%), small bowel involvement (40%) and renal crisis (20%). Anti Scl-70 antibodies are found in 20–30% of diffuse disease cases.

Renal crises are associated with hyperreninaemia, accelerated hypertension, microangiopathic haemolytic anaemia, thrombocytopenia and deteriorating renal function. The hypertension should be treated with ACE inhibitors (which have been shown to improve the prognosis in scleroderma renal crises) and intravenous prostacycline (which may help the microvascular pathology). Up to 50% of patients who require dialysis may improve sufficiently to allow the discontinuation of renal support for up to 2 years following a renal crisis.

Prednisolone doses above 20 mg have been shown in a case control trial to be a risk factor for precipitating a renal crisis in diffuse scleroderma, and should be avoided.

Reference

Mitchell H, Bolster MB, LeRoy EC 1997 Scleroderma and related conditions. Medical Clinics of North America: 81: 129–149

137. HIV infection compared to the normal population

A.T B.F C.F D.T E.T

The B-cell hyperreactivity seen in HIV infection results in a variety of low-titre autoantibodies such as antinuclear antibodies and antineutrophil cytoplasmic antibodies (ANCA). Specific antibodies against extractable nuclear antigens (ENAs) and rheumatoid factors are seen less frequently.

A Sjögren's-like syndrome is seen in graft-versus-host disease, HTLV-1 infection and HIV-1 infection (diffuse infiltrative lymphocytosis syndrome, or DILS). DILS is distinguished from classic Sjögren's syndrome by parotid gland enlargement and an increased incidence of extraglandular involvement, e.g. generalized lymphadenopathy, lymphocytic interstitial pneumonitis and neurological complications. In addition, the salivary gland T-cell infiltrate is predominantly CD8, compared to classic Sjögren's syndrome which is predominantly CD4. Anti-Ro and anti-La antibodies are rarely seen in DILS. Patients with DILS have a lower rate of HIV progression to overt immunodeficiency (e.g. slow CD4 cell decline).

HIV infection is associated with a lower incidence of CD4+ T-cell dependent diseases such as rheumatoid arthritis, and increased remission rates and reduced severity of systemic lupus erythematosus (SLE). Several rheumatic diseases are commonly associated with HIV infection. These include arthralgia and many arthritides, including psoriatic arthritis, which occurs with increased severity and possibly increased frequency. Reiter's disease and other spondyloarthropathies occur with increased incidence in the HIV population. The incidence of myositis is increased due to HIV infection per se, associated bacterial and fungal infections, and as an adverse effect of zidovudine treatment.

Reference

Itescu S 1996 Adult immunodeficiency and rheumatic disease. Rheumatic disease clinics of North America 22: 53–73

138. Mixed cryoglobulinaemia
A.F   B.T   C.T   D.F   E.T

Cryoglobulinaemia is the presence in the serum of immunoglobulins that precipitate reversibly at temperatures below 37°C.

Type 1 cryoglobulinaemia is characterized by monoclonal cryoglobulins and is found in multiple myeloma, Waldenström's macroglobulinaemia and lymphoproliferative disorders. Type II cryoglobulinaemia is characterized by mixed monoclonal and polyclonal cryoglobulins. The monoclonal cryoglobulin is usually IgM rheumatoid factor. Type II cryoglobulinaemia is associated with the hepatitis viruses, particularly hepatitis C (HCV), autoimmune rheumatic diseases, lymphoproliferative disorders and porphyria cutanea tarda. It may be idiopathic, when it is known as essential mixed cryoglobulinaemia. Type III cryoglobulinaemia is a polyclonal cryoglobulinaemia and is found in infections, autoimmune rheumatic disease and primary biliary cirrhosis, and can also be idiopathic (essential mixed).

Mixed cryoglobulinaemia typically presents with purpura (leucocytoclastic vasculitis), weakness and arthralgia. A non-erosive arthritis is sometimes seen. Various other organ involvement may occur, including glomerulonephritis and peripheral neuropathy. Clinical features of the underlying cause, e.g. HCV, may also be seen. IgM rheumatoid factors and low C4 complement levels are often found. HCV infection is the commonest identified cause (>70% cases) and predisposes to an increased risk of subsequent B-cell non-Hodgkin's lymphoma.

Treatment of HCV-associated cryoglobulinaemia involves antiviral therapy, adding immunosuppressive agents if required. One randomized study found that response to treatment with antiviral therapy (interferon-α) was similar whether or not prednisolone was added to the regimen, although in the corticosteroid-treated group viral loads (detected by HCV RNA) rose. This suggests corticosteroids should be avoided if possible in hepatitis C-associated cryoglobulinaemia

Reference

Ferri C, La Civita L, Longombardo G et al. 1998 Mixed cryoglobulinaemia: a crossroad between autoimmune disease and lymphoproliferative disorders. Lupus 7: 275–279

139. Poor prognostic markers in rheumatoid arthritis

A.F B.F C.T D.T E.T

Poor prognostic markers in rheumatoid arthritis include low social class, immunogenetic factors and certain disease characteristics. The latter include the persistence of joint inflammation after treatment, early X-ray evidence of joint erosions, persistently raised inflammatory markers (ESR and CRP), and rapid early disability in the patient.

Most prognostic markers are not sensitive or specific enough to identify which patients to target for aggressive immunosuppressive therapy in an attempt to prevent long-term damage from the disease.

Patients with HLA DRB1 genes that code a discrete structural element within the HLA DR molecule known as the rheumatoid 'shared' epitope have an increased susceptibility and an increased severity of rheumatoid arthritis. This sequence is exposed on the surface of the HLA DR molecule in a location that is in contact with both the T-cell receptor and antigenic peptides bound by the HLA molecule itself. All HLA DR molecules that carry the shared epitope (particularly DR4, DR1 and DR6 subtypes) are associated with rheumatoid arthritis.

Screening for the rheumatoid shared epitope in combination with other prognostic markers may be clinically useful for identifying patients to treat aggressively if such therapies can be shown to alter the long-term outcome of the disease.

References

Nepom GT, Gersuk V, Nepom BS 1996 Prognostic implications of HLA genotyping in the early assessment of patients with rheumatoid arthritis. Journal of Rheumatology 23: 5–9

Wolfe F 1997 The prognosis of rheumatoid arthritis: assessment of disease activity and disease severity in the clinic. American Journal of Medicine 103 (6A): 12S–18S

140. Bone mineral density

A.F B.T C.F D.T E.T

Bone mass increases with age, reaching a peak at the end of the third decade and declining gradually thereafter. Women achieve 30% lower peak bone mass than men, and caucasian women 8% lower than Afro-Caribbean women, because of their smaller bone size. Bone mass gradually reduces from the fourth decade, although the rate of loss accelerates in women in the 5–10 years following the menopause.

In clinical practice bone mass measured as bone mineral density (BMD) is most commonly estimated using dual-energy X-ray absorptometry (DEXA), although other techniques such as quantitative CT and ultrasound may become more widely used in the future.

BMD in young healthy adults shows a normal distribution. BMD values are therefore typically expressed in terms of standard deviation units. A T-score refers to the number of standard deviations an individual's BMD differs from the mean peak bone mass of a young, sex-matched reference group. The commonly used WHO criteria define low bone mass (osteopenia) as a T-score that lies between 1 and 2.5 standard deviations, and osteoporosis as a T-score which is greater than 2.5 standard deviations below mean peak bone mass of the reference group.

Cross-sectional and longitudinal studies show that rheumatoid arthritis patients have lower bone mineral density than controls. This is probably due to increased levels of circulating cytokines such as tumour necrosis factor-α, interleukin-1 and interleukin-6. Polycystic ovary syndrome (PCOS) is associated with oligoamenorrhoea but is not associated with a total oestrogen-deficiency state. High androgen levels and excess body mass index may also prevent demineralization in PCOS.

Raloxifene is a selective oestrogen receptor modulator (SERM). Such drugs have both oestrogen agonist and antagonist actions. Raloxifene has oestrogen-like effects on bone (increasing bone mineral density) and lowers serum cholesterol (total and low-density lipoprotein) without stimulating the endometrium. Raloxifene does not appear to increase the incidence of breast cancer, and potentially may reduce it. Such drugs have the potential for reducing postmenopausal morbidity and mortality in the future.

References

Ballard PA, Purdie D 1996 The natural history of osteoporosis. British Journal of Hospital Medicine 55: 503–507

Kanis JA, Delmas P, Burckhardt P et al. 1997 Guidelines for diagnosis and management of osteoporosis. Osteoporosis International 7: 390–406

Delmas PD, Bjarnason NH, Mitlak BH et al. 1997 Effects of raloxifene on bone mineral density, serum cholesterol concentrations, and uterine endometrium in postmenopausal women. New England Journal of Medicine 337: 1641–1647

DERMATOLOGY

141. Acne vulgaris

A.F   B.F   C.T   D.T   E.T

Acne vulgaris is a common disorder of the pilosebaceous unit that affects 95% of boys and 83% of girls at age 16. However, it is becoming increasingly common in the 20–40-year age group, especially in women.

The pathogenesis of acne vulgaris is multifactorial. One factor is excessive sebum production. Sebum secretion is under the control of the androgenic sex hormones and the level of excess sebum secretion generally correlates with the severity of acne. Growth hormone also stimulates sebum secretion, and therefore acne can be a feature of acromegaly. A second factor is abnormal follicular epithelial keratinization. During the normal process of epithelial differentiation fully matured cornified squames are shed from the surface of the skin. However, in acne vulgaris the squames are abnormally retained in the hair follicle orifice, thus forming a keratin plug. This results in the formation of the microcomedo, which is the primary lesion in acne vulgaris. Enlargement of microcomedones gives rise to both open and closed comedones. The third factor is colonization of the pilosebaceous unit by *Propionobacterium acnes*. Protease enzymes produced by *P. acnes* result in the production of proinflammatory mediators which diffuse from the follicle and result in the formation of the inflammatory lesions of acne – the papule, pustule and cyst.

There are many commonly prescribed drugs that can cause acne or acne-like eruptions. These include corticosteroids and anabolic steroids, antiepileptic drugs (phenytoin, phenobarbitone), halogens, antituberculous drugs (isoniazid, rifampicin) and also lithium, quinine and disulfiram. Corticosteroid-induced acne typically results in a monomorphic, predominantly pustular picture.

Apert's syndrome is a rare disorder in which patients manifest heightened sensitivity to circulating androgens. Affected individuals exhibit premature epiphyseal closure of long bones and the skull, and also have acne which is particularly resistant to treatment.

Treatment of acne vulgaris is usually titrated according to the severity of the problem. The antibiotic minocycline is commonly used in moderate cases. It is often used in preference to oxytetracycline because it only needs to be taken once or twice daily and there are no dietary restrictions. A well documented adverse effect of minocycline is a dose-dependent blue-black pigmentation of the skin, mucous membranes and sclerae, which fades slowly after stopping therapy. Other more serious adverse effects include hypersensitivity reactions, a systemic lupus erythematosus-like syndrome (with positive lupus serology) and hepatitis.

The recommended treatment of severe acne is with the vitamin A analogue isotretinoin. It is prescribed at a dose of 0.5–1.0 mg/kg/day for an average of 20 weeks. At the end of the treatment period 40% of patients are cured of their acne and a further 21% require only topical treatment. The most important adverse effect of isotretinoin is teratogenicity, and great care is taken to ensure that women of childbearing age use a reliable method of contraception for 1 month prior to and after the treatment course. Common adverse effects include skin and mucosal dryness, epistaxis, myalgia and reversible hair loss. The drug should not be coadministered with tetracycline because of the increased risk of benign intracranial hypertension. Recently, a suicide was reported in the American press in a young person taking isotretinoin. Psychiatric disturbance has been reported in 5% of patients taking the drug since 1982, and patients should be made aware of this.

Reference

Brown SK, Shalita AR 1998 Acne vulgaris. Lancet 351: 1871–1876

---

142. Alopecia
A.F   B.F   C.F   D.T   E.F

Androgenetic alopecia refers to the extremely common male pattern alopecia. Although the same pathophysiological process also takes place in females, the pattern of hair loss is different. In males there is typically bitemporal recession, loss of the anterior hairline and loss of vaultal hair. In female pattern baldness, vaultal thinning occurs but the anterior hairline is typically retained. Androgenetic alopecia is inherited as an autosomal dominant trait with variable penetrance. The stimulation of susceptible hair follicles by androgens at puberty leads to their progressive miniaturization to form downy vellus hair.

Finasteride, the type two (II) 5_{α}-reductase inhibitor, was approved by the US Food and Drug Administration in late 1997 for treatment of androgenetic alopecia in males. It inhibits the formation of active dihydrotestosterone (DHT) from testosterone within peripheral target cells and results in decreased concentrations of DHT in the scalp over a period of 6–12 months. Clinically this can result in a significant increase in scalp hair counts over this time.

Alopecia areata is thought to have an autoimmune origin and has been found in association with other autoimmune diseases, the commonest of which is autoimmune thyroid disease. It has also been described in patients with pernicious anaemia, systemic lupus erythematosus (SLE), rheumatoid arthritis, vitiligo and myaesthenia gravis. There is also an increased incidence in patients with Down syndrome. The prognosis is worse in patients with onset prior to puberty, involvement of the hairline (ophiasis), total scalp or body hair loss (alopecia totalis and universalis, respectively) and associated atopy. Nail changes are present in 7–66% of patients with alopecia areata. Fine pitting, longitudinal ridges and furrows and transverse lines have been detected but not onycholysis (lifting of the nail from the nailplate). Topical FK506 is one of the novel treatments currently being evaluated for use in alopecia areata.

SLE is one of the causes of cicatricial alopecia with destruction of the hair follicle. Causes include physical injuries, e.g. radiodermatitis, infections (fungal, e.g. kerion; bacterial, e.g. syphilis; viral, e.g. herpes zoster), cutaneous tumours, and other dermatoses such as scleroderma, lichen planus and sarcoidosis.

Causes of diffuse hair loss include malnutrition, zinc and iron deficiency, hypo- and hyperthyroidism, hypopituitarism, hyperparathyoidism, hepatic dysfunction and severe chronic illness, including AIDS. Intake of more than 50 000 units of vitamin A daily gives rise to dry skin, progressive thinning of scalp and body hair, weight loss, fatigue, anaemia and hepatosplenomegaly.

Reference

Schwartz RA, Janniger CK 1997 Alopecia areata. Cutis 59: 238–241

143. Atopic eczema

A.**T** B.**T** C.**T** D.**F** E.**F**

Atopic eczema (AE) is an extremely common skin condition affecting 10–15% of the population. In approximately two-thirds of cases the disease goes into remission by puberty. There is evidence for a genetic predisposition, with many affected individuals reporting a strong family history of atopy, either eczema, asthma or hayfever. The primary underlying defect is thought to be hyperactivity of cell-mediated immunity. Recent studies have suggested that atopy could be linked to genetic polymorphisms in the gene for the β subunit of the IgE receptor on chromosome 11q12–13 (FCεR1). Environmental factors also have a role, i.e. food allergens and house dust mite (*Dermatophagoides pteronyssinus*) sensitivity. Adult-onset AE is relatively unusual. In these case, lesions can resemble the patch stage of mycosis fungoides.

The diagnosis of AE is usually straightforward and is based on the patient's history and clinical features. Investigations, including a skin biopsy and serum IgE level, may be helpful, although the latter is not elevated in all patients.

Human papillomavirus (HPV), poxvirus and herpesvirus frequently complicate atopic eczema. HPV causes stubborn warts and pox virus is the causative agent of molluscum contagiosum. The latter is manifest by cutaneous umbilicated papules, which are particularly widespread in children with AE. Eczema herpeticum and Kaposi's varicelliform eruption are serious complications of herpes simplex and varicella zoster virus infection, respectively. The resulting acute exacerbation of AE produces painful vesicopustules and crusting.

Staphylococcus aureus and β-haemolytic streptococci can colonize or infect the skin of patients with atopic eczema. Stapholococcus aureus is not a usual resident of the skin, but in atopic eczema both lesional and non-lesional skin is heavily colonized. Lesions become infected when the organism density achieves $10^6/cm^2$. A high percentage of Staph. aureus strains isolated from eczematous lesions produce one or more superantigens: staphylococcal enterotoxins A and B and toxic shock syndrome toxin 1. These molecules can nonspecifically activate T cells to release cytokines, which cause inflammation and are thought to have an important role in producing clinical exacerbations of eczema.

The immunological mechanisms underlying the pathogenesis of AE have not as yet been clearly elucidated, although roles for T cells, CD1a-positive Langerhans' cells and dermal dendrocytes have been put forward. T cells can be divided into two groups depending upon their cytokine release profile. Upon stimulation, Th1 cells secrete large volumes of interleukin-2 and γ-interferon, whereas Th2 cells release interleukins 4, 5, 10, 13 and very little γ-interferon. Th2 cells can also induce IgE production by B cells. The T-cell profile predominantly found in lesions of AE is Th2. Current models of AE implicate both Th1 and/ or Th2 cells at different temporal points in the pathogenesis.

Azathioprine is a commonly used oral agent for the treatment of severe AE. Myelosuppression, gastrointestinal upset and hepatotoxicity are well documented adverse effects. The risk of myelosuppression is governed by a genetic polymorphism for the enzyme thiopurine methyltransferase (TPMT). One in 300 people have a homozygous defect in the TPMT gene and this results in an increased risk. Serum levels of TPMT can be used to screen individuals being considered for this treatment.

Reference

Rudikoff D, Lebwohl M 1998 Atopic dermatitis. Lancet 351: 1715–1721

144. Pyoderma gangrenosum
A.T   B.F   C.F   D.T   E.F

Pyoderma gangrenosum (PG) produces destructive ulceration of the skin. The pathogenesis of this condition is as yet unknown, although various abnormal immune responses have been reported in affected patients. There are essentially two patterns of presentation. The first is a typical ragged ulcer with an undermined blue-purple margin which follows the breakdown of a tender erythematous nodule. The second type is a vesicopustular variety. More unusual forms such as the bullous type also exist.

Pathergy is an interesting feature displayed by patients with PG and also Behçet's syndrome. It is manifest by lesions worsening or appearing after minor trauma. Therefore, lesions can occur at sites of burns or venepuncture, for example, and may worsen after surgical intervention. Interestingly, pathergy may also be evident at peristomal sites following bowel surgery in patients with associated inflammatory bowel disease. All lesions typically heal with cribriform scarring.

The lesions of PG vary in their histopathological appearance. There is haemorrhage, necrosis and a cellular infiltrate composed predominantly of neutrophils. There is usually no accompanying neutrophil leucocytosis. However, there may be an associated fever, malaise, myalgia or arthralgia. PG can occasionally mimic a related neutrophilic dermatosis named Sweet's syndrome (acute febrile neutrophilic dermatosis). The latter is typified by tender purplish-red nodules and plaques, fever and neutrophil leucocytosis. Ten per cent of cases of Sweet's syndrome are associated with haematological malignancy. PG and Sweet's syndrome are thought to represent points along a spectrum of skin diseases typified by a neutrophilic skin infiltrate.

Approximately 50% of patients with PG have 'idiopathic' disease. However, the conditions associated with PG are numerous and include: (1) diseases of the gastrointestinal tract, e.g. Crohn's disease and ulcerative colitis, (2) liver disease, e.g. chronic active hepatitis and primary biliary cirrhosis, (3) arthritides, both seropositive and seronegative, (4) haematological disorders, e.g. benign paraproteinaemia (most commonly of the IgA type), (5) malignancy (7.2% of cases), most commonly acute myeloid leukaemia, (6) infectious disease, e.g. AIDS, and (7) a miscellaneous group of systemic lupus erythematosus, sarcoidosis and thyroid disease.

Treatment involves both topical and systemic measures. It is also imperative to actively manage any accompanying underlying condition, as this can result in a more rapid resolution of ulceration. Local measures are aimed primarily at keeping the wound clean and free from infection. Hyperbaric oxygen may also be of benefit. The mainstay of systemic therapy are corticosteroids, although there are reports of several other immunomodulatory drugs which have been successfully used including cyclosporine, azathioprine, cyclophosphamide, tacrolimus and mycophenolate mofetil.

> **Reference**
>
> Callen JP 1998 Pyoderma gangrenosum. Lancet 351: 581–585

145. Mycosis fungoides
A.F   B.F   C.T   D.T   E.T

Mycosis fungoides (MF) is the most common variant of cutaneous T-cell lymphoma (CTCL). Average age of presentation is 50; males are more commonly affected than females and blacks more than whites.

The condition is often described in 'stages'. The initial patch stage can closely resemble an area of discoid eczema, psoriasis, tinea corporis or fixed drug eruption. This stage can persist unchanged for many years without progression. Progress to the plaque stage occurs when these lesions become infiltrated. Advancement to the tumour stage occurs when the lesions develop into the polypoid mushroom-like growths that give this condition its name. Extensive skin necrosis can occur at this more advanced stage, leaving the patient open to infection. Over 50% of deaths from MF are caused by *Pseudomonas aeruginosa* or *Staphylococcus aureus* sepsis. Involvement of lymph nodes and internal organs, typically liver and spleen, is an extremely poor prognostic sign.

In 5% of cases cutaneous T-cell lymphoma can present as a leukaemic variant called Sézary syndrome. These patients present with a pruritic erythroderma, lymphadenopathy (57%) and peripheral circulating Sézary cells with abnormal cerebriform nuclei making up more than 10% of the peripheral lymphocyte count. Other clinical features include hepatomegaly (36%), alopecia (32%), onychodystrophy (32%) and thickening of the skin on the palms and soles. In very advanced disease the patients may develop leonine facies.

Histologically there are collections of abnormal T cells in the dermis. These can also be found in the epidermis as single cells, or in clusters forming Pautrier's microabscesses. The lymphocytes often exhibit abnormal cerebriform nuclei (the same phenotype as those circulating in Sézary syndrome) and are usually of CD3+, CD4+, T-helper cell phenotype.

Molecular biological techniques can be used to aid the diagnosis of cutaneous and disseminated CTCL. These so-called T-cell receptor gene rearrangement studies can detect clonal populations of T cells, i.e. groups of identical cells typically derived from one lymphoid cell. However, the results should be interpreted with care as clonality, although highly suggestive, does not always indicate a malignant T-cell proliferation.

Current treatments for CTCL include topical corticosteroids, phototherapy (PUVA, ultraviolet B radiation), topical chemotherapy (nitrogen mustard, carmustine), systemic chemotherapy, radiotherapy including superficial electron beams, interferons, retinoids, extracorporeal photophoresis and photodynamic therapy. These can be used alone or in combination.

Extracorporeal photophoresis was initially described in 1987 and is currently under formal assessment. It is probably most beneficial for patients with erythrodermic CTCL or Sézary syndrome. It involves oral administration of a psoralen photosensitizer followed by white cell removal. The white cells are then exposed to ultraviolet A radiation and returned to the patient. The antigenically altered T cells are thought to initiate a therapeutic immune response in the host.

Reference

Lorincz AL 1996 Cutaneous T cell lymphoma (mycosis fungoides).
   Lancet 347: 871–876

---

146. Psoriasis

A.F   B.T   C.T   D.F   E.F

Psoriasis is a common disorder affecting 2% of the population. It has long been proposed that there is an inherited predisposition to this disorder. Recent studies suggest that there are broadly two groups of affected individuals. The commonest form usually commences before the age of 40, is clinically more severe, and is associated with a strong family history. The mode of inheritance in this group is thought to be autosomal dominant with variable penetrance and is linked to HLA-Cw6. The less common sporadic form typically presents around the age of 60, is less severe and probably results from multifactorial inheritance. These two forms have been termed types 1 and 2, respectively, although this terminology is not in widespread use.

The most characteristic form of this inflammatory hyperkeratotic disorder is chronic plaque psoriasis, which is typified by well demarcated erythematous scaly plaques on the scalp and extensor surfaces. Other well recognized clinical variants include palmoplantar psoriasis, pustular psoriasis (localized and generalized), erythrodermic psoriasis and guttate psoriasis. The latter typically follows streptococcal infection and is manifest by small 'raindrop'-type lesions. It responds well to ultraviolet B (UVB) radiation therapy. Nail changes are found in 25–50% of cases of psoriasis and are frequently found along with psoriatic arthropathy.

The severity of nail changes varies tremendously from case to case and is independent of the extent of cutaneous disease.

Acute generalized pustular psoriasis of Zumbusch is a life-threatening disease. Complications include hypoalbuminaemia, hypocalcaemia, oliguria and acute renal failure and inflammatory polyarthritis. The pustules of pustular psoriasis are sterile. This condition responds well to oral methotrexate. A rare complication of persistent erythrodermic psoriasis is high-output cardiac failure, which results from a hyperdynamic cutaneous circulation.

Several drugs reportedly lead to an exacerbation of psoriasis. The most commonly reported are lithium, β-blockers, antimalarials, and withdrawal of systemic corticosteroids. Other exacerbating factors include infections (*Streptococcus*, HIV), sunlight and smoking (particularly in palmoplantar psoriasis); excess alcohol intake and stress are thought to have a detrimental effect on the ability to treat and cope with psoriasis. Local injury can lead to the development of new lesions at the affected site – this feature is termed Koebnerization.

There is a multitude of treatments currently in regular use by dermatologists for psoriasis. These include emollients, topical steroids, tar, dithranol, vitamin D analogues, ultraviolet therapy (UVB or PUVA: oral <u>P</u>soralen plus <u>UVA</u> irradiation) and systemic therapies, which include methotrexate, hydroxyurea, retinoids, cyclosporin A and systemic corticosteroids. Tacrolimus (FK506) and anti-CD4 monoclonal antibodies have also been found to be effective.

A new form of phototherapy has recently been introduced, termed TL-01. This provides narrowband UV light at around 311 nm wavelength and is reported to produce longer disease remissions, a lower incidence of burning and possibly a lower incidence of UV-associated carcinogenesis compared to PUVA and UVB.

Reference

Stern RS 1997 Psoriasis. Lancet 350: 349–353

---

147. Effects of ultraviolet radiation on the skin

A.F   B.T   C.T   D.F   E.F

Ultraviolet radiation (UVR) is composed of UVA (wavelength 320–400 nm), UVB (290–320 nm) and UVC (200–290 nm). However, UVC does not reach the earth's surface. UVR below wavelengths of 300 nm are mostly absorbed in the epidermis, but wavelengths above this pass mostly into the dermis. The cutaneous effects of UVR exposure are related to the wavelength and total radiation dose.

Several cutaneous effects result from UVR exposure. Early effects include inflammation, tanning, hyperplasia or thickening of the epidermis, immunological changes and vitamin D synthesis. Photocarcinogenesis and photoageing are later effects. Smoking is thought to lead to premature ageing, possibly as a result of a reduction in cutaneous blood flow. Smoking-related changes are most pronounced on sun-exposed skin.

DNA is the primary site of UVR-induced injury within the skin cells. As a consequence of DNA damage, the levels of p53, a tumour suppressor gene, become elevated within the nucleus. This results in a temporary pause of the cell cycle, which allows the DNA damage to be repaired prior to re-entrance into the cell cycle, or apoptosis (programmed cell death) to occur. p53 exerts some influence over the number of cells containing abnormal DNA within the skin. Consequently, loss of p53 function would be detrimental to the cell.

UVR absorbed by epidermal keratinocyte DNA results in the formation of UV photoproducts, which facilitate the development of UV-specific DNA mutations. Two-thirds of these specific mutations are C–T substitutions and 10% are CC–TT mutations. Both of these have been detected within skin carcinomas. The vast majority of squamous cell carcinomas contain p53 tumour suppressor gene mutations and two-thirds of these are UV-specific. UV specific p53 mutations are also found in 50% of BCC (basal cell carcinomas) and 60% of solar keratoses. Thus, UVR is the commonest carcinogen implicated in the formation of skin cancers.

A skin cell that contains a UVR-induced p53 mutation will have become more resistant to apoptosis secondary to the loss of the tumour suppressor gene function. This cell is able to enter another round of cell division and will possibly accumulate further UVR DNA damage on additional sun exposure. Hence the number of UVR-induced mutations can accumulate, thereby increasing the risk of premalignant change. This is the process of photocarcinogenesis.

Another consequence of UVR-induced DNA damage is the increased production of nuclear transcription factors and cytokines. This results in the production of serum and epidermal interleukins, which ultimately leads to the release of inflammatory mediators and clinical erythema, pain, swelling and heat, i.e. sunburn.

Skin tanning may occur as a result of UVR-induced DNA damage, although the mechanisms have not yet been fully elucidated. The number and size of melanocytes, rate of melanogenesis (melanin production) and rate of melanin transfer to adjacent keratinocytes are all increased.

Immunological effects on the skin include an increase in CD8-positive suppressor T-cell number and a decrease in natural killer cell activity. Langerhans' cell (antigen-presenting cells found mostly in the epidermis) numbers are decreased as are CD4+ helper T cells. These changes modify and suppress the skin's immune response.

Reference

Whittaker S 1996 Sun and skin cancer. British Journal of Hospital Medicine 56: 515–518

148. Skin cancer in organ transplant recipients
A.F   B.F   C.T   D.T   E.F

Most studies of non-melanoma skin cancer (NMSC) in transplant patients have been carried out in those receiving renal allografts. It became evident that as survival in this population of patients was increasing, the incidence of warts and NMSCs was unusually elevated compared to the normal population. This was first noted in the sunny climate of Australia. Even in the UK up to 40% of patients who were transplanted more than 20 years ago have NMSC. Lesions tend to appear up to 30 years earlier and behave much more aggressively than in non-immunosuppressed individuals.

The commonest malignancy in renal transplant recipients is squamous cell carcinoma (SCC), followed by lymphoreticular carcinoma. The ratio of BCC (basal cell carcinoma) to SCC in the normal population is 5:1, but in the transplant population the reverse is true. Carcinomas of the lip and anogenital region are more common in the immunosuppressed group. To date it is not totally clear whether it is the level of immunosuppression or the particular drugs used in different treatment regimens that has the greatest influence on the rate of occurrence of NMSC in different transplant groups.

Other risk factors in addition to immunosuppression are sun exposure and human papillomavirus (HPV) infection. The latter two appear to be acting as cocarcinogens, as skin carcinomas often appear on sun-exposed sites on a background of wart virus infection. Virtually all transplant recipients have clinical warts 5 years post transplant. Various HPV types have been detected within SCCs of transplant patients. These include both 'low-risk' (HPV 1–4, 6, 11) and 'high-risk' (HPV 16, 18) types.

Importantly, patients should be warned immediately post transplant of the risk of skin carcinogenesis. They should be advised to protect their skin from the sun with protective clothing and high-factor sunblocks giving both UVA and UVB protection. Their skin should be examined regularly, including the genital areas. Because of their potential aggressiveness suspicious lesions should be removed promptly. Oral retinoids are of use in preventing the development of new skin carcinomas in those with established disease. However, when the treatment is stopped, rebound worsening of the skin occurs. Thus prevention in the form of early sun protection advice and regular skin surveillance is mandatory in these individuals.

References

Glover M 1998 The increased incidence of skin cancer in organ-transplant recipients. Dermatology in Practice Jan/Feb: 6–8

London NJ, Farmery SM, Will EJ, Davison AM, Lodge JPA 1995 Risk of neoplasia in renal transplant patients. Lancet 346: 403–406

149. Neurocutaneous disorders

A.F B.T C.F D.F E.T

There are two types of neurofibromatosis. Type 1 (NF-1) is the most common. The mode of inheritance is autosomal dominant with 100% penetrance by the age of 5. The rate of new somatic mutations is high owing to the fact that the gene for NF-1 is large (350 kb). It is found on chromosome 17q11.2 and encodes a protein named neurofibromin, which may be involved in the inactivation of the *ras* oncogene. Cutaneous features of NF-1 include six or more café-au lait macules, axillary freckling and multiple cutaneous, subcutaneous or plexiform neurofibromas. Pruritis is a well recognized symptom of NF-1 and this is thought to be a result of the large numbers of mast cells in the skin in this disorder. Café-au-lait macules are the first cutaneous feature to appear in all children; however, 25–40% of normal schoolchildren have between one and five. Café-au-lait macules are present in 35% of individuals with the syndrome. The extent of cutaneous disease gives no clue as to the severity of internal organ involvement. An interesting segmental form of NF-1 has been described and is thought to arise from a somatic mutation of the NF-1 gene.

NF-2 is an autosomal dominant disorder. The gene NF-2 is located on chromosome 22q11-q13 and encodes a tumour suppressor protein named merlin. Skin manifestations of NF-2 are less common than NF-1. Axillary freckling is rare and café-au-lait macules rarely exceed five in number.

Tuberous sclerosis complex (TSC) is an autosomal dominant condition manifested by the formation of tissue hamartomas. Affected families are linked to either chromosome 9 (TSC 1) or 16 (TSC 2). The latter gene encodes a protein named tuberin, which appears to have a function similar to that of neurofibromin. Cutaneous lesions are found in 60–70% of cases and the following are pathognomonic of TSC: angiofibromas, periungual fibromas which appear at or after puberty, the shagreen patch and the ash-leaf macule, forehead plaques and soft fibromas in skin folds. The ash-leaf macule can be detected under Wood's light. The shagreen patch is a skin-coloured plaque of irregular thickness found on the lower back.

Xeroderma pigmentosum is an autosomal recessive condition resulting in abnormal DNA repair. This gives rise to the clinical picture of photosensitivity, pigmentary changes (skin freckling), premature ageing, squamous and basal cell carcinoma, melanoma and neurological manifestations. Skin carcinomas typically develop at sun-exposed sites and ultraviolet light-induced DNA mutations are thought to be important in their pathogenesis. The skin carcinomas will typically begin before the age of 20. Two-thirds of patients die before the age of 20 as result of metastatic squamous cell carcinoma or melanoma. Complete sun avoidance is advocated for these patients, along with early excision of tumours. Prophylactic oral retinoids may reduce the incidence of skin cancers.

Reference

Zvulunov A, Esterly N 1995 Neurocutaneous syndromes associated with pigmentary skin lesions. Journal of the American Academy of Dermatology 32: 915–935

150. Bullous pemphigoid

A.T   B.T   C.F   D.F   E.T

Bullous pemphigoid is an acquired subepidermal blistering disease which occurs most commonly in individuals over 60. In recent years there has been an increased understanding of the ultrastructure of the basal keratinocyte hemidesmosome, the organelle responsible for epidermal adhesion to the basement membrane zone and dermis. Related studies have also led to a greater understanding of other genetic (epidermolysis bullosa) and acquired blistering diseases.

The typical lesions of bullous pemphigoid are tense blisters of varying sizes, usually on an erythematous, sometimes urticated, background. The blisters are tense as their roof is comprised of full-thickness epidermis. This is in contrast to the flaccid blisters and erosions characteristic of pemphigus vulgaris, which have an intraepidermal split so that the blister roof is made up of partial-thickness epidermis. Bullous pemphigoid is associated with oral involvement in 40% of cases.

The clinical differential diagnosis of bullous pemphigoid includes blistering drug eruptions, insect bite reactions, burns, herpes gestationis, bullous lupus erythematosus and bullous erythema multiforme.

Histopathological analysis of an intact blister reveals a subepidermal split accompanied by a varying level of cellular infiltrate in the blister cavity and dermis. The eosinophil is the predominant cell type in the infiltrate. Interestingly, peripheral eosinophilia is found in 50% of cases.

Perilesional skin is most useful for immunofluorescence studies. Direct immunofluoresence reveals linear deposits of IgG and C3 along the epidermal basement membrane, i.e. on the roof of the blister, and circulating IgG antibodies are found in approximately 70% of patients. IgG4 is the predominant subclass detected both in skin and peripheral blood.

Immunoblotting studies have revealed that 50–70% of antibodies in patients' sera recognize a 230 kDa polypeptide, and 30–50% also recognize a 180 kDa polypeptide. Both of these polypeptides are localized to the hemidesmosome, and animal studies have confirmed that they do have a pathogenetic role in blister formation.

Probably the commonest forms of treatment used to control blistering are the oral corticosteroids. Corticosteroid-sparing agents are introduced at an early stage and maintained while the steroids are withdrawn. Azathioprine, cyclophosphamide, cyclosporin A and tetracyclines in combination with nicotinamide are commonly used steroid-sparing therapies. Topical or intralesional steroids are useful in the management of localized blistering. The disease typically goes into remission, with or without treatment, after approximately 4 years.

Reference

Korman NJ 1993 Bullous pemphigoid. Dermatologic Clinics 11: 483–498

Viva questions

BASIC SCIENCE, IMMUNOLOGY AND GENETICS

1. What is the difference between apoptosis and necrosis?
2. How does a flow cytometer work and what can it be used for in clinical medicine?
3. What do you understand by the terms Th1 and Th2 response?
4. What do you understand by the term cytokine? Can you describe the function of any of the cytokines? Do you know of any diseases associated with an excess or deficiency of any cytokines?
5. What are chemokines?
6. I am a 25-year-old asthmatic. I have just read on the Internet that I can be cured if I have a course of allergen immunotherapy. Could you give me some more information?
7. What is the Human Genome Project?
8. What does the term genetic imprinting refer to?
9. What scientific methods are available to detect a genetically inherited disease?
10. How would you advise a 20-year-old man with a family history of Huntington's disease? Would your advice change with the age of your patient?
11. What prothrombotic mutations have been identified?

PHARMACOLOGY AND DRUG DEVELOPMENT

12. What is meta-analysis and when can it be useful? How does a meta-analysis differ from a systematic review?
13. What is a type I/ type II error?
14. How can you avoid positive publication bias?
15. What is a case-control study, and what is it useful for? What is a cohort study?
16. In what sort of disease is it useful to describe incidence rather than prevalence?

17. What do you understand by the term phase 1 trial? How does a phase 3 trial differ from a phase 2 trial?

18. How can drugs interact?

19. What drugs inhibit cytochrome P450?

20. What resources are available for investigating a suspected adverse drug reaction?

THERAPEUTICS

21. What are the known medical complications of Ecstasy use?

22. What are the harmful effects of the social use of cannabis?

23. Which drugs prolong the QT interval?

24. What are the symptoms of depression? What are the treatment options?

25. What do you know about donezepil as a treatment for Alzheimer's disease?

26. What new epilepsy drugs have you read about? Do you know of any serious adverse effects associated with lamotrogine or vigabatrin treatment?

NEUROLOGY

27. A 25-year-old woman presents with a left hemiparesis. What are the causes of stroke in a young adult?

28. How would you manage a 35-year-old man who has been brought into hospital by ambulance and is still fitting despite having been given 20 mg of i.v. diazepam?

29. Tell me what you know about the genetic mutation responsible for Friedreich's ataxia. What are the clinical features of this disease?

30. Diabetes mellitus is the most common cause of peripheral neuropathy in the west. What different types of peripheral neuropathy does it cause?

31. What are the adverse effects of L-dopa treatment?

32. Tell me about the different drug and surgical treatments for Parkinson's disease. Do you know of any new treatments?

33. What does the term trinucleotide repeat disorder refer to?

34. What do you know about the clinical features and management of migraine?

35. What do you know about analgesia-induced headache?

RESPIRATORY MEDICINE

36. What do you understand by the term 'brittle asthma'?

37. What do you understand by the term 'slow relaxing substance of anaphylaxis'? Are there any agents that can modify its activity to treat patients with asthma?

38. Do you know of any new therapies for the treatment of asthma?

39. Describe the genetic mechanisms underlying disease due to α_1-antitrypsin deficiency?

40. I have cryptogenic fibrosing alveoitis – what are the treatment options and how successful might they be?

41. What surgical therapies are available to treat emphysema?

42. Discuss the postoperative treatment options following lung transplantation.

43. Discuss the limitations of lung transplantation as a treatment for chronic pulmonary disease.

ENDOCRINOLOGY

44. A 20-year-old woman attends your clinic complaining of excessive facial hair. What is your differential diagnosis? What would make you suggest imaging of the abdomen and pelvis?

45. How would you approach the medical management of a 30-year-old woman with suspected polycystic ovary syndrome?

46. You see a 33-year-old man in casualty with a blood pressure of 190/110. What is your differential diagnosis and management?

47. A 42-year-old woman presents complaining of excessive sweating and palpitations and has a blood pressure of 220/120. What is your differential diagnosis, and tell me about your management?

48. A 55-year-old man with a blood pressure of 190/110 and occasional headaches is seen by you in casualty. What is your differential diagnosis and management?

49. You see a 56-year-old woman with acromegaly for the first time. She tells you her mother had the same problem but she had forgotten to tell your consultant. If you are allowed to perform one test, what would it be and why?

50. What do you understand by the term multiple endocrine neoplasia? Describe the features of the syndrome.

51. Do you think there is any advantage in obtaining tight blood glucose control in type II diabetics?

52. You admit a patient with type II diabetes and an acute myocardial infarction: do you have any special considerations regarding their management?

53. How would you distinguish between primary hypothyroidism, secondary hypothyroidism and subclinical hypothyroidism? What are the causes of hypothyroidism?

CARDIOLOGY

54. What advice would you give a hypertensive patient about salt intake?

55. A patient is admitted with worsening congestive cardiac failure and ischaemic dilated cardiomyopathy is suspected. In addition to diuretics and an ACE inhibitor, what therapies would you consider and why?

56. Discuss the treatment of hypertension in pregnancy.

57. After myocardial infarction what strategies would you offer a patient as secondary prevention?

58. Would you treat a blood pressure recording of 145/90?

59. How would you manage a patient admitted with a wide complex-tachycardia and a blood pressure of 100/60?

60. What strategies do you know for the treatment of atrial fibrillation?

61. What functions does the vascular endothelium have, and how may endothelial dysfunction contribute to acute coronary syndromes?

62. Do women have the same risk of ischaemic heart disease as men? What is the role of hormone replacement therapy in cardiovascular risk reduction in women?

GASTROENTEROLOGY

63. A patient who had a bowel resection for Crohn's disease 6 months ago and did not attend follow-up presents to A+E with renal failure. He is severely dehydrated on examination and further questioning reveals that he has suffered recurrent severe diarrhoea since his discharge. What is your immediate management and differential diagnosis of the diarrhoea? How would you go about investigating the likely causes?

64. A 25-year-old woman goes to see her GP after her mother's death from primary biliary cirrhosis. She complains of lethargy. What would you advise the GP to do?

65. What is your opinion regarding population screening for Barrett's oesophagus?

66. What would you recommend a patient with Wilson's disease to tell their family with regard to testing?

67. How do you investigate a patient presenting with acute abdominal pain and jaundice?

68. Discus the advantages and disadvantages of initiating a screening programme of the general population for coeliac disease.

69. Is undernutrition important in the general medical setting?

70. If you were to audit the nutritional care of general medical inpatients in your hospital how would you go about it?

71. A 43-year-old female patient with Crohn's disease and three previous operations is admitted to your casualty department. She has not 'felt right' since discharge from your surgical unit 3 weeks ago, and feels dizzy and has a ringing in the ears. What is your differential diagnosis, what are the key points you would like to pursue further in the history and examination, and what are the key emergency investigations?

NEPHROLOGY

72. What are the non-renal complications of the nephrotic syndrome?

73. What are the recognized adverse effects of cyclosporin treatment?

74. What factors would you consider when deciding how to treat a patient with atheromatous renal artery stenosis?

75. How would you investigate a patient with recurrent renal calculi?

76. What are the mechanisms by which NSAIDs can cause acute renal failure?

77. What are the complications of long-term haemodialysis?

78. What are the causes of rhabdomyolysis?

79. What infections are patients at risk of developing following solid organ transplantation?

80. What are the bad prognostic indicators for a patient with IgA nephropathy?

INFECTIOUS DISEASES

81. How would you manage a case of severe malaria?

82. What is the difference between tuberculoid and lepromatous leprosy?

83. What antimalarial advice would you give a traveller to the tropics?

84. In what infections are corticosteroids a useful treatment?

85. Tell me about new diagnostic methods in infectious diseases.

86. How would you investigate someone with fever who has recently returned from the tropics?

87. How would you investigate someone for syphilis?

88. How would you investigate eosinophilia?
89. Tell me about a vector-borne disease.
90. What is the lifecycle of the malaria parasite?
91. Tell me the lifecycle of a gut worm.
92. What can you tell me about amoebic disease?
93. What can you tell me about schistosomiasis?
94. Which bacterial diseases are mediated by toxins?

HIV

95. A 22-year-old man presents with a 1-week history of headache, fever, macular papular rash and oral ulceration, and has leucopenia and thrombocytopenia on his blood film. What is your differential diagnosis and what is the most likely diagnosis? Discuss the relevant investigations.
96. Is there any evidence to suggest that treating early HIV disease is beneficial?
97. Are you aware of any guidelines regarding antiretroviral treatment in HIV disease?
98. Reverse transcriptase is important in the pathogenesis of HIV disease – do you know of any agents that inhibit this enzyme?
99. What do you understand by the term HAART (highly active antiretroviral therapy)?
100. What do you understand by the term immune reconstitution?
101. What is the importance of reservoirs of HIV infection?
102. Do you know any adverse effects of antiretroviral therapy?
103. Is drug resistance still important in HIV disease with the advent of HAART?
104. A 33-year-old man has an HIV RNA viral load of 20 000 and a CD4 count of 350 cell/ml. What advice can you give him regarding the options for therapy?

ONCOLOGY

105. Describe what measures can be taken to palliate a patient with non-small cell lung cancer and recurrent haemoptysis.
106. Hormonal manipulation has an important role in the treatment of metastatic breast cancer. List the three main classes of drugs used for hormone manipulation in this disease and describe their adverse effects.

107. A 39-year-old woman complains of feeling non-specifically unwell and gives a history of rigors. She is pyrexial and hypotensive. She was given her first cycle of adjuvant chemotherapy for localized breast cancer 10 days ago. Discuss your management.

108. What options are available for pain control in a 54-year-old man with locally advanced pancreatic cancer?

109. A 43-year-old man from Africa is referred to you with a history of weight loss. Clinically he has hepatomegaly and ultrasound reveals a large single mass in the right lobe of the liver. What investigations would you request in order to make a diagnosis? If malignancy is confirmed, what is the role of surgery in this patient?

110. A 70-year-old man with known metastatic non-small cell lung cancer arrives in casualty with a 3-day history of increasing confusion. He has widespread bone metastases and requires opiates for pain control. List your differential diagnoses and discuss your management of each.

111. A 60-year-old woman who underwent mastectomy for localized breast cancer 10 years ago presents to casualty with a 6-week history of lower back pain and, over the last 3 days, increasing difficulty walking. Clinically she has upper motor neuron signs in her legs and a sensory level at T10. What urgent investigation are you going to request and what are the treatment options?

112. Discuss the rationale behind cervical screening and describe the difficulties that there have been in implementing this in the UK.

113. What are the different histological subclasses of Hodgkins' disease and how do they affect prognosis? Define B symptoms and describe what investigations are required to stage a patient with Hodgkin's disease.

114. A 30-year-old man presents with shortness of breath and clinical signs of superior vena cava obstruction. Chest X-ray shows a large mediastinal mass. What is the differential diagnosis and what investigations would you request? What simple urine test may provide the diagnosis? This test proves to be negative and he starts to deteriorate before a diagnosis can be made; what are your treatment options?

HAEMATOLOGY

115. What screening tests are performed on donated blood products?

116. What are the criteria for the diagnosis of multiple myeloma? What treatment options are available for a 45-year-old woman who is newly diagnosed with this condition?

117. A patient presents with pancytopenia. What are the possible causes? Describe any special measures that should be introduced.

118. What criteria are available to make the diagnosis of antiphospholipid antibody syndrome?

119. Describe the features of thrombotic thrombocytopenic purpura. What do you know about the pathogenesis? Outline treatment options.

120. What prophylactic measures are recommended for the asplenic patient?

121. What do you understand by the term 'graft-versus-leukaemia'? In which diseases has it been demonstrated?

122. What are colony-stimulating factors? Describe their use.

123. What are the causes of disseminated intravascular coagulation? Describe its treatment.

RHEUMATOLOGY

124. How would you classify the subtypes of scleroderma and do you feel this distinction is of academic or clinical relevance? Are there any tests to help distinguish between these subtypes?

125. A 35-year-old woman suffers from symptomatic Raynaud's phenomenon, acid reflux, and scleroderma of the forearms, face, neck and on the lower legs below the knees. What is her prognosis and what would you tell her?

126. How would you treat a patient with renal crisis and diffuse scleroderma? What is the prognosis following this complication?

127. Do you think HIV disease can influence the clinical course of any of the rheumatic diseases?

128. How would you classify the cryoglobulinaemias?

129. A patient with hepatitis C virus infection presents with purpura, weakness, arthralgia and a rising creatinine. What do you think is the most likely diagnosis? What tests would you recommend?

130. A 32-year-old woman with a history of two previous fetal losses presents to casualty with a low platelet count and a reticular rash. What is the most likely diagnosis? What tests would you perform and how would you interpret them? Are there any treatments which have been shown to reduce fetal loss?

131. A 54-year-old female presents to you with classic features of rheumatoid arthritis – she is particularly concerned about her prognosis. What prognostic markers do you know and how could you advise the patient?

132. What do you understand by oestrogen receptor modulators (SERM) and do you think they might be clinically useful?

133. What is the WHO classification of osteoporosis?

DERMATOLOGY

134. Can you describe the dermatological manifestations of diabetes mellitus?

135. What do you understand by the term Koebnerization and which skin conditions manifest this phenomenon?

136. The presence of which dermatological conditions could raise the suspicion of HIV infection?

137. How would you go about investigating and managing an erythrodermic patient? If you suspect drugs as a cause, which would be the most likely culprits?

138. Can you describe the process of sentinel node biopsy and how it is applicable to the management of a patient with malignant melanoma?

139. A young patient presents to your clinic concerned about the number of cutaneous naevi that she has. She mentions that other family members have numerous naevi and that one of her grandparents may have had a melanoma. What features would you look for if considering the diagnosis of atypical mole syndrome, and what advice would you give her regarding the possibility of developing malignant melanoma?

140. What cutaneous features could be found in a patient with sarcoidosis?

141. A patient with generalized pruritus also describes weight loss: which systemic conditions might you consider?

142. When faced with a patient with leg ulceration, how would you go about excluding non-venous causes of ulceration?

143. A 23-year-old woman presents with occasional bouts of diarrhoea , a general feeling of tiredness and crops of intensely itchy blisters over the scalp and buttocks. Which diagnoses would you consider and how would you investigate this patient?

144. Which parts of the hair cycle do anagen, catagen and telogen describe? Which class of drugs are a common cause of acute anagen hair loss?

145. You are confronted with a woman who has severe psoriasis; she warrants systemic therapy. What are your considerations for treatment?

References

BASIC SCIENCE, IMMUNOLOGY AND GENETICS

Adams DH, Lloyd AR 1997 Chemokines: leucocyte recruitment and activation cytokines, Lancet 349: 490–495

Allen KM, Walsh C 1996 Shaking down new epilepsy genes. Nature Medicine 2: 516–518

Ambrus J L, Sridhar N R 1997 Immunological aspects of renal disease. Journal of the American Medical Association 278: 1938–1945

Anon. 1996 Malnourished inpatients: overlooked and undertreated. Drug and Therapeutics Bulletin 34: 57–59

Auwerx J, Staels B 1998 Leptin. Lancet 351: 737–742

Baggiolini M 1998 Chemokines and leucocyte traffic. Nature 392: 565–568

Boulet LP, Chapman KR, Cole J et al. 1997 Inhibitory effects of an anti-IgE antibody E25 on allergen-induced early asthmatic response. American Journal of Respiratory and Critical Care Medicine 155: 1835–1840

Bousquet J, Michel FB 1994 Specific immunotherapy in asthma; is it effective? Journal of Allergy and Clinical Immunology 94: 1–11

Brice A 1998 Unstable mutations and neurodegenerative disorders. Journal of Neurology 245: 505–510

Burke W, Thomson E, Khoury et al. 1998 Hereditary haemochromatosis. Gene discovery and its implications for population based screening. Journal of the American Medical Association 280: 172–178

Cairns JS, D'Souza MP 1998 Chemokines and HIV-1 second receptors: the therapeutic connection. Nature Medicine 4: 563–568

Cambridge G 1998 Anti-neutrophil cytoplasmic antibodies. Arthritis and Rheumatism Council Topical Reviews series 3, no.13

Dudley J, Kai-Lik So A 1998 T cells and related cytokines. Current Opinion in Rheumatology 10: 207–211

Fahy JV, Fleming HE, Wong HH et al. 1997 The effect of an anti-IgE monoclonal antibody on the early and late phase responses to allergen inhalation in asthmatic subjects. American Journal of Respiratory and Critical Care Medicine 155: 1828–1834

Feder JN, Gnirke A, Thomas W et al. 1996 A novel MHC class 1–like gene is mutated in patients with hereditary haemochromatosis. Nature Genetics 13: 399–408

Garred P 1998 Chemokine-receptor polymorphisms: clarity or confusion for HIV-1 prognosis? Lancet 351: 2–3

Hardy J, Gwinn-Hardy K 1998 Genetic classification of primary neurodegenerative disease. Science 282: 1075–1079

Hoffman GS, Specks U 1998 Antineutrophil cytoplasmic antibodies. Arthritis and Rheumatism 41: 1521–1537

Johns DR 1996 The other human genome: mitochondrial DNA and disease. Nature Medicine 2(10): 1065–1068

Jordan E, Collins FS 1996 A march of genetic maps. Nature 380: 111–112

Keverne EB 1997 Genomic imprinting in the brain. Current Opinion in Neurobiology 7: 463–468

Kinloch RA, Treherne JM, Furness LM, Hajimohamadreza I 1999 The pharmacology of apoptosis. Trends in Pharmacological Sciences 20: 35–42

Lemon SM, Thomas DL 1997 Vaccines to prevent viral hepatitis. New England Journal of Medicine 336: 196–204

Li TS, Tubiana R, Karlama C, Calvez V, Ait Mohand H, Autran B 1998 Long-lasting recovery in CD4 T-cell function and viral-load reduction after highly active antiretroviral therapy in advanced HIV-1 disease. Lancet 351: 1682–1686

Lo JC, Mulligan K, Tai VW, Algren H, Schambelan M 1998 'Buffalo hump' in men with HIV-1 infection. Lancet 351: 867–870

Loveday C, Devereux H 1998 Clinical implications of antiretroviral drug resistance. Journal of HIV Therapy.3: 48–54

Luster AD 1998 Chemokines – chemotactic cytokines that mediate inflammation. New England Journal of Medicine 338: 436–445

Male D, Cooke A, Owen M, Trowsdale J, Champion B 1996 Advanced Immunology 3rd edn. Times Mirror International Publishers Ltd. London

Martinelli I, Sacchi E, Landi G et al. 1998 High risk of cerebral vein thrombosis in carriers of a prothrombin-gene mutation and in users of oral contraceptives. New England Journal of Medicine 338: 1793–1797

Miossec P, Van den Berg W 1997 Th1/Th2 cytokine balance in arthritis. Arthritis and Rheumatism 40: 2105–2115

Miller KD, Jones E, Yanovski JA, Shankar R, Feuerstein I, Fallon J 1998 Visceral abdominal-fat accumulation associated with the use of indinavir. Lancet 351: 871–875

Mosman TR, Sad S 1996 The expanding universe of T cell subsets: Th1,Th2 and more. Immunology Today 17: 138–146

Muraille E, Leo O 1998 Revisiting the Th1/Th2 paradigm. Scandinavian Journal of Immunology 47: 1–9

Mutsaers SE, Foster ML, Chambers RC, Laurent GJ, McAnulty RJ 1998 Increased endothelin-1 and Its localization during the development of bleomycin-induced pulmonary fibrosis in rats. American Journal of Respiratory Cell Molecular Biology 18: 611–619

Ophoff RA, Terwindt GM, Vergouwe MN et al. 1996 Familial hemiplegic migraine and episodic ataxia type-2 are caused by mutations in the Calcium channel gene CACNL1N4. Cell 87: 543–552

Ormerod MG 1994 Flow cytometry. BIOS Scientific Publishers, Oxford

Paulson HL, Fischbeck KH 1996 Trinucleotide repeats in neurodegenerative disorders. Annual Reviews in Neuroscience 19: 79–107

Payne-James JJ 1995 Enteral nutrition. European Journal of Gastroenterology and Hepatology 7: 501–506

Poort SR, Rosenthal FR, Reitsma PH et al. 1996 A common genetic variant in the 3'-untranslated region of the prothrombin gene is associated with elevated prothrombin levels and an increase in venous thrombosis. Blood 88: 3698–3707

Powderly WG, Landay A, Lederman MM 1998 Recovery of the immune system with antiretroviral therapy. The end of opportunism? Journal of the American Medical Association 280: 72–77

Roquet A, Dahlen B, Kumlin M et al. 1997 Combined antagonism of leukotrienes and histamine produces predominant inhibition of allergen induced early and late airway obstruction in asthmatics. American Journal of Respiratory and Critical Care Medicine 155: 1856–1863

Rosenberg SA 1997 Cancer vaccines based on the identification of genes encoding cancer regression antigens. Immunology Today 18: 175–182

Schrager LK, D'Souza PD 1998 Cellular and anatomical reservoirs of HIV-1 in patients receiving potent antiretroviral combination therapy. Journal of the American Medical Association 280: 67–71

Secrist H, Chelen CJ, Wen Y, Marshall JD, Umetsu DT 1993 Allergen immunotherapy decreases interleukin-4 production in CD4+ T cells from allergic individuals. Journal of Experimental Medicine 178: 2123–2130

Silk D 1995 Nutrition for gastroenterologists: when, how and for how long? European Journal of Gastroenterology and Hepatology 7: 491–500

Steinlein OK et al. 1995 A missense mutation in the neuronal nicotinic acetylcholine receptor alpha4 subunit is associated with autosomal dominant nocturnal frontal lobe epilepsy. Nature Genetics 11: 201–203

Vandenbroucke JP 1998 Cerebral sinus thrombosis and oral contraceptives. British Medical Journal 317: 483–484

WHO/IUIS Working Group Report 1989 The current status of allergen immunotherapy (hyposensitisation). Allergy 44: 369–379

PHARMACOLOGY AND DRUG DEVELOPMENT

Arlett P, Hooker M, Lee E, Darbyshire J, Breckenridge A 1997 Reporting adverse drug reactions in HIV infection. Genitourinary Medicine 73: 335

Bailey DG, Malcolm J, Arnold O, Spence J D 1998 Grapefruit–drug interactions. British Journal of Clinical Pharmacology 46: 101–110

Barker DJP, Rose G 1990 Epidemiology in medical practice. 4th edn. Churchill Livingstone, Edinburgh

Bates DW 1998 Drugs and adverse drug reactions – how worried should we be? Journal of the American Medical Association 279: 1216–1217

Cairns JS, D'Souza MP 1998 Chemokines and HIV-1 second receptors: the therapeutic connection. Nature Medicine 4: 563–568

Coggon D 1995 Statistics in clinical practice. BMJ Publishing, London

Harman RJ 1999 The drug development process – introduction and overview. Pharmaceutical Journal 262: 334–337

Henry K, Melroe H, Huebsch J et al. 1998 Severe premature coronary artery disease with protease inhibitors. Lancet 351: 1328

Kelton JG, Warkentin TE 1998 Heparin-induced thrombocytopenia: an overview of the diagnosis, natural history and treatment options. Postgraduate Medicine 103: 169–171, 175–178

Lazarou J, Pomeranz BH, Corey PN 1998 Incidence of adverse drug reactions in hospitalised patients; a meta-analysis of prospective studies. Journal of the American Medical Association 279: 1200–1205

Naylor CD 1997 Meta-analysis and the meta-epidemiology of clinical research. British Medical Journal 315: 617–619

Routledge P 1998 150 years of pharmacovigilance. Lancet 351: 1200–1201

Shenfield G, Gross A 1999 The cytochrome P450 system and adverse drug reactions. Adverse Drug Reaction Bulletin 194: 739–742

Styrt BA, Piazza-Hepp TD, Chikami GK 1996 Clinical Toxicity of antiretroviral nucleoside analogs. Antiviral Research. 31: 121–135

Tanaka E 1998 Clinically important pharmacokinetic drug–drug interactions: role of cytochrome P450 enzymes. Journal of Clinical Pharmacy and Therapeutics 23: 403–416

THERAPEUTICS

Adachi JD, Benson WA, Brown J et al. 1997 Intermittent cyclical etidronate therapy in the prevention and treatment of corticosteroid induced osteoporosis. New England Journal of Medicine 337: 382–387

American College of Rheumatology Task Force on Osteoporosis Guidelines. 1996 Recommendations for the prevention and treatment of glucocorticoid induced osteoporosis. Arthritis and Rheumatism 39: 1791–1801

Angulo P, Batts KP, Therneau TM, Jorgensen RA, Dickson ER, Lindor KD 1999 Long-term ursodeoxycholic acid delays histological progression in primary biliary cirrhosis. Hepatology 29: 644–647

Anon 1996. Stopping status epilepticus. Drug and Therapeutics Bulletin 34 (10): 73–75

Anon 1997 Donepezil for Alzheimer's disease? Drug and Therapeutics Bulletin 35 (10): 75–76

Anon 1997 Paclitaxel and docetaxel in breast and ovarian cancer. Drug and Therapeutics Bulletin 35: 43–46

Anon 1998 Management of unstable angina. Drug and Therapeutics Bulletin 36(5): 36–39

Anon 1998 Managing migraine. Drug and Therapeutics Bulletin 36: 41–44

Anon 1998 Donepezil update. Drug and Therapeutics Bulletin 36 (8): 60–61

Anon 1998 Sildenafil for erectile dysfunction. Drug and Therapeutics Bulletin 36: 81–84

Anon 1998 Reboxetine – another new antidepressant. Drug and Therapeutics Bulletin 36 (11): 86–88

Anon 1999 Mirtazapine – another new class of antidepressant. Drug and Therapeutics Bulletin 37 (1): 1–3

Anon 1999 Ursodeoxycholic acid for primary biliary cirrhosis. Drug and Therapeutics Bulletin 37: 30–32

Berenson JR, Lichtenstein A, Porter L et al. 1996 Efficacy of pamidronate in reducing the skeletal events in patients with advanced multiple myeloma. New England Journal of Medicine 334: 488–493

Bonn D 1997 Getting to the heart of the long QT syndrome. Lancet 349: 408

Bone RC 1996 Why sepsis trials fail. Journal of the American Medical Association 276: 565–566

Canalis E 1996 Mechanisms of glucocorticoid action in bone: implications for glucocorticoid induced osteoporosis. Journal of Endocrinology and Metabolism 81: 3441–3447

Cave A, Arlett P, Lee E 1999 An assessment of the potential for inhaled and nasal corticosteroids to cause systemic adverse effects. Pharmacology and Therapeutics 83: 153–179

Charache S, Terrin ML, Moore RD et al. 1995 Effect of hydroxyurea on the frequency of painful crises in sickle cell anaemia. New England Journal of Medicine 332: 1317–1332

Connolly HM, Crary JL, McGoon MD et al. 1997 Valvular heart disease associated with fenfluramine-phentermine. New England Journal of Medicine 337: 581–588

Cumming RG, Mitchell P, Leeder SR 1997 Use of inhaled corticosteroids and the risk of cataracts. New England Journal of Medicine 337: 8–14

Cunningham D, Pyrhonen S, James RD et al. 1998 Randomised trial of irinotecan plus supportive care versus supportive care alone after fluorouracil failure for patients with metastatic colorectal cancer. Lancet 352: 1413–1418

Delmas PD, Bjarnason NH, Mitlak BH et al. 1997 Effects of raloxifene on bone mineral density, serum cholesterol concentrations, and uterine endometrium in postmenopausal women. New England Journal of Medicine 337: 1641–1647

Devita VT, Hellman S, Rosenberg SA 1997 Cancer, principles and practice of oncology. 5th edn. Lippincott-Raven, Philadelphia

Drazen JM, Israel E, O'Byrne PM 1999 Treatment of asthma with drugs modifying the leukotriene pathway New England Journal of Medicine 340: 197–206

Ernst A, Zibrak JD 1998 Carbon monoxide poisoning. New England Journal of Medicine 339: 1603–1608

Farthing MJG 1996 The role of somatostatin analogues in the treatment of refractory diarrhoea. Digestive Diseases. 57 (Suppl 1): 107–113

Feely M 1999 Drug treatment of epilepsy. British Medical Journal 318: 106–109

First M R 1998 Clinical Applications of immunosuppressive agents in renal transplantation. Surgical Clinics of North America 78: (1): 61–76

Flexner C 1998 HIV-Protease Inhibitors. New England Journal of Medicine 338: 1281–1292

Flicker L 1999 Acetylcholinesterase inhibitors for Alzheimer's disease. British Medical Journal 318: 615–616

Fox K 1998 The role of the antithrombins in improving outcome in unstable angina. British Journal of Cardiology 5 (2): S2–S11

Garbe E, LeLorier J, Boivin JF, Suissa S 1997 Inhaled and nasal glucocorticoids and the risk of ocular hypertension or open angle glaucoma. Journal of the American Medical Association 277: 722–727

Garg R, Gorhin R, Smith T et al. 1997 DIG (effect of digoxin on mortality and morbidity in patients with heart failure). New England Journal of Medicine 336: 525–533

Gent M, Beaumont D, Blanchard J et al. 1996 CAPRIE randomised blinded trial of clopidrogel versus aspirin in patients at risk of ischaemic events. Lancet 348: 1229–1239

Gennari J 1998 Hypokalaemia. New England Journal of Medicine 339: 451–458

Goldstein I, Lew TS, Padma-Nathan H, Rosen RC, Steers WD, Wicker PA 1998 Oral sildenafil in the treatment of erectile dysfunction. New England Journal of Medicine 338: 1397–1404

Gore S, Healey CJ, Sutton R, Eyre-Brook IA, Gear MWL, Shepherd NA, Wilkinson SP 1993 Regression of columnar lined (Barrett's) oesophagus with continuous omeprazole therapy. Alimentary Pharmacology and Therapy 7: 623–628

Hale AS 1997 Depression (ABC of mental health). British Medical Journal 315: 43–45

Hall W, Solowij N 1998 Adverse effects of cannabis. Lancet 352: 1611–1616

Halperin ML, Kamel KS 1998 Potassium. Lancet 352: 135–140

Hammer SM, Squires KE, Hughes MD for the AIDS Clinical Trials Group 320 Study Team 1997 A controlled trial of two nucleoside analogues plus indinavir in persons with human immunodeficiency virus infection and CD4 cell counts of 200 per cubic millimeter or less. New England Journal of Medicine 337: 725–733

Hawkey CJ 1999 COX-2 inhibitors. Lancet 353: 307–314

Heidreich P 1997 Effect of β blockade on mortality in heart failure (a meta-analysis). Journal of the American College of Cardiologists.30: 27–34

Inzucchi SE, Maggs DG, Spollett et al. 1998 Efficacy and metabolic effects of metformin and troglitazone in type 2 diabetes mellitus. New England Journal of Medicine 338: 867–872

Joint Council for Clinical Oncology Report 1998 The current role of paclitaxel in the first-line chemotherapy of ovarian cancer. Royal College of Physicians, London

Khan MA, Herzog CA, St Peter JV et al. 1998 The prevalence of cardiac valvular insufficiency assessed by transthoracic echocardiography in obese patients treated with appetite-suppressant drugs. New England Journal of Medicine 339: 713–718

Leach JP, Brodie MJ 1998 Tiagabine. Lancet. 351: 203–207

McLaughlin VV, Genthner DE, Panella MM, Rich S 1998 Reduction in pulmonary vascular resistance with long term epoprostenol (prostacyclin) therapy in primary pulmonary hypertension. New England Journal of Medicine 338: 273–277

Marson AG, Kadir ZA, Chadwick DW 1996 New antiepileptic drugs: a systematic review of their efficacy and tolerability. British Medical Journal 313: 1169–1173

MCA/CSM 1998 The safety of inhaled and nasal corticosteroids. Current Problems in Pharmacovigilance 24: 8

MCA/CSM 1999 In focus: Donepezil. Current Problems in Pharmacovigilance 25: 7

MCA/CSM 1999 Vigabatrin (Sabril): visual field defects. Current Problems in Pharmacovigilance 25: 13

MCA/CSM 1999 Withdrawal of tolcapone. Current Problems in Pharmacovigilance 25 (Feb): 2

Milroy CM 1999 Ten years of 'Ecstasy'. Journal of the Royal Society of Medicine 92: 68–72

Moran N 1998 Novel antiplatelet agents. British Journal of Cardiology 5(8): 413–21

Nutt JG 1998 Catechol-O-methyltransferase inhibitors for the treatment of Parkinson's disease. Lancet 351: 1221–1222

O' Bryne PM 1997 Leukotrienes in the pathogenesis of asthma. Chest 111/2 (Supp) 27S–34S

O'Callaghan C, Cant M, Robertson C 1994 Delivery of beclomethasone dipropionate from a spacer device: what dose is available for inhalation? Thorax 49: 961–964

Okudaira H 1997. Challenge studies of a leukotriene receptor antagonist. Chest 111/2 (Supp) 46S–51S

Packer M, Bristow M 1996 The effect of carvedilol on morbidity and mortality in patients with chronic heart failure. New England Journal of Medicine 334: 1349–1355

Packer M, Gheorghiade M, Young J et al. 1993 RADIANCE (withdrawal of digoxin from patients with CHF treated with ACE inhibitors). New England Journal of Medicine 329: 1–7

Pederson T, Kjekshus J, Berg K et al. 1994 Scandinavian Simvastatin Survival Study. Randomised trial of cholesterol lowering in 4444 patients with coronary heart disease. Lancet 344: 1383–1389

Pitt B, Segal R, Martinez F et al. 1997 ELITE (randomised trial of losartan vs. captopril in patients over 65 with heart failure. Lancet 349: 747–752

Reijers MHE, Weverling GJ, Jurriaans S, et al. 1998 Maintenance therapy after quadruple induction therapy in HIV-1 infected individuals: Amsterdam Duration of Antiretroviral Medication (ADAM) study. Lancet 352: 185–190

Remme W 1998 β blockade in congestive heart failure: time for consideration. Heart 79 (Supp.): 2

Rendell MS, Rajfer J, Wicker PA, Smith MD 1999 Sildenafil for treatment of erectile dysfunction in men with diabetes. Journal of the American Medical Association 281: 421–426

Rogers SL, Farlow MR, Doody RS, Mohs R, Friedhoff LT and the Donepezil Study Group 1998 A 24-week, double-blind, placebo-controlled trial of donepezil in patients with Alzheimer's disease. Neurology 50: 136–145

Rosler M, Anand R, Cicin-Sain A et al. 1999 Efficacy and safety of rivastigmine in patients with Alzheimer's disease: international, randomised controlled trial. British Medical Journal 318: 633–640

Rougier P,Van Cutsem E, Bajetta E et al. 1998 Randomised trial of irinotecan versus fluorouracil by continuous infusion after fluorouracil failure in patients with metastatic colorectal cancer. Lancet 352: 1407–1412

Sacks F, Pfeffer M, Moye L et al. 1996 CARE (effect of pravastatin on coronary events after MI in patients with average cholesterol levels). New England Journal of Medicine 335: 1001–1009

Schoenen J 1997 Acute migraine therapy: the newer drugs. Current Opinion in Neurology 10: 237–243

Simoons M, Rutsch W, Vahanian A et al. 1997 CAPTURE randomised placebo controlled trial of abciximab before and during coronary intervention during coronary intervention in refractory unstable angina. Lancet 349: 1429–1435

Singal PW, Iliskovic N 1998 Doxorubicin induced cardiomyopathy. New England Journal of Medicine 339: 900–905

Sjostrom L, Rissanen A, Andersen T et al. 1998 Randomised placebo-controlled trial of orlistat for weight loss and prevention of weight regain in obese patients. Lancet 352: 167–173

Stephen LJ, Maxwell JE, Brodie MJ 1999 Transient hemiparesis with topirimate. British Medical Journal 318: 845

Theroux P, Pelletier G, Davies R et al. 1998 PRISM PLUS Inhibition of glycoprotein IIb/IIIa receptor with unstable angina and Non-Q wave MI. New England Journal of Medicine 338: 1488–1497

Thomas SHL 1997 Drugs and the QT interval. Adverse Drug Reaction Bulletin 182: 691–694

Tibbles PM, Edelsberg JS 1996 Hyperbaric oxygen therapy. New England Journal of Medicine 334: 1642–1648

Topol E, Califf R, Simoons M et al. 1998 PURSIT Inhibition of platelet glycoprotein IIb/IIIa with eptifibrate in patients with acute coronary syndrome. New England Journal of Medicine 339: 436–443

Tran TH, Day NP, Nguyen MD et al. 1996 A controlled trial of artemether or quinine in Vietnamese adults with severe falciparum malaria. New England Journal of Medicine 335: 76–83

Urtsky B, Young J, Shahidi F et al. 1993 PROVED (randomised study assessing effect of digoxin withdrawal in patients with mild- moderate CCF). Journal of the American College of Cardiology 22: 955–962

Vandenbroucke JP 1998 Cerebral sinus thrombosis and oral contraceptives. British Medical Journal 317: 483–484

White NJ 1996 The treatment of malaria. New England Journal of Medicine 335: 800–806

White NJ, Dung NM, Vinh H, Bethell D, Hien TT 1996 Fluoroquinolones in children with multi-drug resistant typhoid. Lancet 348: 547

Woosley RL 1996 Cardiac actions of antihistamines. Annual Review of Pharmcology and Toxicology 36: 233–252

Yeomans ND, Cook GA, Giraud AS 1998 Selective COX-2 inhibitors: are they safe for the stomach? Gastroenterology 115: 227–229

NEUROLOGY

Allen KM, Walsh C 1996 Shaking down new epilepsy genes. Nature Medicine 2: 516–518

Anon 1996 Stopping status epilepticus. Drug and Therapeutics Bulletin 34 (10): 73–75

Anon 1997 Donezepil for Alzheimer's disease? Drug and Therapeutics Bulletin 35 (10): 75–76

Anon 1998 Managing migraine. Drug and Therapeutics Bulletin 36: 41–44

Anon 1998 Donezepil update. Drug and Therapeutics Bulletin 36 (8): 60–61

Anon 1998 Reboxetine – another new antidepressant. Drug and Therapeutics Bulletin 36 (11): 86–88

Anon 1999 Mirtazapine – another new class of antidepressant. Drug and Therapeutics Bulletin 37 (1): 1–3

Boulton AJ 1998 Guidelines for diagnosis and outpatient management of diabetic peripheral neuropathy. European Association for the Study of Diabetes, Neurodiabetes Diabetes Metabolism 94 (3): 55–65

Brice A 1998 Unstable mutations and neurodegenerative disorders. Journal of Neurology. 245 (8): 505–510

Delanty N, Vaughan CJ, French JA 1998 Medical causes of seizures (seminar). Lancet 352: 383–390

Feely M 1999 Drug treatment of epilepsy. British Medical Journal 318: 106–109

Ferrari MD 1998 Migraine. Lancet 351: 1043–1051

Flicker L 1999 Acetylcholinesterase inhibitors for Alzheimer's disease. British Medical Journal 318: 615–616

Goadsby PJ 1997 Bench to bedside: what have we learnt recently about headache? Current Opinion in Neurology 10: 215–220

Golbe LI 1998 Pallidotomy for Parkinson's disease: hitting the target? Lancet 351: 998–999

Hale AS 1997 Depression (ABC of mental health). British Medical Journal 315: 43–45

Hardy J, Gwinn-Hardy K 1998 Genetic classification of primary neurodegenerative disease. Science 282: 1075–1079

Headache Classification Committee of the International Headache Society 1988 Classification and diagnostic criteria for headache disorders, cranial neuralgias and facial pain. Cephalgia 8 (Suppl 7): 1–96

Hughes RAC 1994 Neurological emergencies. BMJ Publishing, London

Hussain M, Brooks DJ 1999 Case Report: ataxia and ophthalmoplegia. CPD Bulletin Neurology 1: 25–27

Keverne EB 1997 Genomic imprinting in the brain. Current Opinion in Neurobiology 7: 463–468

Leach JP, Brodie MJ 1998 Tiagabine. Lancet. 351: 203–207

Lindvall O 1999 Cerebral implantation in movement disorders: state of the art movement disorders. 14 (2): 201–205

Lowenstein DH, Alldredge BK 1998 Status Epilepticus [review]. New England Journal of Medicine 338: 970–978

Markus HS, Hambley H 1998 Neurology and the blood: haematological abnormalities in ischaemic stroke. Journal of Neurology, Neurosurgery and Psychiatry 64: 150–159

Marson AG, Kadir ZA, Chadwick DW 1996 New antiepileptic drugs: a systematic review of their efficacy and tolerability. British Medical Journal 313: 1169–1173

Martinelli I, Sacchi E, Landi G et al. 1998 High risk of cerebral vein thrombosis in carriers of a prothrombin-gene mutation and in users of oral contraceptives. New England Journal of Medicine 338: 1793–1797

MCA/CSM 1999 Vigabatrin (Sabril): visual field defects. Current Problems in Pharmacovigilance 25: 13

MCA/CSM 1999 Withdrawal of tolcapone. Current Problems in Pharmacovigilance 25 (Feb): 2

MCA/CSM 1999 In focus: Donepezil. Current Problems in Pharmacovigilance 25: 7

Nutt JG 1998 Catechol-O-methyltransferase inhibitors for the treatment of Parkinson's disease. Lancet 351: 1221–1222

Ophoff RA, Terwindt GM, Vergouwe MN et al. 1996 Familial hemiplegic migraine and episodic ataxia type-2 are caused by mutations in the calcium channel gene CACNL1N4. Cell 87: 543–552

Paulson HL, Fischbeck KH 1996 Trinucleotide repeats in neurodegenerative disorders. Annual Reviews in Neuroscience 19: 79–107

Quinn N, Bhatia K 1998 Functional neurosurgery for Parkinson's disease. British Medical Journal 316: 1259–1260

Rogers SL. Farlow MR, Doody RS, Mohs R, Friedhoff LT and the Donepezil Study Group 1998 A 24-week, double-blind, placebo-controlled trial of donepezil in patients with Alzheimer's disease. Neurology 50: 136–145

Rosler M, Anand R, Cicin-Sain A et al. 1999 Efficacy and safety of rivastigmine in patients with Alzheimer's disease: international, randomised controlled trial. British Medical Journal 318: 633–640

Schapira AHV 1999 Science, medicine and the future: Parkinson's disease. British Medical Journal 318: 311–314

Schoenen J 1997 Acute migraine therapy: the newer drugs. Current Opinion in Neurology 10: 237–243

Steinlein OK et al. 1995 A missense mutation in the neuronal nicotinic acetylcholine receptor alpha4 subunit is associated with autosomal dominant nocturnal frontal lobe epilepsy. Nature Genetics 11: 201–203

Stephen LJ, Maxwell JE, Brodie MJ 1999 Transient hemiparesis with topirimate. British Medical Journal 318: 845

Thomas PK 1997 Clinical features and investigation of diabetic somatic peripheral neuropathy. Clinical Neuroscience 4 (6): 341–345

Warlow C 1991 Handbook of neurology. Blackwell Scientific publications, Oxford

Younger DS, Rosoklija G, Hays AP 1998 Diabetic peripheral neuropathy. Seminars in Neurology. 18 (1): 95–104

Zvulunov A, Esterly N 1995 Neurocutaneous syndromes associated with pigmentary skin lesions. Journal of the American Academy of Dermatology 32: 915–935

RESPIRATORY MEDICINE

Ayres JG, Miles JF, Barnes PJ 1998 Brittle asthma. Thorax. 53: 315–321

Boulet LP, Chapman KR, Cole J et al. 1997 Inhibitory effects of an anti-IgE antibody E25 on allergen-induced early asthmatic response. American Journal of Respiratory and Critical Care Medicine 155: 1835–1840

Bousquet J, Michel FB 1994 Specific immunotherapy in asthma; is it effective? Journal of Allergy and Clinical Immunology 94: 1–11

Benditt JO, Albert RK 1997 Surgical options for patients with advanced emphysema. Clinics in Chest Medicine 18: 577–593

Bisgaard H, Dolovich M 1997 Nebulizer technology: the way forward. European Respiratory Review 7: 378–392

Brantigan OC, Mueller E 1957 Surgical treatment of pulmonary emphysema. American Surgeon 23: 789

Cave A, Arlett P, Lee E 1999 An assessment of the potential for inhaled and nasal corticosteroids to cause systemic adverse effects. Pharmacology and Therapeutics 83: 153–179

Cooper JD, Trulock EP, Triantafillou AN et al. 1995 Bilateral pneumectomy (volume reduction) for chronic obstructive pulmonary diseases. Journal of Thoracic and Cardiovascular Surgery 109: 106

Cumming RG, Mitchell P, Leeder SR 1997 Use of inhaled corticosteroids and the risk of cataracts. New England Journal of Medicine 337: 8–14

Drazen JM, Israel E, O'Byrne PM 1999 Treatment of asthma with drugs modifying the leukotriene pathway. New England Journal of Medicine 340: 197–206

Egan JJ, Stewart JP, Hasleton PS, Arrand JR, Carroll KB, Woodcock AA 1995 Epstein–Barr virus replication within pulmonary epithelial cells in cryptogenic fibrosing alveolitis. Thorax 50: 1234–1239

Fahy JV, Fleming HE, Wong HH et al. 1997 The effect of an anti-IgE monoclonal antibody on the early and late phase responses to allergen inhalation in asthmatic subjects. American Journal of Respiratory and Critical Care Medicine 155: 1828–1834

Garbe E, LeLorier J, Boivin JF, Suissa S 1997 Inhaled and nasal glucocorticoids and the risk of ocular hypertension or open angle glaucoma. Journal of the American Medical Association 277: 722–727

Haworth SG 1998 Primary pulmonary hypertension. Journal of the Royal College of Physicians of London. 32: 187–190

Herve P, Launay JM, Scrobohaci ML et al. 1995 Increased plasma serotonin in primary pulmonary hypertension. American Journal of Medicine 99: 249–254

Hosenpud JD, Bennett LE, Keck BM et al. 1998 Effect of diagnosis on survival benefit of lung transplantation for end-stage lung disease. Lancet 351: 24

Hubbard R, Johnston I, Britton J 1997 Survival in patients with cryptogenic fibrosing alveolitis. Chest 113: 396–400

Hutchison DC, Hughes MD 1997 Alpha-1-antitrypsin replacement therapy: will its efficacy ever be proved? European Respiratory Journal 10: 2191–2193

Keenan RJ, Landreneau FJ, Sciurba FC et al. 1996 Unilateral thoracoscopic surgical approach for diffuse emphysema. Journal of Thoracic and Cardiovascular Surgery 111: 308

Levine SM, Bryan CL 1995 Bronchiolitis obliterans in lung transplant recipients: the "thorn in the side" of lung transplantation. Chest 107: 894

Macbeth F 1996 Radiotherapy in the treatment of lung cancer. British Journal of Hospital Medicine 55: 639–642

McLaughlin VV, Genthner DE, Panella MM, Rich S 1998 Reduction in pulmonary vascular resistance with long term epoprostenol (prostacyclin) therapy in primary pulmonary hypertension. New England Journal of Medicine 338: 273–277

MCA/CSM 1998 The safety of inhaled and nasal corticosteroids. Current Problems in Pharmacovigilance 24: 8

Mutsaers SE, Foster ML, Chambers RC, Laurent GJ, McAnulty RJ 1998 Increased endothelin-1 and Its localization during the development of bleomycin-induced pulmonary fibrosis in rats. American Journal of Respiratory Cell Molecular Biology 18: 611–619

Non Small Cell Lung Cancer Collaborative Group 1995 Chemotherapy in non small cell lung cancer: a meta-analysis using updated data on individual patients from 52 randomised clinical trials. British Medical Journal 311: 899–909

O' Byrne PM 1997 Leukotrienes in the pathogenesis of asthma. Chest 111/2 (Supp): 27S–34S

O'Callaghan C, Cant M, Robertson C 1994 Delivery of beclomethasone dipropionate from a spacer device: what dose is available for inhalation? Thorax 49: 961–964

O'Driscoll BRC, Ruffles SP, Ayres JG, Cochrane GM 1988 Long term treatment of severe asthma with subcutaneous terbutaline. British Journal of Diseases of the Chest 82: 360–365

Okudaira H 1997 Challenge studies of a leukotriene receptor antagonist. Chest 111/2 (Supp): 46S–51S

PORT Meta-analysis Trialists Group 1998 Postoperative radiotherapy in non-small cell lung cancer: systematic review and meta-analysis of individual patient data from nine randomised controlled trials. Lancet 352: 257–263

Rich S, Dantzker DR, Ayres SM 1987 Primary pulmonary hypertension; a national retrospective study. Annals of Internal Medicine 107: 216–223

Roquet A, Dahlen B, Kumlin M et al. 1997 Combined antagonism of leukotrienes and histamine produces predominant inhibition of allergen induced early and late airway obstruction in asthmatics. American Journal of Respiratory and Critical Care Medicine 155: 1856–1863

Saunders M, Dische S, Barrett A et al. 1997 Continuous hyperfractionated radiotherapy (CHART) versus conventional radiotherapy in non small cell lung cancer: a multicentre randomised trial. Lancet 350: 161–165

Seersholm N, Wencker M, Banik N et al. 1997 Does alpha1-antitrypsin augmentation therapy slow the annual decline in FEV in patients with severe hereditary alpha1-antitrypsin deficiency? European Respiratory Journal 10: 2260–2263

Trulock EP 1997 Lung transplantation. American Journal of Respiratory and Critical Care Medicine 155: 789

Wehner JH, Kirsch CM 1997 Pulmonary manifestations of strongyloides Seminars in Respiratory Infections 12: 122–129

ENDOCRINOLOGY

Al Zahrani A, Levine MA 1997 Primary hyperparathyroidism. Lancet 349: 1233–1238

Caplin ME, Buscombe JR, Hilson AJ, Jones AL, Watkinson AF, Burroughs AK 1998 Carcinoid tumour. Lancet 352: 799–805

Cleland SJ, Connell JMC 1998 Endocrine hypertension. Journal of the Royal College of Physicians of London 32: 104–108

Diabetes Control and Complication Trial Research Group 1993 The effect of intensive treatment of diabetes on the development and progression of long-term complications in insulin-dependent diabetes mellitus. New England Journal of Medicine 329 (14): 977–986

Dunaif A 1997 Insulin resistance and the polycystic ovary syndrome: mechanism and implications for pathogenesis. Endocrine Reviews 18: 774–800

Eng C, Clayton D, Schuffenecker I et al. 1996 The relationship between specific RET proto-oncogene mutations and disease phenotype in multiple endocrine neoplasia type 2 Journal of the American Medical Association 276: 1575–1579

Expert Committee on the Diagnosis and Classification of Diabetes Mellitus Report 1998 Diabetes Care. 21: S5– S19

Franks S 1995 Polycystic ovary syndrome. New England Journal of Medicine 333: 853–861

Ganguly A 1998 Primary aldosteronism. New England Journal of Medicine 339: 1828–1834

Halford S, Waxman J 1998 The management of carcinoid tumours. Quarterly Journal of Medicine 91: 795–798

Inzucchi SE, Maggs DG, Spollett et al. 1998 Efficacy and metabolic effects of metformin and troglitazone in type 2 diabetes mellitus. New England Journal of Medicine 338: 867–872

Labram EK, Wilkin TJ 1995 Growth hormone deficiency in adults and its response to growth hormone replacement. Quarterly Journal of Medicine 88: 391–399

Lazarus JH 1997 Hyperthyroidism. Lancet 349: 339–343

Lindsay RS, Toft AD 1997 Hypothyroidism. Lancet 349: 413–417

MacDougall IC, Isles CG, Stewart H, Inglis GC 1998 Overnight clonidine suppression tests in the diagnosis and exclusion of phaeochromocytoma. American Journal of Medicine 84: 993–1000

Malmberg K 1997 Prospective randomised study of intensive insulin treatment on long term survival after acute myocardial infarction in patients with diabetes mellitus DIGAMI Study Group. British Medical Journal 314: 1512–1515

Monson JP 1998 Adult growth hormone deficiency. Journal of the Royal College of Physicians of London 32: 19–22

Rittmaster RS 1997 Hirsutism. Lancet 349: 191–195

Ross EJ, Griffith DNW 1989 The clinical presentation of phaeochromocytoma. Quarterly Journal of Medicine. 71: 485–496.

Schlumberger MJ 1998 Papillary and follicular thyroid carcinoma. New England Journal of Medicine 338: 297–306

Thakker R V 1997 Multiple endocrine neoplasia medicine 25: 86–88

Thomas PK 1997 Clinical features and investigation of diabetic somatic peripheral neuropathy. Clinical Neuroscience 4 (6): 341–345

Tweed MJ, Roland JM 1998 Haemochromatosis as an endocrine cause of subfertility. British Medical Journal 316: 915–916

UK Prospective Diabetes Study Group 1998 Efficacy of atenolol and captopril in reducing risk of macrovascular and microvascular complications in type 2 diabetes. British Medical Journal 317: 13–20

UK Prospective Diabetes Study Group 1998 Tight blood pressure control and risk of macrovascular and microvascular complications in type 2 diabetes. British Medical Journal 317: 703–713

Vanderpump PM, Ahlquist JAO, Franklyn JA, Clayton RN 1996 Consensus statement for good practice and audit measures in the management of hypothyroidism and hyperthyroidism. British Medical Journal 313: 539–544

Younger DS, Rosoklija G, Hays AP 1998 Diabetic peripheral neuropathy. Seminars in Neurology. 18 (1): 95–104

CARDIOLOGY

Adgey A 1998 Approaches to modern management of cardiac arrest. Heart 80: 397–414

Anon 1996 Malnourished inpatients: overlooked and undertreated. Drug and Therapeutics Bulletin 34: 57–59

Anon 1998 Management of unstable angina. Drug and Therapeutics Bulletin 36(5): 36–39

Assmann G 1996 Hypertrigliceridaemia and elevated lipoprotein(a) are risk factors for major coronary events. American Journal of Cardiology 77: 1179–1184

Assmann G, Cullen P, Schulte H et al. 1998 The Munster heart study. PROCAM. European Heart Journal 19 (Supp A): A2–11

Bonn D 1997 Getting to the heart of the long QT syndrome. Lancet 349: 408

Bowers T, O'Neill WW, Grines C et al. 1998 Effect of reperfusion on biventricular function and survival after right ventricular infarction. New England Journal of Medicine 338: 933–940

Cohen M, Demers M, Gerfinkel M et al. 1997 ESSENCE study group. New England Journal of Medicine 337: 447–452

Connolly HM, Crary JL, McGoon MD et al. 1997 Valvular heart disease associated with fenfluramine-phentermine. New England Journal of Medicine 337: 581–588

Dell'Italia L 1998 Reperfusion for right ventricular infarction. New England Journal of Medicine 338: 978–980

European Resuscitation Council 1998 Guidelines for adult advanced life support. Resuscitation 37(2): 81–90

Fontaine G 1998 Arrhythmogenic right ventricular cardiomyopathies. Circulation 97: 1532–1535

Fox K 1998 The role of the antithrombins in improving outcome in unstable angina. British Journal of Cardiology 5 (2): S2–S11

Garg R, Gorhin R, Smith T et al. 1997 DIG (effect of digoxin on mortality and morbidity in patients with heart failure). New England Journal of Medicine 336: 525–533

Gent M, Beaumont D, Blanchard J et al. 1996 CAPRIE randomised blinded trial of clopidrogel versus aspirin in patients at risk of ischaemic events. Lancet 348: 1229–1239

Heidreich P 1997 Effect of β blockade on mortality in heart failure (a meta-analysis). Journal of the American College of Cardiologists.30: 27–34

Khan MA, Herzog CA, St Peter JV et al. 1998 The prevalence of cardiac valvular insufficiency assessed by transthoracic echocardiography in obese patients treated with appetite-suppressant drugs. New England Journal of Medicine 339: 713–718

McKenna W 1994 Diagnosis of arrhythmogenic right ventricular dysplasia/cardiomyopathy. British Heart Journal 71: 215–219

Malmberg K 1997 Prospective randomised study of intensive insulin treatment on long term survival after acute myocardial infarction in patients with diabetes mellitus DIGAMI Study Group. British Medical Journal 314: 1512–1515

Mayet J, Foale R A 1998 Diastolic dysfunction. Cardiology News 1(3): 6–10

Moran N 1998 Novel antiplatelet agents. British Journal of Cardiology 5(8): 413–21

Nygard O, Nordrehaug JE, Refsum H et al. 1997 Plasma homocysteine levels and mortality in patients with coronary artery disease. New England Journal of Medicine 337: 230–236

Packard C 1998 End of triglicerides in cardiovascular risk assessment? British Medical Journal 7158: 553–554

Packer M, Bristow M 1996 The effect of carvedilol on morbidity and mortality in patients with chronic heart failure. New England Journal of Medicine 334: 1349–1355

Packer M, Gheorghiade M, Young J et al. 1993 RADIANCE (withdrawal of digoxin from patients with CHF treated with ACE inhibitors). New England Journal of Medicine 329: 1–7

Pederson T, Kjekshus J, Berg K et al. 1994 Scandinavian Simvastatin Survival Study. Randomised trial of cholesterol lowering in 4444 patients with coronary heart disease. Lancet 344: 1383–1389

Pitt B, Segal R, Martinez F et al. 1997 ELITE (randomised trial of losartan vs. captopril in patients over 65 with heart failure). Lancet 349: 747–752

Remme W 1998 β blockade in congestive heart failure: time for consideration. Heart 79 (Supp.): 2

Sacks F, Pfeffer M, Moye L et al. 1996 CARE (effect of pravastatin on coronary events after MI in patients with average cholesterol levels). New England Journal of Medicine 335: 1001–1009

Shepard J, Cobbe S M, Ford I et al. (for the West of Scotland Coronary Prevention Study) 1995 Prevention of coronary heart disease with pravastatin in men with hypercholesterolaemia. New England Journal of Medicine 333: 1301–1307

Simoons M, Rutsch W, Vahanian A et al. 1997 CAPTURE randomised placebo controlled trial of abciximab before and during coronary intervention during coronary intervention in refractory unstable angina. Lancet 349: 1429–1435

Struthers A 1998 Angiotensin II receptor antagonists for heart failure. Heart 80: 5–6

Theroux P, Pelletier G, Davies R et al. 1998 PRISM PLUS Inhibition of glycoprotein IIb/IIIa receptor with unstable angina and Non-Q wave MI. New England Journal of Medicine 338: 1488–1497

Thomas S H L 1997 Drugs and the QT interval. Adverse Drug Reaction Bulletin 182: 691–694

Topol E, Califf R, Simoons M et al. 1998 PURSIT Inhibition of platelet glycoprotein IIb/IIIa with eptifibrate in patients with acute coronary syndrome. New England Journal of Medicine 339: 436–443

Topol E, Lincoff A, Califf R et al. 1998 EPISTENT randomised placebo control and balloon PTCA trial to assess safety of coronary stenting with GP IIb/IIIa blockade. Lancet 352: 87–92

Toss H, Lindahl B, Wallentin L et al. 1996 FRISC Study group. Lancet 347: 561–568

Urtsky B, Young J, Shahidi F et al. 1993 PROVED (randomised study assessing effect of digoxin withdrawal in patients with mild– moderate CCF). Journal of the American College of Cardiology 22: 955–962

Vos J, de Feyter P, Kingma J et al. 1997 Evolution of coronary atherosclerosis in patients with mild coronary artery disease studied by serial quantitative coronary angiography at 2 and 4 year follow up. The multicenter anti-atheroma study MAAS. European Heart Journal 18(7): 1081–1089

Wheeldon N, Clarkson P 1994 Diastolic heart failure. European Heart Journal 15: 1689–1697

Woosley RL 1996 Cardiac actions of antihistamines. Annual Review of Pharmcology and Toxicology 36: 233–252

Zipes D, Wyse D, Friedman P et al. 1997 AVID The antiarrhythmics versus implantable defibrillators investigators. New England Journal of Medicine 337: 1576–1583

GASTROENTEROLOGY

Adams PC, Deugnier Y, Moirand R, Brissot P 1997 The relationship between iron overload, clinical symptoms and age in 410 patients with hemochromatosis. Hepatology 25: 162–166

Angulo P, Batts KP, Therneau TM, Jorgensen RA, Dickson ER, Lindor KD 1999 Long-term ursodeoxycholic acid delays histological progression in primary biliary cirrhosis. Hepatology 29: 644–647

Anon 1996 Malnourished inpatients: overlooked and undertreated. Drug and Therapeutics Bulletin 34: 57–59

Anon 1998 Why and how should adults lose weight? Drug and Therapeutics Bulletin 36: 89–92

Anon 1999 Ursodeoxycholic acid for primary biliary cirrhosis. Drug and Therapeutics Bulletin 37: 30–32

Auwerx J, Staels B 1998 Leptin. Lancet 351: 737–742

Bacon BR 1997 Diagnosis and management of hemochromatosis. Gastroenterology 113: 995–999

Bailey T, Biddlestone L, Shepherd NA, Barr H, Warner P, Jankowski J 1998 Altered cadherin and catenin complexes in the Barrett's esophagus dysplasia–adenocarcinoma sequence: correlation with disease progression and dedifferentiation. American Journal of Pathology 152: 135–144

Barham CP, Jones RL, Biddlestone LR, Hardwick RH, Shepherd NA, Barr H 1997 Photothermal laser ablation of Barrett's oesophagus: endoscopic and histological evidence of squamous reepithelialization. Gut 41: 281–284

Barr H, Shepherd NA, Dix A, Roberts DJ, Tan WC, Krasner N 1996 Eradication of high-grade dysplasia in columnar-lined (Barrett's) oesophagus by photodynamic therapy with endogenously generated protoporphyrin IX. Lancet 348: 561–562

Biddlestone LR, Barham CP, Wilkinson SP, Barr H, Shepherd NA 1998 The histopathology of treated Barrett's oesophagus: squamous reepithelialization after acid suppression and laser photodynamic therapy. American Journal of Surgical Pathology 22: 239–245

Burke W, Thomson E, Khoury et al. 1998 Hereditary haemochromatosis. Gene discovery and its implications for population based screening. Journal of the American Medical Association 280: 172–178

Connolly HM, Crary JL, McGoon MD et al. 1997 Valvular heart disease associated with fenfluramine-phentermine. New England Journal of Medicine 337: 581–588

Farthing MJG 1996 The role of somatostatin analogues in the treatment of refractory diarrhoea. Digestive Diseases. 57 (Suppl 1): 107–113

Feder JN, Gnirke A, Thomas W et al. 1996 A novel MHC class 1-like gene is mutated in patients with hereditary haemochromatosis. Nature Genetics 13: 399–408

Ferguson A 1999 The coeliac iceberg. CME Journal Gastroenterology, Hepatology and Nutrition 2: 52–56

Folsch UR, Nitsche R, Ludtke R, Hilgers RA, Creutzfeld W 1997 Early ERCP and papillotomy compared with conservative treatment for acute biliary pancreatitis. New England Journal of Medicine 336: 237–242

Galmiche JP, Letessier E, Scarpignato C 1998 Treatment of gastro-osophageal disease in adults. British Medical Journal 316: 1720–1723

Gore S, Healey CJ, Sutton R, Eyre-Brook IA, Gear MWL, Shepherd NA, Wilkinson SP 1993 Regression of columnar lined (Barrett's) oesophagus with continuous omeprazole therapy. Alimentary Pharmacology and Therapy 7: 623–628

Hardcastle JD, Chamberlain JO, Robinson MHE et al. 1996 Randomised controlled trial of faecal-occult-blood screening for colorectal cancer. Lancet 348: 1472–1477

Hawkey CJ 1999 COX-2 inhibitors. Lancet 353: 307–314

Hill MD, McIntyre AS 1998 Coeliac disease: modern clinical practice. CME Journal Gastroenterology, Hepatology and Nutrition 1: 36–41

Holmes GKT, Prior P, Lane MR et al. 1989 Malignancy in coeliac disease – effect of gluten free diet. Gut 30: 333–338

Holscher AH, Bollschweiler E, Schneider PM, Siewert JR 1997 Early adenocarcinoma in Barrett's oesophagus. British Journal of Surgery 84: 1470–1473

Johnson CD 1998 Severe acute pancreatitis: a continuing challenge for the intensive care team. British Journal of Intensive Care 8: 130–136

Kaplan MM 1996 Primary biliary cirrhosis. New England Journal of Medicine 335: 1570–1580

Kerr DJ, Gray R 1996 Adjuvant chemotherapy for colorectal cancer. British Journal of Hospital Medicine 55: 259–266

Khan MA, Herzog CA, St Peter JV et al. 1998 The prevalence of cardiac valvular insufficiency assessed by transthoracic echocardiography in obese patients treated with appetite-suppressant drugs. New England Journal of Medicine 339: 713–718

Koff RS 1998 Hepatitis A. Lancet 351: 1643–1649

Kronberg O, Fenger C, Olsen J et al. 1996 Randomised study of screening for colorectal cancer with faecal-occult-blood test. Lancet 348: 1467–1471

Lean MEJ, Han TS, Siedel JC 1998 Impairment of health and quality of life in people with large waist circumference. Lancet 351: 853–856

McMillan SA, Watson RP, McCrum EE et al. 1996 Factors associated with serum antibodies to reticulin, endomysium and gliadin in adult population. Gut 39: 43–47

Maki M 1997 Tissue transglutaminase as the autoantigen of coeliac disease. Gut 41: 565–566

Mergener K, Baillie J 1998 Acute pancreatitis. British Medical Journal 316: 44–48

Metcalf JV, Mitchison HC, Palmer JM, Jones DE, Bassendine MF, James OFW 1996 Natural history of primary biliary cirrhosis. Lancet 348: 1399–1402

Nandurkar S, Talley NJ, Martin CJ, Ng TH, Adams S 1997 Short segment Barrett's oesophagus: prevalence, diagnosis and associations. Gut 40: 710–715

Neuberger J 1997 Primary biliary cirrhosis. Lancet 350: 875–879

Nightingale J 1995 The short bowel syndrome. European Journal of Gastroenterology and Hepatology 7: 514–520

Payne-James JJ 1995 Enteral nutrition. European Journal of Gastroenterology and Hepatology 7: 501–506

Reithmuller GS, Schlimck G. 1994 Randomized trial of monoclonal antibody for adjuvant therapy of resected Dukes C colorectal carcinoma. Lancet 343: 1177

Silk D 1995 Nutrition for gastroenterologists: when, how and for how long? European Journal of Gastroenterology and Hepatology 7: 491–500

Sjöstrom L, Rissanen A, Andersen T et al. 1998 Randomised placebo-controlled trial of orlistat for weight loss and prevention of weight regain in obese patients. Lancet 352: 167–173

Spechler S, Goyal RK 1986 Barrett's Oesophagus. New England Journal of Medicine 315: 362–371

Taubro S, Astrup A 1997 Randomised comparison of diets for maintaining obese subjects' weight after major weight loss: ad lib, low fat, high carbohydrate diet v fixed energy intake. British Medical Journal 314: 29–34

Tweed MJ, Roland JM 1998 Haemochromatosis as an endocrine cause of subfertility. British Medical Journal 316: 915–916

van der Burgh A, Dees J, Hop WC, van Blankenstein M 1996 Oesophageal cancer is an uncommon cause of death in patients with Barrett's oesophagus. Gut 39: 5–8

Wils J 1998 The establishment of a large collaborative trial programme in the adjuvant treatment of colon cancer. British Journal of Cancer 77(S2): 23–28

Wright TA 1997 High-grade dysplasia in Barrett's oesophagus. British Journal of Surgery 84: 760–766

Yeomans ND, Cook GA, Giraud AS 1998 Selective COX-2 inhibitors: are they safe for the stomach? Gastroenterology 115: 227–229

NEPHROLOGY

Ambrus JL, Sridhar NR 1997 Immunological aspects of renal disease. Journal of the American Medical Association 278: 1938–1945

Bywaters EG, Beall D 1998 Crush injuries with impairment of renal function 1941 [classic article]. Journal of the American Society of Nephrology 9(2): 322–332

Eggers PW 1990 Mortality rates amongst dialysis patients in Medicare's end-stage renal disease program. American Journal of Kidney Diseases 15: 414–421

First MR 1998 Clinical Applications of immunosuppressive agents in renal transplantation. Surgical Clinics of North America 78: (1): 61–76

Fishman JA, Rubin RH 1998 Infection in organ-transplant recipients. New England Journal of Medicine 338: 1741–1751

Ganguly A 1998 Primary aldosteronism. New England Journal of Medicine 339: 1828–1834

Gennari J 1998 Hypokalaemia. New England Journal of Medicine 339: 451–458

Glover M 1998 The increased incidence of skin cancer in organ-transplant recipients. Dermatology in Practice Jan/Feb: 6–8

Halperin ML, Kamel KS 1998 Potassium. Lancet 352: 135–140

Harper L, Savage COS 1999 Treatment of IgA nephropathy. Lancet 353: 860–862

Hricik DE, Chung-Park M, Sedor JR 1998 Glomerulonephritis. New England Journal of Medicine 339: 888–899

Ifudu O 1998 Care of patients undergoing haemodialysis. New England Journal of Medicine 339: 1054–1062

Jungers P, Chauveau D 1997 Pregnancy in renal disease. Kidney International 52: 871–885

Klahr S, Miller SB 1998 Acute oliguria. New England Journal of Medicine 338: 671–675

National High Blood Pressure Education Working Group 1996 1995 Update of the Working Group reports on chronic renal failure and renovascular hypertension. Archives of Internal Medicine 156: 1938–1947

New DI, Barton IK 1996 Prevention of acute renal failure. British Journal of Hospital Medicine 55: 162–166

Newstead CG 1998 Assessment of risk of cancer after renal transplantation. Lancet 351: 610–611

Nicholls A 1997 Renovascular disease: the fifth frontier. Journal of the Royal Society of Medicine 90: 315–318

Orth SR, Ritz E 1998 The nephrotic syndrome. New England Journal of Medicine 338(17): 1202–1211

Pak CYC 1998 Kidney stones. Lancet 351: 1797–1801

Paller MS 1998 Hypertension in pregnancy. Journal of the American Society of Nephrology 9: 314–321

Pastan S, Bailey J 1998 Dialysis Therapy. New England Journal of Medicine 338: 1428–1437

Saklayen MG 1997 Medical management of nephrolithiasis. Medical Clinics of North America 81: 785–799

Slater MS, Mullins RJ 1998 Rhabdomyolysis and myoglobinuric renal failure in trauma and surgical patients: a review. Journal of the American College of Surgeons 186: 693–716

Szewczyk D, Ovadia P, Abdullah F, Rabinovici R 1998 Pressure induced rhabdomyolysis and acute renal failure. Journal of Trauma 44: 384–388

Turney J H 1996 Acute renal failure [editorial]. Journal of the American Medical Association 15: 275: 19

Vella JP, Sayegh MH 1997 Maintenance pharmacological strategies in renal transplantation. Post-Graduate Medical Journal 73: 386–390

INFECTIOUS DISEASES

Bone RC 1996 Why sepsis trials fail. Journal of the American Medical Association 276: 565–566

Burnham G 1998 Onchocerciasis. Lancet 351: 1341–1346

Chiodini PL 1998 Non-microscopic methods for the diagnosis of malaria. Lancet 351: 80–81

Cobb JP, Danner RL 1996 Nitric oxide and septic shock. Journal of the American Medical Association 275: 1193–1196

Conte JE 1997 A novel approach to preventing insect-borne diseases. New England Journal of Medicine 337: 785–786

Fishman J A, Rubin R H 1998 Infection in organ-transplant recipients. New England Journal of Medicine 338: 1741–1751

Gonzalez-Ruiz A, Wright SG 1998 Disparate amoebae. Lancet 351: 1672–1673

Karonga Prevention Trial Group 1996 Randomised controlled trial of single BCG, repeated BCG, or combined BCG and killed *Mycobacterium leprae* vaccine for prevention of leprosy and tuberculosis in Malawi. Lancet 348: 17–24

Koff RS 1998 Hepatitis A. Lancet 351: 1643–1649

Lemon SM, Thomas DL 1997. Vaccines to prevent viral hepatitis. New England Journal of Medicine 336: 196–204

Marshall BG, Shaw RJ 1996 New technology in the diagnosis of tuberculosis. British Journal of Hospital Medicine 55: 491–494

Nandwani R 1996 Modern diagnosis and management of acquired syphilis. British Journal of Hospital Medicine 55: 399–403

Ong RK, Doyle RL 1998 Tropical pulmonary eosinophilia. Chest 113: 1673–1679

Rothenberg ME 1998 Eosinophilia. New England Journal of Medicine 338: 1592–1600

Russo R, Nigro LC, Minniti S et al 1996 Visceral leishmaniasis in HIV infected patients: treatment with high dose liposomal amphotericin. British Journal of Infection 32: 133–137

Sanchez JL, Taylor DN 1997 Cholera. Lancet 349: 1825–1830

Sarinas PS, Chitkara RK 1997 Ascariasis and hookworm. Seminars in Respiratory Infections 12: 130–137

Schneider JH, Rogers AI 1997 Strongyloides: the protean parasitic infection. Postgraduate Medicine 102: 177–192

Stout JE, Yu VL 1997 Current concepts – Legionellosis. New England Journal of Medicine 337: 682–688

Tran TH, Day NP, Nguyen MD et al.1996 A controlled trial of artemether or quinine in Vietnamese adults with severe falciparum malaria. New England Journal of Medicine 335: 76–83

Wehner JH, Kirsch CM 1997 Pulmonary manifestations of strongyloides. Seminars in Respiratory Infections 12: 122–129

White NJ 1996 The treatment of malaria. New England Journal of Medicine 335: 800–806

White NJ, Dung NM, Vinh H, Bethell D, Hien TT 1996 Fluoroquinolones in children with multi-drug resistant typhoid. Lancet 348: 547

Whitty CJM 1997 Malaria prophylaxis for the 1990's and beyond. British Journal of Hospital Medicine 58: 545–546

Whitty CJM, Lockwood DNL 1999 Leprosy – new perspectives on an old disease. Journal of Infection 36: 38

Zenilman JM 1997 Typhoid fever. Journal of the American Medical Association 278: 847–850

HIV

Arlett P, Hooker M, Lee E, Darbyshire J, Breckenridge A 1997 Reporting adverse drug reactions in HIV infection. Genitourinary Medicine 73: 335

BHIVA Guidelines Co-ordinating Committee 1997 British HIV Association guidelines for antiretroviral treatment of HIV seropositive individuals. Lancet 349: 1086–1092

Cairns JS, D'Souza MP 1998 Chemokines and HIV-1 second receptors: the therapeutic connection. Nature Medicine 4: 563–568

Carpenter CCJ, Fischi MA, Hammer SM et al. 1998 Antiretroviral therapy for HIV infection in 1998. Updated recommendations of the international AIDS Society – USA Panel. Journal of the American Medical Association 280: 76–86

Carr A, Samaras K, Burton S et al. 1998 A syndrome of peripheral lipodystrophy, hyperlipidaemia and insulin resistance in patients receiving HIV protease inhibitors. AIDS 12: F51–58

Cohen OJ, Fauci AS 1998 HIV/AIDS in 1998 – gaining the upper hand? Journal of the American Medical Association 280: 87–88

Flexner C 1998 HIV-protease Inhibitors. New England Journal of Medicine 338: 1281–1292

Garred P 1998 Chemokine-receptor polymorphisms: clarity or confusion for HIV-1 prognosis? Lancet 351: 2–3

Gazzard B, Moyle G on behalf of the BHIVA Guidelines Writing Committee 1998 1998 revision to the British HIV Association guidelines for antiretroviral treatment of HIV seropositive individuals. Lancet 352: 314–316

Hammer SM, Squires KE, Hughes MD for the AIDS Clinical Trials Group 320 Study Team 1997 A controlled trial of two nucleoside analogues plus indinavir in persons with human immunodeficiency virus infection and CD4 cell counts of 200 per cubic millimeter or less. New England Journal of Medicine 337: 725–733

Hecht FM, Grant RM, Petropoulos CJ et al. 1998 Sexual transmission of an HIV-1 variant resistant to multiple reverse-transcriptase and protease inhibitors. New England Journal of Medicine 339: 307–311

Henry K, Melroe H, Huebsch J et al. 1998 Severe premature coronary artery disease with protease inhibitors. Lancet 351: 1328

Hogg RS, Heath KV, Yip B for the EuroSIDA Study Group 1998 Changing patterns of mortality across Europe in patients infected with HIV-1. Lancet 352: 1725–1730

Kahn JO, Walker BD 1998 Acute human immunodeficiency virus infection. New England Journal of Medicine 339: 33–39

Li TS, Tubiana R, Karlama C, Calvez V, Ait Mohand H, Autran B 1998 Long-lasting recovery in CD4 T-cell function and viral-load reduction after highly active antiretroviral therapy in advanced HIV-1 disease. Lancet 351: 1682–1686

Lo JC, Mulligan K, Tai VW, Algren H, Schambelan M 1998. 'Buffalo hump' in men with HIV-1 infection. Lancet 351: 867–870

Loveday C, Devereux H 1998 Clinical implications of antiretroviral drug resistance. Journal of HIV Therapy 3: 48–54

Miller KD, Jones E, Yanovski JA, Shankar R, Feuerstein I, Fallon J 1998 Visceral abdominal-fat accumulation associated with the use of indinavir. Lancet 351: 871–875

Montaner JSG 1998 Improved survival among HIV-infected individuals following initiation of antiretroviral therapy. Journal of the American Medical Association 279: 450–454

Powderly WG, Landay A, Lederman MM 1998 Recovery of the immune system with antiretroviral therapy. The end of opportunism? Journal of the American Medical Association 280: 72–77

Quinn TC 1997 Grand round at the Johns Hopkins Hospital. Acute primary HIV infection. Journal of the American Medical Association 278: 58–62

Reijers MHE, Weverling GJ, Jurriaans S, et al. 1998 Maintenance therapy after quadruple induction therapy in HIV-1 infected individuals: Amsterdam Duration of Antiretroviral Medication (ADAM) study. Lancet 352: 185–190

Rettig MB, Ma HJ, Vescio RA et al. 1997 Kaposi's sarcoma associated herpes virus infection of bone marrow dendritic cells from myeloma patients. Science 276: 1851–1854

Sepkoitz KA 1998 Editorial: effects of HAART on natural history of AIDS-related opportunistic disorders. Lancet 351: 228–230

Schrager LK, D'Souza PD 1998 Cellular and anatomical reservoirs of HIV-1 in patients receiving potent antiretroviral combination therapy. Journal of the American Medical Association 280: 67–71

Styrt BA, Piazza-Hepp TD, Chikami GK 1996 Clinical Toxicity of antiretroviral nucleoside analogs. Antiviral Research 31: 121–135

Vella S 1998 Prevention and detection of resistance: what does the future hold? Journal of HIV Therapy 3: 31–32

Wainberg MA, Friedland G 1998 Public health implications of antiretroviral therapy and HIV drug resistance. Journal of the American Medical Association 279: 1977–1991

ONCOLOGY

Anon 1997 Late complications of radiotherapy. Drug and Therapeutics Bulletin 35: 13–16

Anon 1997 Paclitaxel and docetaxel in breast and ovarian cancer. Drug and Therapeutics Bulletin 35: 43–46

Charatan FB 1998 Prostate cancer screening reduces deaths. British Medical Journal 316: 1625

Cunningham D, Pyrhonen S, James RD et al. 1998 Randomised trial of irinotecan plus supportive care versus supportive care alone after fluorouracil failure for patients with metastatic colorectal cancer. Lancet 352: 1413–1418

Delmas PD, Bjarnason NH, Mitlak BH et al. 1997 Effects of raloxifene on bone density, serum cholesterol concentrations, and uterine endometrium in postmenopausal women. New England Journal of Medicine 337: 1641–1686

DeVita VT, Hellman S, Rosenberg SA 1997 Cancer, principles and practice of oncology. 5th edn. Lippincott-Raven

Diel IJ, Solomayer EF, Costa S et al. 1998 Reduction in new metastases in breast cancer with adjuvant clodronate treatment. New England Journal of Medicine 339: 357–363

EBCTCG 1998 Tamoxifen for early breast cancer: an overview of the randomised trials. Lancet 351: 1451–1467

EBCTCG 1998 Polychemotherapy for early breast cancer: an overview of randomised trials. Lancet 352: 930–942

Eng C, Clayton D, Schuffenecker I et al. 1996 The relationship between specific RET proto-oncogene mutations and disease phenotype in multiple endocrine neoplasia type 2 Journal of the American Medical Association 276: 1575–1579

Gallo RC 1995 A surprising advance in the treatment of viral leukaemia. New England Journal of Medicine 332: 1783–1784

Glover M 1998 The increased incidence of skin cancer in organ-transplant recipients. Dermatology in Practice Jan/Feb: 6–8

Grob JJ, Dreno B, de la Salmoniere P et al. 1998 Randomised trial of interferon α-2a as adjuvant therapy in resected primary melanoma thicker than 1.5 mm without clinically detectable node metastases. Lancet 351: 1905–1910

Hardcastle JD,Chamberlain JO, Robinson MHE et al. 1996 Randomised controlled trial of faecal-occult-blood screening for colorectal cancer. Lancet 348: 1472–1477

Holmes GKT, Prior P, Lane MR et al. 1989 Malignancy in coeliac disease – effect of gluten free diet. Gut 30: 333–338

Hortobagyi GN, Theriault RL, Porter L et al. 1996 Efficacy of pamidronate in reducing skeletal complications in patients with breast cancer and lytic bone metastases. New England Journal of Medicine 335: 1785–1791

Hortobagyi GN 1998 Treatment of breast cancer. New England Journal of Medicine 339: 974–984

Howell A, Dowsett M 1997 Recent advances in endocrine therapy of breast cancer. British Medical Journal 315: 863–866

Johansson JE, Holmberg L, Johansson S et al. 1997 Fifteen year survival in prostate cancer, a prospective, population-based study in Sweden. Journal of the American Medical Association 277: 467–471.

Joint Council for Clinical Oncology Report 1998 The current role of paclitaxel in the first-line chemotherapy of ovarian cancer. Royal College of Physicians, London

Kaminski MS, Fenner MC, Estes J et al.1996 Phase 1/2 trial results of I131 anti-B-1 (anti- CD20) non-myeloablative radioimmunotherapy for refractory B cell lymphoma. Proceedings of the American Society for Clinical Oncology 15: 1266

Kirkwood JM, Strawderman MH, Ernstoff MS et al. 1996 Interferon Alfa-2b adjuvant therapy of high risk resected cutaneous melanoma: the eastern cooperative oncology group trial EST 1684. Journal of Clinical Oncology 14: 7–17.

Kerr DJ, Gray R 1996 Adjuvant chemotherapy for colorectal cancer. British Journal of Hospital Medicine 55: 259–266

Kronberg O, Fenger C, Olsen J et al. 1996 Randomised study of screening for colorectal cancer with faecal-occult-blood test. Lancet 348: 1467–1471

London NJ, Farmery SM, Will EJ, Davison AM, Lodge JPA 1995 Risk of neoplasia in renal transplant patients. Lancet 346: 403–406

Lorincz AL 1996 Cutaneous T cell lymphoma (mycosis fungoides). Lancet 347: 871–876

Macbeth F 1996 Radiotherapy in the treatment of lung cancer. British Journal of Hospital Medicine 55: 639–642

Miller TP, Dahlberg S, Cassady JR et al. 1998 Chemotherapy alone compared with chemotherapy plus radiotherapy for localized intermediate and high grade non-Hodgkin's lymphoma. New England Journal of Medicine 339: 21–26

Newstead C G 1998 Assessment of risk of cancer after renal transplantation. Lancet 351: 610–611

Non-Small Cell Lung Cancer Collaborative Group 1995 Chemotherapy in non-small cell lung cancer: a meta-analysis using updated data on individual patients from 52 randomised clinical trials. British Medical Journal 311: 899–909

O'Neill B, Fallon M 1997 ABC of palliative care: principles of palliative care and pain control. British Medical Journal 315: 801–804

Pettengell R 1996 High-dose therapy for aggressive non-Hodgkin's lymphoma. British Journal of Hospital Medicine 56: 5215–5228

PORT Meta-analysis Trialists Group 1998 Postoperative radiotherapy in non-small cell lung cancer: systematic review and meta-analysis of individual patient data from nine randomised controlled trials. Lancet 352: 257–263

Powles T, Eeles R, Ashley S et al. 1998 Interim analysis of the incidence of breast cancer in the Royal Marsden tamoxifen randomised chemoprevention trial. Lancet 352: 98–101

Press OW, Eary JF, Appelbaum FR et al. 1995 Phase 2 trial of I131 B1 (anti CD20) antibody therapy with autologous stem cell transplantation for relapsed B cell lymphomas. Lancet 346: 336–340.

Reithmuller GS, Schlimck G 1994 Randomized trial of monoclonal antibody for adjuvant therapy of resected Dukes C colorectal carcinoma. Lancet 1994: 343: 1177

Rodenhuis S, Richel DJ, van der Wall E et al. 1998 Randomised trial of high dose chemotherapy and haemopoietic progenitor-cell support in operable breast cancer with extensive axillary lymph node involvement. Lancet 352: 515–521

Rosenberg SA 1997 Cancer vaccines based on the identification of genes encoding cancer regression antigens. Immunology Today 18: 175–182

Rougier P, Van Cutsem E, Bajetta E et al. 1998 Randomised trial of irinotecan versus fluorouracil by continuous infusion after fluorouracil failure in patients with metastatic colorectal cancer. Lancet 352: 1407–1412

Saunders M, Dische S, Barrett A et al. 1997 Continuous hyperfractionated radiotherapy (CHART) versus conventional radiotherapy in non-small cell lung cancer: a multicentre randomised trial. Lancet 350: 161–165

Schlumberger MJ 1998 Papillary and follicular thyroid carcinoma. New England Journal of Medicine 338: 297–306

Singal PW, Iliskovic N 1998 Doxorubicin induced cardiomyopathy. New England Journal of Medicine 339: 900–905

Sox HC 1998 Benefit and harm associated with screening for breast cancer. New England Journal of Medicine 338: 1145–1146

Sykes J, Johnson R, Hanks GW 1997 ABC of palliative care: difficult pain problems. British Medical Journal 315: 867–869

Thakker R V 1997 Multiple endocrine neoplasia medicine 25: 86–88

van der Burgh A, Dees J, Hop WC, van Blankenstein M 1996 Oesophageal cancer is an uncommon cause of death in patients with Barrett's oesophagus. Gut 39: 5–8

Veronesi U, Maisonneuve P, Costa A et al. 1998 Prevention of breast cancer with tamoxifen: preliminary findings from the Italian randomised trial among hysterectomised women. Lancet 352: 93–97

Vijayakumar S, Hellman S 1997 Advances in radiation oncology. Lancet 349: (Suppl 2): 1–3

Whittaker S 1996 Sun and skin cancer. British Journal of Hospital Medicine 56: 515–518

Wils J 1998 The establishment of a large collaborative trial programme in the adjuvant treatment of colon cancer. British Journal of Cancer 77(S2): 23–28

HAEMATOLOGY

Bataille R, Harousseau JL 1997 Multiple Myeloma. New England Journal of Medicine 336: 1657–1664

Berenson JR, Lichtenstein A, Porter L et al. 1996 Efficacy of pamidronate in reducing the skeletal events in patients with advanced multiple myeloma. New England Journal of Medicine 334: 488–493

Burnett AK, Goldstone AH, Stevens RMF et al. 1998 Randomized comparison of addition of autologous bone-marrow transplantation to intensive chemotherapy for acute myeloid leukaemia in first remission: results of MRC AML 10 trial. Lancet 351: 700–708

Cahill MR, Colvin BT 1997 Haemophilia. Postgraduate Medical Journal. 73: 201–206

Charache S, Terrin ML, Moore RD et al. 1995 Effect of hydroxyurea on the frequency of painful crises in sickle cell anaemia. New England Journal of Medicine 332: 1317–1332

Ferreira OC, Planelles V, Rosenblatt JD 1997 Human T-cell leukaemia viruses: epidemiology, biology, and pathogenesis. Blood Reviews 11: 91–104

Gallo RC 1995 A surprising advance in the treatment of viral leukaemia. New England Journal of Medicine 332: 1783–1784

Greaves MR 1997 Aetiology of acute leukaemia. Lancet 349: 344–349

Guilhot F, Chastang C, Michallat M et al. 1997 Interferon alpha-2b combined with cytarabine versus interferon alone in chronic myelogenous leukaemia. New England Journal of Medicine 337: 223–229

Hansen JA, Gooley TA, Martin PJ et al. 1998 Bone marrow transplants from unrelated related donors for patients with chronic myeloid leukaemia. New England Journal of Medicine 338: 962–968

Harrison CN, Linch DC, Machin SJ 1998 Desirability and problems of early diagnosis of essential thrombocythaemia. Lancet 351: 846–847

Hollsberg P, Hafler DA 1993 Pathogenesis of diseases induced by human lymphotropic virus type I infection. New England Journal of Medicine 328: 1173–1182

Kaminski MS, Fenner MC, Estes J et al.1996 Phase 1/2 trial results of I131 anti-B-1 (anti- CD20) non-myeloablative radioimmunotherapy for refractory B cell lymphoma. Proceedings of the American Society for Clinical Oncology 15: 1266

Kelton JG, Warkentin TE 1998 Heparin-induced thrombocytopenia: an overview of the diagnosis, natural history and treatment options. Postgraduate Medicine 103: 169–171, 175–178

Leisner RJ, Goldstone AH 1997 The acute leukaemias. British Medical Journal 314: 733–736

Lorincz AL 1996 Cutaneous T cell lymphoma (mycosis fungoides). Lancet 347: 871–876

Malinow MR, Duell PB, Hess DL et al. 1998 Reduction of plasma homocysteine levels by breakfast cereal fortified with folic acid in patients with coronary heart disease. New England Journal of Medicine 338: 1009–1015

Markus HS, Hambley H 1998 Neurology and the blood: haematological abnormalities in ischaemic stroke. Journal of Neurology, Neurosurgery and Psychiatry 64: 150–159

Messinezy M, Pearson TC 1997 Polycythaemia, primary (essential) thrombocythaemia and myelofibrosis. British Medical Journal 314: 587–590

Miller TP, Dahlberg S, Cassady JR et al. 1998 Chemotherapy alone compared with chemotherapy plus radiotherapy for localized intermediate and high grade non-Hodgkin's lymphoma. New England Journal of Medicine 339: 21–26

Nygard O, Nordrehaug JE, Refsum H et al. 1997 Plasma homocysteine levels and mortality in patients with coronary artery disease. New England Journal of Medicine 337: 230–236

Pettengell R 1996 High-dose therapy for aggressive non-Hodgkin's lymphoma. British Journal of Hospital Medicine 56: 5215–5228

Poort SR, Rosenthal FR, Reitsma PH et al. 1996. A common genetic variant in the 3'-untranslated region of the prothrombin gene is associated with elevated prothrombin levels and an increase in venous thrombosis. Blood 88: 3698–3707

Press OW, Eary JF, Appelbaum FR et al.1995. Phase 2 trial of I131 B1 (anti CD20) antibody therapy with autologous stem cell transplantation for relapsed B cell lymphomas. Lancet 346: 336–340.

Rettig MB, Ma HJ, Vescio RA et al. 1997 Kaposi's sarcoma associated herpes virus infection of bone marrow dendritic cells from myeloma patients. Science 276: 1851–1854

Rothenberg ME 1998 Eosinophilia. New England Journal of Medicine 338: 1592–1600

Serjeant GR 1997 Sickle cell disease. Lancet 350: 725–730

Singer CRJ 1997 Multiple myeloma and related conditions. British Medical Journal 314: 960–996

Vandenbroucke JP 1998 Cerebral sinus thrombosis and oral contraceptives. British Medical Journal 317: 483–484

Vichinsky EP, Charles MH et al. 1995 A comparison of conservative and aggressive transfusion regimens in the perioperative management of sickle cell disease. New England Journal of Medicine 333: 206–213

Walters MC et al. 1996 Bone marrow transplantation for sickle cell disease. New England Journal of Medicine 335: 369–376

RHEUMATOLOGY

Adachi JD, Benson WA, Brown J et al. 1997 Intermittent cyclical etidronate therapy in the prevention and treatment of corticosteroid induced osteoporosis. New England Journal of Medicine 337: 382–387

American College of Rheumatology Task Force on Osteoporosis Guidelines. 1996 Recommendations for the prevention and treatment of glucocorticoid induced osteoporosis. Arthritis and Rheumatism 39: 1791–1801

Ballard PA, Purdie D 1996 The natural history of osteoporosis. British Journal of Hospital Medicine. 55: 503–507

Cambridge G 1998 Anti-neutrophil cytoplasmic antibodies. Arthritis and Rheumatism Council Topical Reviews series 3, no.13

Canalis E 1996 Mechanisms of glucocorticoid action in bone: implications for glucocorticoid induced osteoporosis. Journal of Endocrinology and Metabolism 81: 3441–3447

Delmas PD, Bjarnason NH, Mitlak BH et al. 1997 Effects of raloxifene on bone mineral density, serum cholesterol concentrations, and uterine endometrium in postmenopausal women. New England Journal of Medicine 337: 1641–1647

Dudley J, Kai-Lik So A 1998 T cells and related cytokines. Current Opinion in Rheumatology 10: 207–211

Ferri C, La Civita L, Longombardo G et al 1998 Mixed cryoglobulinaemia: a crossroad between autoimmune disease and lymphoproliferative disorders. Lupus 7: 275–279

Hoffman GS, Specks U 1998 Antineutrophil cytoplasmic antibodies. Arthritis and Rheumatism 41: 1521–1537

Itescu S 1996 Adult immunodeficiency and rheumatic disease. Rheumatic Disease Clinics of North America 22: 53–73

Kanis JA, Delmas P, Burckhardt P et al. 1997 Guidelines for diagnosis and management of osteoporosis. Osteoporosis International 7: 390–406

Miossec P, Van den Berg W 1997 Th1/Th2 cytokine balance in arthritis. Arthritis and Rheumatism 40: 2105–2115

Mitchell H, Bolster MB, LeRoy EC 1997 Scleroderma and related conditions. Medical Clinics of North America 81: 129–149

Nepom GT, Gersuk V, Nepom BS 1996 Prognostic implications of HLA genotyping in the early assessment of patients with rheumatoid arthritis. Journal of Rheumatology 23: 5–9

Wolfe F 1997 The prognosis of rheumatoid arthritis: assessment of disease activity and disease severity in the clinic. American Journal of Medicine 103 (6A): 12S–18S

DERMATOLOGY

Brown SK, Shalita AR 1998 Acne vulgaris. Lancet 351: 1871–1876

Callen JP 1998 Pyoderma gangrenosum. Lancet 351: 581–585

Glover M 1998 The increased incidence of skin cancer in organ-transplant recipients. Dermatology in Practice Jan/Feb: 6–8

Grob JJ, Dreno B, de la Salmoniere P et al. 1998 Randomised trial of interferon a-2a as adjuvant therapy in resected primary melanoma thicker than 1.5 mm without clinically detectable node metastases. Lancet 351: 1905–1910

Kirkwood JM, Strawderman MH, Ernstoff MS et al. 1996 Interferon Alfa-2b adjuvant therapy of high risk resected cutaneous melanoma: the eastern cooperative oncology group trial EST 1684. Journal of Clinical Oncology 14: 7–17.

Korman NJ 1993 Bullous pemphigoid. Dermatology Clinics 11: 483–498

London NJ, Farmery SM, Will EJ, Davison AM, Lodge JPA 1995 Risk of neoplasia in renal transplant patients. Lancet 346: 403–406

Lorincz AL 1996 Cutaneous T cell lymphoma (mycosis fungoides). Lancet 347: 871–876

Rudikoff D, Lebwohl M 1998 Atopic dermatitis. Lancet 351: 1715–1721

Schwartz RA, Janniger CK 1997 Alopecia areata. Cutis 59: 238–241

Stern RS 1997 Psoriasis. Lancet 350: 349–353

Whittaker S 1996 Sun and skin cancer. British Journal of Hospital Medicine 56: 515–518

Zvulunov A, Esterly N 1995 Neurocutaneous syndromes associated with pigmentary skin lesions. Journal of the American Academy of Dermatology 32: 915–935

Abbreviations

AAAD	Aromatic amino acid decarboxylases
AAT	Alpha 1-antitrypsin
ACE	Angiotensin-converting enzyme
ACEI	Angiotensin converting enzyme inhibitors
ACTH	Adrenocorticotrophin
AD	Alzheimer's disease
ADAS	Alzheimer's disease assessment scale
ADH	Anti-diuretic hormone
ADL	Activities of daily living
ADR	Adverse drug reaction
AE	Atopic eczema
AIDS	Acquired immunodeficiency syndrome
AMA	Antimitochondrial antibodies
AML	Myeloid leukaemia
ANCA	Anti-neutrophil cytoplasmic antibodies
APL	Acute promyelocytic leukaemia
ARF	Acute renal failure
ARVD	Atheromatous renovascular disease
ARVD	Arrhythmogenic right ventricular dysplasia
AST	Aspartate transaminase
ATL	Adult T-cell leukaemia/lymphoma
ATRA	All-trans retinoic acid
BCC	Basal cell carcinomas
BCG	Bacille Calmette-Guerin
BHIVA	British HIV Association
BMD	Bone mineral density
BMI	Body mass index
BMR	Basal metabolic rate
BMT	Bone marrow transplant
BNF	British national formulary
Brdu	Bromodeoxyuridine
CAMP	Cyclic adenosine monophosphate
CAPD	Continuous ambulatory peritoneal dialysis
CADASIL	Cerebral autosomal dominant arteriopathy with subcortical infarction and leucoencephalopathy
CCF	Congestive cardiac failure
CCR	cc chemokine receptor
CFA	Cryptogenic fibrosing alveolitis
CHART	Continuous hyperfractionated accelerated radiotherapy

CHOP	Cyclophosphamide, doxorubicin, vincristine and prednisolone chemotherapy
CML	Chronic myeloid leukaemia
CO	Cardiac output
COMT	Catechol-O-methyl transferase
CGMP	Cyclic guanine monophosphate
CK	Creatinine kinase
CNS	Central nervous system
CREST	Calcinosis, Raynaud's, oesophagus, scleroderma and telangiectasia
CSD	Cortical spreading depression
CSF	Cerebrospinal fluid
CTCL	Cutaneous T cell lymphoma
CMF	Cyclophosphamide, methotrexate, 5 fluorouracil
CMV	Cytomegalovirus
COPD	Chronic obstructive pulmonary disease
COX	Cyclo-oxygenase
CSM	Committee of safety of medicines
CXCR	CXC chemokine receptor
CYP	Cytochrome P450
DCCT	Diabetes Control and Complications Trial
DCM	Dilated cardiomyopathy
DEXA	Dual-energy X-ray absorptiometry
DILS	Diffuse infiltrative lymphocytosis syndrome
DHT	Dihydrotestosterone
DIG	Digitalis Investigation Group
DLI	Lymphocyte infusions obtained from the donor
DNA	Deoxynucleic acid
DRE	Digital rectal examination
dUMP	5 uridine monophosphate
dTMP	Thymidine 5 monophosphate
EATCL	Enteropathy associated T-cell lymphoma
EBV	Epstein–Barr virus
ECG	Electrocardiogram
EEG	Electroencephalogram
ELISA	Enzyme linked immunosorbent assay
ENAs	Extractable nuclear antigens
ER	Oestrogen receptor
ERCP	Endoscopic retrograde cholangiopancreatogram
ESPGAN	European Society for Paediatric Gastroenterology and Nutrition
ESR	Erythrocyte sedimentation rate
ESSENCE	Efficacy and safety of subcutaneous enoxaparin in non-Q wave coronary events
ET	Essential thrombocythaemia
ETEC	Enterotoxigenic E. coli
FBC	Full blood count
FDCs	Follicular dendritic cells
FDA	Food and Drug Administration
FdUMP	Fluoro-2-deoxyuridine monophoasphate
FEV_1	Forced expiratory volume in one second
FISH	Fluorescent in situ hybridisation

FRISC trial	Fragmin during instability in coronary artery disease
FSH	Follicle stimulating hormone
FTA	Fluorescent treponemal antibody absorbed
5-FU	5-fluorouracil
GABA	Gamma amino butyric acid
G-CSF	Granulocyte colony stimulating factor
GM-CSF	Granulocyte–monocyte colony stimulating factor
GFR	Glomerular filtration rate
GH	Growth hormone
GHD	Growth hormone deficiency
GI	Gastrointestinal
GORD	Gastro-oesophageal reflux disease
GP120	HIV viral envelope protein 120
G6PD	Glucose-6-phosphate dehydrogenase deficiency
GTN	Glycerol trinitrate
GSM	Glucocorticoid-suppressible hyperaldosteronism
GVHD	Graft versus host disease
HAART	Highly active antiretroviral therapy
HAMA	Human antibodies against mouse antibodies
HAM/TSP	HTLV-I-associated myelopathy/tropical spastic paraparesis
HAV	Hepatitis A virus
Hb F	Fetal haemoglobin
HBIG	Hepatitis B immunoglobulin
HbsAg	Hepatitis B surface antigen positive
HBV	Hepatitis B virus
HCV	Hepatitis C virus
HDL	High-density lipoprotein
HELLP	Haemolysis, Elevated Liver enzymes, Low Platelets
HHV8	Human herpes virus 8
5-HIAA	5-hydroxyindoleacetic acid
HITS	Heparin induced thrombocytopenia
HPA	Hypothalamic–pituitary axis
HPV	Human papillomavirus
H-1 receptor	Histamine type 1 receptor
5-HT	5-hydroxytryptamine
HTLV-1	Human T-cell lymphotrophic virus-1
HU	Hydroxyurea
ICD	Internal cardioverter defibrillator
IDDM	Insulin dependent diabetes mellitus
IFN-α	α-interferon
IgE	Immunoglobulin E
IHD	Ischaemic heart disease
IIF	Indirect immunofluorescence
II	Interleukin
IL6	Interleukin 6
Ip-10	Interferon inducible protein 10 interleukin
I-TAC	IFN-inducible T-cell alpha chemoattractant
ITU	Intensive care unit
IVDUs	Intravenous drug-users
IVP	Intravenous pyelogram
JVP	Jugular venous pressure
LBBB	Left bundle branch block

LDH	Lactate dehydrogenase
LDL	Low density lipoprotein
L-dopa	L-dihydroxyphenylalanine
LFTs	Liver function tests
LH	Luteinising hormone
LHON	Leber's hereditary optic neuropathy
LMWH	Low molecular weight heparin
5-LO	5-lipoxygenase
LVRS	Lung volume reduction surgery
LTD4	Leukotriene D4
LV	Left ventricular
LVEF	Left ventricular ejection fraction
MALT	Mucosa associated lymphoid tissue
MCA	Medicines Control Agency
MCP-1	Monocyte chemotactic protein-1
MDIs	Metered dose inhalers
MDMA	3,4-methylenedioxy-methamphetamine
MDR	Multidrug resistance
MELAS	Mitochondrial encephalomyopathy, lactic acidosis and stroke-like episodes
MEN	Multiple endocrine neoplasia
MF	Mycosis fungoides
MHC	Major histocompatibility complex
MI	Myocardial infarction
MIBG	Metaiodobenzylguanidine
MIG	Monokine induced by interferon gamma
MIP 1alpha	Macrophage inflammatory protein
MM	Multiple myeloma
MMF	Mycophenylate mofetil
MRC	Medical Research Council
MTC	Medullary thyroid cancer
M-Tropic	Macrophage tropic
MUGA	Multi-gate acquisition
NCEP	National Cholesterol Education Programme
NF-1.	Neurofibromatosis type 1
NF-2	Neurofibromatosis type 2
NIDDM	Non-insulin dependent diabetes mellitus
NMSC	Non melanoma skin carcinoma
NNRTIs	Non-nucleoside analogue reverse transcriptase inhibitors
NRTIs	Nucleoside analogue reverse transcriptase inhibitors
NSAID	Non-steroidal anti-inflammatory drugs
OCP	Oral contraceptive pill
PAI-1	Plasminogen-activator inhibitor type 1
PBC	Primary biliary cirrhosis
PCOS	Polycystic ovary syndrome
PCP	*Pneumocystis carinii* pneumonia
PCR	Polymerase chain reaction
PD	Parkinson's disease
PDE3	Phosphodiesterase isoenzyme three
PEFR	Peak expiratory flow rate
PEG	Percutaneous endoscopic gastrostomy
PF4	Platelet factor 4

PG	Pyoderma gangrenosum
POEMS	Polyneuropathy, organomegaly, endocrinopathy, M-protein band from plasmacytoma and skin pigmentation
Pi type	Serum proteinase phenotype
PiZZ	Homozygotes for the Z allele of the alpha-1-antitrypsin gene
PPH	Primary pulmonary hypertension
PPI	Proton pump inhibitor
PSA	Prostate specific antigen
PTCA	Percutaneous transarterial coronary angioplasty
PTH	Parathyroid hormone
PUVA	Psoralen plus UVA irradiation
QBC	Fluorescent microscopy
QTc	Corrected QT interval (corrected for heart rate)
REE	Resting energy expenditure
RANTES	Regulated-on-activation normal T-expressed and secreted genes
RV	Right ventricular
SCAs	Spinocerebellar ataxias
SCC	Squamous cell carcinoma
SDF-1	Stromal cell derived factor-1 (chemokine)
SERM	Selective oestrogen receptor modulator
SLE	Systemic lupus erythematosus
SLPI	Secretory leucoproteinase inhibitor
S phase	Synthetic phase
SR	Sarcoplasmic reticulum
SRS-A	Slow relaxing substance of anaphylaxis
STS	Sequence tagged site
SSRIs	Selective serotonin reuptake inhibitors
TB	Tuberculosis
TEE	Total energy expenditure
TEW	Thermic effect of muscle
TF	Tissue factor
TG	Triglycerides
TGF-β	Transforming growth factor-β
Th1	T-helper 1 response
Th2	T helper 2 response
THC	δ-9-tetrahydrocannabinol
TIPSS	Transjugular intrahepatic portosystemic shunting
TNF	anti-Tumour necrosis factor
TNM	Tumour, nodes, metastases staging system
TPHA	*Treponema pallidum* haemagglutination assay
TPMT	Thiopurine methyltransferase
TRH	Thyrotropin releasing hormone
TSC	Tuberous sclerosis complex
TSH	Thyroid stimulating hormone
T-tropic	T lymphocyte-tropic
UDCA	Ursodeoxycholic acid
UFH	Unfractionated heparin
UKPDS	United Kingdom Prospective Diabetes Study
UPDRS	Unified Parkinson's Disease Rating Scores
UVB	Ultraviolet B

UVR	Ultraviolet radiation
VATS	Video assisted thoracoscopy
VDRL	Venereal disease reference laboratory
VT	Ventricular tachycardia
WHO	World Health Organisation

Index